SECOND EDITION

Demystifying
Opioid
Conversion
Calculations

A GUIDE
FOR
EFFECTIVE
DOSING

Mary Lynn McPherson, PharmD, MA, MDE, BCPS, CPE

Professor, Executive Director
  Advanced Post-Graduate Education in Palliative Care
Program Director, Online Master of Science and Graduate
  Certificates in Palliative Care
University of Maryland School of Pharmacy
Baltimore, Maryland

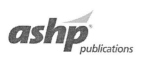

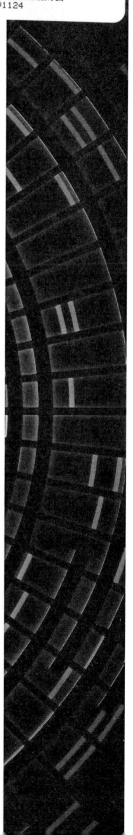

Any correspondence regarding this publication should be sent to the publisher, American Society of Health-System Pharmacists, 4500 East-West Highway, Bethesda, MD, 20814, attention: Special Publishing.

The information presented herein reflects the opinions of the contributors and advisors. It should not be interpreted as an official policy of ASHP or as an endorsement of any product.

Because of ongoing research and improvements in technology, the information and its applications contained in this text are constantly evolving and are subject to the professional judgment and interpretation of the practitioner due to the uniqueness of a clinical situation. The author and editors and ASHP have made reasonable efforts to ensure the accuracy and appropriateness of the information presented in this document. However, any user of this information is advised that the editors and ASHP are not responsible for the continued currency of the information, for any errors or omissions, and/or for any consequences arising from the use of the information in the document in any and all practice settings. Any reader of this document is cautioned that ASHP makes no representation, guarantee, or warranty, express or implied, as to the accuracy and appropriateness of the information contained in this document and specifically disclaims any liability to any party for the accuracy and/or completeness of the material or for any damages arising out of the use or non-use of any of the information contained in this document.

Vice President, Publishing: Daniel J. Cobaugh, PharmD, DABAT, FAACT
Editorial Project Manager, Special Publishing: Ruth Bloom, BA
Production Manager: Johnna Hershey, BA
Cover & Page Design: David Wade, BA

Library of Congress Cataloging-in-Publication Data

Names: McPherson, Mary Lynn, author. | American Society of Health-System
  Pharmacists, issuing body.
Title: Demystifying opioid conversion calculations : a guide for effective dosing /
  Mary Lynn McPherson.
Description: Second edition. | Bethesda, MD : American Society of Health-System
  Pharmacists, [2019] | Includes bibliographical references and index.
Identifiers: LCCN 2018023233 | ISBN 9781585284290 (pbk.)
Subjects: | MESH: Analgesics, Opioid—administration & dosage | Analgesics,
  Opioid—therapeutic use | Drug Dosage Calculations
Classification: LCC RM328 | NLM QV 89 | DDC 615.7/822—dc23
LC record available at https://lccn.loc.gov/2018023233

Printed in Canada.

ISBN: 978-1-58528-429-0

Dedication

This book is dedicated to

My husband, *Jim*, for his ceaseless love and support;

and

Our daughter, *Alexandra*, a brilliant palliative care pharmacist, who makes us proud every single day.

Contents

Foreword

Mathematics and biologic systems can be at times incompatible or at least conflictual. Mathematics deals with the logical, the predictable, and the precise, while biologic systems are intrinsically changing, often unpredictable and imprecise. To bring it home, a single answer for equianalgesia between two drugs given to different individuals will be imprecise. Should one, therefore, consider a range of equianalgesia with confidence intervals considering the population and its biologic heterogeneity or be precise using a single number to express equivalents but with footnotes for population considerations and the multitude of clinical contexts? Dr. McPherson has tirelessly and meticulously worked, putting in long hours with blood, sweat, and tears, to give us an evidence-based table that provides opioid equivalents in an easily understood format but with all the considerations of population and clinical differences (see Table 1-1 and the inside cover). I believe this table is the most useful equianalgesic table published. As an aside, the table should not be mistaken for a "conversion" table because such a table does not exist. Dr. McPherson asks you to put away your "conversion calculators" and use your cognitive abilities and clinical skills to make the *right* opioid choice for the *right* patient at the *right* dose at the *right* time.

This text, in its second edition, addresses questions of route conversions, dosing strategies, and opioid switches in its opening chapters. The section on dosing strategies is clinically quite useful. The middle chapters contain an in-depth discussion on fentanyl, methadone, and patient-controlled analgesia. The patient-controlled analgesia chapter is rather pragmatic because the literature is a bit "messy" as most studies on the subject contain low-grade evidence from case series. The chapter on methadone provides up-to-date dosing schedules that are safe and a plethora of important considerations when using methadone to avoid the unique problems and pitfalls associated with methadone. Dr. McPherson has included information on buprenorphine and nalbuphine, which are presently being substituted for the usual potent opioids because of national shortages of parenteral morphine, hydromorphone, and fentanyl. Nalbuphine and buprenorphine have unique properties and should be considered as first-line opioids for certain patients and clinical circumstances.

So why buy this volume if you have the 2009 edition? Well, practice has changed; important data have been published in the basic sciences that have bearing on opioid choices and dosing. We have become more knowledgeable clinically in part due to mistakes that have generated an opioid epidemic. Importantly, opioids have received national attention from the growing number of opioid-related deaths, not all of which are related to heroin; some of the deaths are related to a lack of understanding about opioid pharmacology, equivalents, and poor opioid prescribing habits due to misinformation. Therefore, the information in this book is critical for anyone who wants to practice opioid therapy safely.

The book is full of humor and common sense. As usual, Dr. McPherson makes it fun and enjoyable to learn. The case presentations give body to theory and will help clinicians solve difficult pain problems through evidence-based opioid dosing strategies and choices. Lynn provides pearls of wisdom, so if you don't buy this text, it will be a great loss to yourself and to the patients whom you serve.

Mellar P. Davis, MD, FCCP, FAAHPM
Director of Palliative Services
Geisinger Medical System
Danville, PA

Preface

I started the preface to the first edition of this book by saying that writing a book such as this one is like purposely walking around with a bull's eye painted on your forehead. I speculated that if you ask five opioid conversion "experts" about a specific calculation, you'd probably get 15 different answers! I admitted freely that the equianalgesic table was constructed using a few facts, many more semisolid facts, and a significant amount of "this is how we've always done it!" In writing the second edition, I struggled with the equianalgesic table just as mightily as I did with the first edition. However, this time around, there were better data to guide me. Thanks to the work of clinical researchers, we now have better equianalgesic data to make well-informed decisions in patient care that allow us to achieve pain relief quickly and safely, while minimizing adverse effects.

Note: The equivalencies and notes in the equianalgesic table (Table 1-1 and the inside cover) in this edition are a little different from the first edition, those charts widely used in practice today, and the equivalencies that drives conversion calculator apps. This may cause a bit of a stir, but as Laurel Thatcher Ulrich said, "Well-behaved women seldom make history." I'm not trying to be a trouble-maker, rather to provide guidance for best practices in opioid conversion calculations!

What else has informed the development of this second edition? World events to be sure. Everyone reading this knows that we are struggling with two competing public health crises—poorly managed pain (acute and chronic) and an opioid crisis. *So, what do opioid conversion calculations have to do with these problems? Everything.* Indisputably, pain management has, and will continue to, require the use of opioids in some capacity. Unfortunately, it seems that the pendulum has swung to the far left, and prescribers are increasingly loathe to use opioids. In many cases, this may be appropriate; but in other cases, the underprescribing and underdosing of opioids may cause needless suffering. Opioid dosing, like dosing most medications, is not "one size fits all." For example, sending a postoperative patient home on day 2 with 10 Percocet is not always the answer; it may increase suffering and actually increase the risk for the development of chronic pain. This text will help learners how to transition a patient appropriately from one opioid to a different opioid, convert between routes of administration, and safely titrate opioid doses up and down.

What else can I tell you about the second edition? It's chock FULL of goodies! This book holds great appeal for acute care practitioners, those caring for chronic noncancer pain patients, and clinicians working with patients at the end of life. It's written in a conversational tone (like we were besties having lunch) while including the latest evidence possible. Contemporary issues such as explaining WHY you cannot increase a continuous infusion opioid before 8 to 12 hours are addressed.

The book contains several new and updated features!

- *"Could I Get That to Go, Please?"* at the end, highlighting the most important summary points of the chapter.

- Where applicable, chapters contain breakout boxes titled, "Can We Be Steadies?" discussing recent research that reflects steady-state opioid conversion calculations.

- The ever-popular *pearls, pitfalls,* and *fast facts* from the first edition remain, updated and added to as appropriate.

- A new chapter, "Lagniappe: A Little Something Extra in Conversion Calculations," has been added, featuring a discussion of less commonly used opioids (the fentanyls, levorphanol, and nalbuphine) and a baker's dozen of opioid conversion MIScalulations! These cases will be of great use to staff development professionals and teachers in all practice settings.

Feel free to use the practice cases throughout all the chapters, especially in Chapter 9, as teaching tools.

Last, I would like to share any success this book has achieved or will achieve with the clinicians I have worked with over the years, in doing a million or so opioid conversion calculations, particularly professionals in training who struggle so earnestly to master this skill. Most especially, I am humbled by the patients who have allowed me to share in their final journey, which may have included the need for an opioid conversion calculation.

If you would like to email me any thoughts, corrections, or suggestions please feel free to do so at marylynnmcphersonocc@gmail.com.

Mary Lynn McPherson
August 2018

Reviewers

Nancy A. Alvarez, PharmD, BCPS, FAPhA

Assistant Dean, Experiential Education and Continuing Professional Development
Assistant Professor of Pharmacy Practice
Chapman University School of Pharmacy
Irvine, California

Rabia S. Atayee, PharmD, BCPS

Associate Dean for Admissions and Outreach
Associate Professor of Clinical Pharmacy
Palliative Care Pharmacist Specialist
University of California San Diego Skaggs School of Pharmacy and Pharmaceutical Sciences
University of California San Diego Health
San Diego, California

Ryan C. Costantino, PharmD, BCPS

Pharmacy Officer
United States Army
Baltimore, Maryland

Mellar P. Davis, MD, FCCP, FAAHPM

Director of Palliative Services
Geisinger Medical System
Danville, Pennsylvania

Leslie Dixon, PharmD

Pharmacy Clinical Manager
Baton Rouge General
Baton Rouge, Louisiana

Maria Foy, PharmD, BCPS, CPE

Pharmacy Care Coordinator, Palliative Care
Abington Hospital-Jefferson Health
Abington, Pennsylvania

Chris Herndon, PharmD, CPE, FASHP

Professor
Department of Pharmacy Practice
Edwardsville School of Pharmacy
Southern Illinois University
Edwardsville, Illinois

Holly M. Holmes, MD, MS, AGSF

Associate Professor and Division Director
McGovern Medical School
The University of Texas Health Science Center at Houston
Division of Geriatric and Palliative Medicine
Houston, Texas

Karen Snow Kaiser, PhD, RN

Formerly, Clinical Practice Coordinator
Clinical Quality and Safety
University of Maryland Medical Center
Baltimore, Maryland

Leonette O. Kemp, PharmD, CPE

Clinical Pharmacy Specialist, Oncology and Palliative Care
Methodist University Hospital
Memphis, Tennessee

Robin Moorman Li, PharmD, BCACP, CPE

Clinical Associate Professor
Assistant Director, Jacksonville Campus
University of Florida College of Pharmacy
Jacksonville, Florida

Kasey L. Malotte, PharmD, BCPS

Advanced Practice Pharmacist
Supportive Care Medicine
Cedars-Sinai Medical Center
Los Angeles, California

Ronald Manning, MD, HMDC

Assistant Medical Director
Unity Hospice
Green Bay, Wisconsin

Eric Prommer, MD, FAAHP, HMDC

Director UCLA/VA Hospice and Palliative Medicine Fellowship Training Program
Director Inpatient Hospice Unit/Greater Los Angeles Healthcare
Associate Professor of Medicine
UCLA School Medicine
Los Angeles, California

Laura Scarpaci, PharmD, BCPS

Palliative Care Consultant
Haddonfield, New Jersey

Richard Wheeler, PharmD, BCPS

Pharmacy Clinical Manager
Clinical Pharmacy Specialist
Pain Management
Mercy Hospital
Oklahoma City, Oklahoma

Suzanne Wortman, BS, PharmD, BCPS

Clinical Pharmacy Specialist
Penn Highlands DuBois
Johnstown, Pennsylvania

Acknowledgments

Writing a book of this nature is a daunting prospect.

- Thanks to the *administration and staff at the University of Maryland School of Pharmacy* for encouraging me to indulge in this adventure.
- Thanks also to *Ruth Bloom* at ASHP, a most agreeable editor!
- I am exceedingly grateful to the exhaustive efforts of the reviewers—individuals spent hours and hours combing over every chapter and providing thoughtful feedback. Each reviewer provided a different perspective, and the book is immeasurably stronger thanks to their careful consideration.
- Thank you to the "fact checkers" who slaved over checking my math so I can stay out of jail!
- I must call out one reviewer in particular—*Dr. Mellar P. Davis*—seriously the smartest person I know. He reviewed every chapter and gave me detailed feedback (tough love is indeed a beautiful thing). Dr. Davis demanded the very best work I could possibly produce, and the book is so much stronger for it. He also wrote the lovely foreword to this edition!
- Thanks to my family and friends, who remain convinced that I am not in full possession of my faculties for writing another book.
- Thanks to colleagues who have given me solicited and unsolicited feedback since the first edition was published, which I faithfully saved and used in crafting the second edition.

CHAPTER 1

Introduction to Opioid Conversion Calculations

INTRODUCTION

Consider these scenarios:

- MJ is a 72-year-old woman with breast cancer who has grown too weak to swallow her MS Contin tablets. How do you convert her to oral morphine solution? How often is it administered? What happens when she can't swallow the oral morphine solution?

- WE is a 54-year-old man with an end-stage malignancy referred to hospice with an implanted intrathecal pump, which is delivering 1 mg of morphine per day. The hospice nurse calls you and wants to know what would be an appropriate dose of oral morphine to give the patient for breakthrough pain?

OBJECTIVES

After reading this chapter, the participant will be able to:

1. Identify common clinical scenarios that are appropriate for opioid conversion.

2. Compare and contrast the concepts of potency and equianalgesia.

3. Explain the principles used to develop an Equianalgesic Opioid Dosing table and describe the limitations of this tool.

4. Use a five-step process to switch a patient from one opioid to a different opioid.

- SA is a 94-year-old woman with dementia and severe osteoarthritis. She has been maintained on a transdermal fentanyl patch for the past year, but she now weighs 72 pounds and doesn't seem to be receiving the expected continued benefit. How do you convert her to oral oxycodone solution? When do you start the oral oxycodone solution relative to removing the transdermal fentanyl patch?

- WP is a 48-year-old man recently diagnosed with lung cancer, status-post open lung resection. Three days after surgery, WP has received 8 mg of intravenous hydromorphone in the 12 hours prior to discharge. His surgeon writes an order for oxycodone 5 mg/acetaminophen 325 mg, 1 tablet every 4 hours as needed for pain on discharge. Twenty-four hours later, WP's wife is on the phone with the surgeon's office staff, demanding more pain medication. The office staff are concerned about drug-seeking behavior. What's the scoop?

- JR is a 68-year-old man with prostate cancer with significant metastatic disease. He is referred to your outpatient palliative care clinic for a pain consult. He is receiving oral MS Contin 100 mg every 12 hours, oral hydromorphone 4 mg every 4 hours as needed (prn) (using about 5 doses per day), a transdermal fentanyl patch 100 mcg/hr applied every 3 days, and a morphine subcutaneous infusion at 1 mg/hr with 0.5 mg bolus (using about 12 per day). His physician asks your advice on converting all this to a simpler regimen, specifically using methadone. Where do you start?

Ah, . . . drug math. Those two little words can make a strong healthcare professional clench their bowels and want their mommy. But, this doesn't have to be the case! Armed with an understanding of conversion calculations, some semisolid facts about equivalencies, and a healthy sense of "Does that *look* right?" you'll be just fine! Just like much of healthcare, there is both science and art involved in performing opioid conversion calculations. This book is designed to teach you how to do opioid conversion calculations safely and effectively. Jump in; the water's fine!

Opioids are the mainstay of pain management in patients with moderate-to-severe pain. Morphine is practically mother's milk to practitioners who work with patients with advanced illness due to its familiarity, availability of multiple dosage formulations, low cost, and proven effectiveness. However, morphine is not always the answer. For example, we know that up to 30% of cancer patients show poor responsiveness to a given opioid such as morphine during routine administration.[1] This is only one reason why healthcare practitioners must be able to transition patients from one opioid to another, which may require changing the route of administration and/or dosage formulation. A recent multicenter study conducted with palliative care patients showed that 12% of patients required a change to a different opioid (not counting a change in route of administration) for reasons including lack of pain control (64%), development of adverse effects (51%), and medication application problems (22%).[2] Let's take a closer look at the clinical situations that result in the need to switch a patient from one opioid to another.

REASONS FOR CHANGING OPIOIDS

Lack of Therapeutic Response

If the patient's pain is not responding adequately to the opioid and a repeat assessment indicates that opioid therapy continues to remain appropriate, a dose increase would be the most likely intervention. The increase in pain may be due to disease progression or the development of opioid analgesic tolerance. If the patient cannot tolerate an increase in dose due to the development of adverse effects or an increase in dose does not produce a satisfactory reduction in pain, switching to a different opioid may be beneficial.

Occasionally, a patient is receiving a combination analgesic (e.g., Percocet, which contains oxycodone and acetaminophen), and an increase would exceed the maximum recommended daily dose of acetaminophen (4 g). In this case, switching to a tablet or capsule containing just oxycodone would be appropriate, with subsequent dosage titration.

Development of Adverse Effects

If the patient develops an adverse effect to an opioid, the healthcare professional must consider plan B.

Opioid-induced adverse effects are well recognized and include the following:

- Gastrointestinal (nausea, vomiting, constipation)
- Autonomic (xerostomia, urinary retention, postural hypotension)
- Cutaneous (pruritus, sweating)

- Central nervous system (sedation, confusion, dizziness, hallucinations, delirium, myoclonus, hyperalgesia, seizures, and respiratory depression)
- Rarely, opioid allergy (rash, hives, difficulty breathing) may occur.

Faced with an opioid-induced adverse effect, management options include the following:

- Reduction of opioid dose if pain adequately controlled (monitor patient response carefully)
- Aggressive management of the opioid-induced toxicity
- Addition of a nonpharmacologic intervention or co-analgesic to allow reduction of the opioid dose
- Switching to a different route of administration to minimize adverse effect
- Switching to a different opioid that will hopefully be better tolerated and at least as effective

Change in Patient Status

As patients with advanced illness decline, they may not be able to tolerate or use their current opioid formulation or route of administration. For example, a patient may develop difficulty swallowing (dysphagia) or pain with swallowing (odynophagia). Although somewhat controversial, patients who are very cachectic or who have poor peripheral circulation may not receive the fully-expected benefit of a transdermally delivered opioid. On the other hand, a transdermal patch may be more convenient for, and acceptable to, the patient or family, and switching would enhance quality of life.

A patient may require a very high dose of an oral, rectal, or transdermal opioid, necessitating a change to parenteral therapy. Conversely, a patient being discharged home who is able to swallow would likely prefer oral opioid therapy over parenteral.

Other Considerations

Availability of the opioid and/or particular formulation at the patient's pharmacy, cost, and formulary issues may influence prescribing. Medication insurance does not cover all opioid formulations, so a switch may be necessary.

Patients, families, and caregivers may hold healthcare beliefs about certain opioids that affect prescribing such as a previous bad experience with a particular opioid (e.g., severe nausea or vomiting) or a stigma associated with a particular opioid (e.g., "Isn't morphine just for dying patients?" or "Isn't methadone only used by drug addicts?").

An unfortunate reality of practice today is that of drug shortages, which necessitates a switch to a therapeutic alternative. In addition, community pharmacies may unexpectedly reach their monthly allocation of a particular opioid from the wholesaler before reaching the end of the month. If the patient is unable to find their particular opioid, this may require a switch as well.

Drug abuse and diversion is also a harsh reality in today's society, by the patient, a family member, or a visitor to the patient's home. In home-based hospice, for example, practitioners often need to switch to a hopefully less-abused opioid formulation such as transdermal fentanyl and limit quantities kept in the home. This is one example of a risk mitigation strategy.

In an attempt to stem prescription drug abuse and diversion, particularly opioids, many states have imposed a "suggested" maximum daily dose of morphine (e.g., 100 mg a day or morphine milligram equivalents [MME]). The Centers for Disease Control and Prevention (CDC) recommends clinicians prescribe the lowest effective opioid dose after careful consideration, reassess benefits and risks when approaching 50-mg MME per day, and avoid increasing to greater than 90-mg MME (or carefully justify use ≥90-mg MME per day).[3] The CDC has provided guidance on how to calculate the MME, but it's important to remember that this guidance is to *prevent overdose and toxicity, not as a guide to the clinical care of patients.*

Practitioners must be able to calculate the MME of an opioid regimen if the patient is receiving an opioid other than morphine to determine if the patient is approaching or has surpassed the suggested daily dosage limit. Research has shown, however, that practitioners are not consistent in doing these calculations. Rennick and colleagues conducted a survey of physicians, nurse practitioners, physician assistants, and pharmacists, asking participants to calculate the MME of five different opioid regimens (hydrocodone, fentanyl, methadone, oxycodone, and hydromorphone).[4] Three hundred and nineteen participants completed the survey, and there was quite a large standard deviation, indicating a significant variation in mean MME calculations. There was no significant difference between disciplines. I bet all 319 respondents wished they'd had this book!

OPIOID SWITCHING VERSUS ROTATION

Historically, moving a patient from one opioid to a different opioid has been referred to as *opioid rotation.* Other terms include *opioid switching* or *opioid substitution.*[5] These terms are used interchangeably, although some practitioners use the term *opioid rotation* to describe one or sequential trials of opioid therapy to maximize analgesia while minimizing adverse effects. Regardless of the term that is used, getting the job done will require a calculation; hence, the name of this book—*Opioid Conversion Calculations*!

Regardless of what we call it, the big question is, "**Does it work?**" A Cochrane review published in 2004 concluded "the effectiveness of opioid switching to manage pain relief inadequacies and intolerable side effects could not be assessed because of a lack of randomized controlled trials."[6] This review has been withdrawn from the Cochrane database and an update is pending. The European Palliative Care Research Collaborative conducted a systematic review of studies published from 2004 to 2010 to determine more recent outcomes from opioid switching trials.[7] The authors were similarly critical of study design limitations, but concluded that pain intensity was significantly reduced in the majority of studies reviewed, and serious adverse effects were improved. More recently, Mercadante and Bruera reported that satisfactory pain control and reduction in adverse effects after opioid switching is achieved in 50% to 90% of patients.[8]

Several studies published since the European Palliative Care Research Collaborative review found favorable results with opioid switching. Gatti and associates reviewed opioid switching in chronic pain patients from one sustained-release opioid to a different sustained-release opioid (with a transitional respite using an immediate-release opioid).[9] Their conclusion after 326 rotations was the majority of patients experienced improved pain control. Mercadante and colleagues conducted a retrospective review of opioid switching in advanced cancer patients followed at home.[10] Two hundred and one patients were switched, often to parenteral morphine, with good results. Most recently, Gonzalez-Barboteo and associates evaluated 75 opioid rotations in 67 cancer patients.[11] The primary reason for switching was poor pain control; post-switch, average pain intensity decreased by ≥2 points (on a 0–10 numeric rating scale) in 75.4% of cases, and average breakthrough pain intensity decreased by ≥2 points in 57.8% of cases. Their conclusion was that opioid rotation is safe and effective in managing persistent and breakthrough pain.

EQUIANALGESIC OPIOID DOSING

OK, so we want to switch from one opioid to another. How do we get from point A to point B? To understand that, we must first explore several definitions. *Opioid responsiveness* has been defined as "the degree of analgesia achieved as the dose is titrated to an endpoint defined either by intolerable side effects or the occurrence of acceptable analgesia."[12] Obviously, we want a high degree of opioid responsiveness so the patient can achieve pain relief. Can opioid responsiveness be determined solely by opioid potency? What is potency?

Potency refers to the intensity of analgesic effect for a given dose and is dependent on access to the opioid receptor and binding affinity (or "fit") at the receptor site.[12] Several **physicochemical** and **pharmacokinetic** properties affect the access of the opioid to the receptor, which accounts for differing potency among opioid agonists. **Physicochemistry** describes the physical and chemical processes of a drug binding to a receptor (what the drug "does" to the body). The term **pharmacokinetics** describes what the human body "does" to the drug: how we absorb, distribute, metabolize, and excrete a drug.

Two different opioids can be made **equipotent** (have equivalent potency), resulting in an **equianalgesic** effect (the two opioids provide the same degree of pain relief). Equipotent doses of opioids can be determined by accounting for these physicochemical and pharmacokinetic differences through dosage corrections and different routes of administration.[13] Therefore, the potency of an opioid does not solely define opioid responsiveness or efficacy. For opioids that are less "potent," we can simply increase the dose of the drug to get similar efficacy to a more potent opioid. For example, oral oxycodone is generally considered more potent than oral morphine. One commonly used conversion ratio is that 25 (or 30) mg of oral morphine will achieve approximately the same degree of pain relief as 20 mg of oral oxycodone. By knowing this, we can switch from oxycodone to morphine (or vice versa) and achieve a similar clinical outcome by adjusting the dose to allow for this difference.

Doses of two different opioids (or two different routes of administration of the same opioid) are considered **equianalgesic** if they provide approximately the same degree of pain relief. Table 1-1, Equianalgesic Opioid Dosing, lists opioid doses that provide *approximately* the same analgesic response based on potency and bioavailability.[8,14-19] The term **bioavailability** refers to the percentage of drug that is detected in the systemic circulation after its administration and is available to relief. For a drug administered intravenously, the bioavailability is 100%. istered by other routes of administration, such as the oral route, may l bioavailability because the drug must be absorbed through the gut and ough the liver, where it may be subject to metabolism, prior to entering the systemic circulation.

Table 1-1
Equianalgesic Opioid Dosing

| Drug | Equianalgesic Doses (mg) | | Considerations |
	Parenteral	Oral	
Morphine	10	25	A
Codeine	100	200	B
Fentanyl	0.15	NA	C
Hydrocodone	NA	25	D
Hydromorphone	2	5	E
Meperidine	100	300	F
Methadone	See Chapter 6.		G
Oxycodone	10*	20	H
Oxymorphone	1	10	I
Tapentadol	NA	100	J
Tramadol	100*	120	K

*Not available in the United States.

Equianalgesic data presented in this table are that which are most commonly used by healthcare practitioners, and based on best evidence available, but they are still approximate. The clinician is urged to read the following considerations, along with the information in this text, and use good clinical judgment at all times.

Remember, these are NOT opioid DOSES for individual patient use; this is equivalency information.

Considerations:

A. The average oral bioavailability of morphine is 38% (range 15% to 75%).[14,20] With chronic morphine dosing, the average relative potency of IV or sub-Q morphine to oral morphine is between 1:2 and 1:3 (e.g., 20–30 mg of morphine by mouth is equianalgesic to 10 mg IV or sub-Q).[21,22] Oral:rectal morphine bioavailability is considered to be approximately equivalent.[23,24]

B. Codeine is a prodrug, metabolized to morphine by the liver. It is falling out of favor in clinical practice due to limited efficacy, potential toxicity, and variable metabolism. Conversion data are provided here primarily to assist with conversions *from* codeine to a different opioid.

C. Fentanyl is a pure mu-opioid agonist shown to be 75 to 100 times more potent than oral morphine on a molar basis.[25] If we accept that parenteral morphine is 2 to 3 times the potency of oral morphine, then we may assume fentanyl is minimally 30 times more potent than parenteral morphine. In practice, we have seen the parenteral morphine:parenteral fentanyl range described as ranging from 15:1 to 112.5:1. Equivalency theoretically ranges from 10:0.1 mg (IV morphine:IV fentanyl) to 10:0.3. Many clinicians use an equivalency of 4-mg/hr IV morphine equivalent to 100-mcg/hr parenteral or transdermal fentanyl (TDF) (this would be a 10:0.25 IV morphine:IV fentanyl conversion).[1,14,26] Research has shown that the conversion from IV to transdermal fentanyl is approximately 1:1.[27] The bioavailability of transdermal fentanyl ranges from 60% to 84%.[28] Assuming bioavailability of 60%, and using published standards of oral morphine:transdermal fentanyl conversions, this calculates to an equivalency of IV morphine:fentanyl of 10:0.15. When administered as a single IV bolus, fentanyl has a redistribution-limited short duration of action. With prolonged exposure to fentanyl, elimination is clearance limited.[29] For these reasons, a more conservative morphine:fentanyl conversion is used in this equianalgesic table (10:0.15).

A few studies have evaluated switching from parenteral fentanyl to TDF and vice versa.[14] A 1:1 conversion has been shown to be generally safe and effective when switching from IV to TDF, but switching from sub-Q to TDF may result in a somewhat higher fentanyl serum concentration.[27,30,31]

TDF patch (used for chronic pain) dosed in micrograms, is roughly equivalent to 50% of the total daily dose of oral morphine in milligrams (e.g., TDF 25-mcg patch is roughly equal to 50 mg oral morphine per day).[32] Reddy suggests that the median opioid rotation ratio from transdermal fentanyl (mg/day) to morphine equivalent daily dose is 100, and from transdermal fentanyl (mcg/hr) to morphine equivalent daily dose is 2.4.[33] Refer to Chapter 5 for additional information on dosing transdermal fentanyl.

D. Oral hydrocodone equivalence to oral morphine is not clearly defined, but generally thought to be equal to or less potent than oxycodone.[34] Reddy reported a hydrocodone-dose dependent median opioid rotation ratio from hydrocodone to morphine equivalent daily dose from 1.1 to 2.25.[35]

E. Oral bioavailability of hydromorphone may be as high as 60%, particularly with chronic dosing, with ranges from 29% to 95%.[36-38] Equianalgesic tables have long cited a 1:5 ratio for parenteral to oral hydromorphone, but we must remember the very large range in bioavailability. This likely is a reflection of the tremendous differences between populations studied (healthy, ill, young, old, etc.). A 1:5 (parenteral to oral) ratio may result in underdosing or overdosing, depending on which way you are converting. Data from steady-state conversions from parenteral to oral hydromorphone suggest a ratio of 1:2.5 (parenteral:oral hydromorphone) is more appropriate, and is reflected in our Equianalgesic Table.[39] Refer to Chapter 2 for greater discussion about conversion ratios observed from steady-state dosing.

Research has shown a lower dose ratio and a directional influence seen when converting between morphine and hydromorphone. It is suggested that when switching from morphine (M) to hydromorphone (HM) (using the same route of administration; e.g., sub-Q to sub-Q or oral to oral), a conversion ratio of 5:1 (M:HM) when switching from morphine to hydromorphone and a dose ratio of 3.7:1 (M:HM) when switching from hydromorphone to morphine (again, using the same route of administration).[40]

Oral:rectal bioavailability is approximately equal; the dosing interval approved by the Food and Drug Administration (FDA) for rectal hydromorphone is every 6 hours.

F. Meperidine has fallen out of favor clinically due to toxicity of the metabolite, *normeperidine*. Conversion data are provided here primarily to assist with conversions *from* meperidine to a different opioid.

G. Methadone dosing is highly variable, and conversion to/from other opioids is *not* linear; refer to Chapter 6 for additional information on methadone dosing.

H. Because of the variations in bioavailability between morphine (range 15% to 75%) and oxycodone (60% or more), the equianalgesic ratio for oral morphine:oxycodone ranges from 1:1 to 2:1, partially dependent on the patient's ability to absorb the opioid.[41,42]

Parenteral oxycodone is not available in the United States. According to manufacturer's information [Mundipharma New Zealand Limited, distributed by Pharmaco (NZ) Ltd] 2 mg of oral oxycodone is approximately equivalent to 1-mg parenteral oxycodone.[43] This ratio may be somewhat conservative because the oral bioavailability of oxycodone has been shown to be 60% or greater.[42]

I. Conversion from oral morphine or oral oxycodone to oxymorphone has been reported as 30:10 and 20:10, respectively per package labeling. Some data suggest the conversion ratio when switching to oxymorphone is closer to 18:10 for morphine (18-mg oral morphine = 10-mg oral oxymorphone), and 12:10 for oxycodone (12-mg oral oxycodone = 10-mg oral oxymorphone), especially once at steady state.[44]

J. Conversion to and from tapentadol from other opioids, expressed in oral morphine equivalents, is suggested to be 1:3.3 (morphine:tapentadol).[45]

K. Tramadol has multiple mechanisms of action; binding to the mu opioid receptor is only one mechanism. Thus, there are additional considerations when determining equianalgesic beyond bioavailability. Parenteral tramadol has been shown to be approximately equipotent to parenteral morphine in a 10:1 (tramadol:morphine) ratio.[46] With chronic dosing, oral tramadol achieves between 90% and 100% bioavailability.[47] Despite bioavailability data, equipotent use of oral morphine and oral tramadol ranges from 1:4 to 1:10 (morphine:tramadol). Therefore, using an equivalence of 120 mg oral tramadol may be very conservative.[48] Importantly, tramadol may be more potent when being used to treat neuropathic pain, as opposed to nociceptive pain.[49]

****

Looking at Table 1-1, doses listed *across* a row for a given opioid show equipotent doses (e.g., 25-mg oral morphine provides *approximately* the same analgesic as 10-mg parenteral morphine—hey, I did promise you *semi-solid facts!*). In this case, *parenteral* refers to both intravenous (IV) and subcutaneous (sub-Q) dosing. (*Note:* We voted intramuscular [IM] off the island; an IM analgesic is an oxymoron, although if you insist, it's close enough to throw in with sub-Q and IV.) Doses for different opioids in a *column* are also equipotent (e.g., 10-mg parenteral morphine is approximately equivalent to 2-mg parenteral hydromorphone). We can even use this table to look at equivalent doses between opioids *and* routes of administration (e.g., 10-mg parenteral morphine is approximately equivalent to 20-mg oral oxycodone). You will learn more about actually using this table in subsequent chapters. Even though we have just spoken in terms of equivalent *doses*, we're really referring to equivalencies or ratios. The values in this table are *not* patient-specific doses, nor are they recommended starting doses. For example, even though "10 mg" is shown in the "parenteral morphine" box in Table 1-1, this does *not* mean it is necessarily the appropriate *dose* for a given patient.

For completeness sake, it is important to remember that a patient's response to an opioid (the **pharmacodynamic effect**: what the drug does to the body), despite our very best estimate of equianalgesic dosing, may be different from expected. We are created as unique individuals; how we react to drugs varies from person to person based on our genetics and other factors.

ONE SIZE FITS ALL AND OTHER URBAN LEGENDS: THE PROBLEM WITH "THOSE TABLES"

All the left-brain thinkers are no doubt delighted with Table 1-1, Equianalgesic Opioid Dosing. It makes so much sense, doesn't it? Someone figured out the potency differences, put it in this table, we do the math, and we're home free with our opioid conversion calculations! *Well, it's not quite that simple! Unfortunately, there are some caveats to "those tables" such as the one noted previously.*

Early equianalgesic dosing ratios were largely derived from single-dose studies, but questions surfaced about the clinical applicability of the data.[14] When the Equianalgesic Opioid Dosing table was written for the first edition of this book, a lot of head banging was going on. With the publication of equianalgesic data from well-designed trials using a crossover design, the utility of an equianalgesic dosing table has been called into question, warranting this author feeling the need for an anxiolytic while writing the second edition! Parts of the chart still reflect data from older, single-dose studies, while more current data reflect preferred methodology. I'll go get the Ativan while you read more about inherent sources of error in an Equianalgesic Opioid Dosing table!

Source of Equianalgesic Data

As stated above, much of the data in this table were obtained from single-dose crossover studies in opioid-naïve patients with acute pain. An example would be a clinical trial where a healthy volunteer or patient received one dose of Opioid A and the clinical response was observed. Then the volunteer received one dose of Opioid B and the clinical response was observed and compared to the dose of Opioid A. Obviously these individuals had limited opioid exposure (both duration and dose). Very few studies have evaluated equianalgesia in chronic pain patients, and we know that accumulation of opioids and/or their metabolites may contribute to the overall effectiveness of the opioid. For example, with repeated dosing, the analgesic properties of the active metabolite of morphine (morphine-6-glucuronide) become clinically apparent.

Patient-Specific Variables

Patient-related variables such as age, sex, pharmacogenomics (polymorphism of opioid receptors), quantitative and qualitative differences among individuals in cytochrome P450 function, organ function (liver and kidney), level and stability of pain control, duration and extent of opioid exposure, interacting medications, and comorbid conditions have not been considered in putting together a table such as the one shown above. No consideration has been given as to why the patient is no longer responding to the original opioid or the influence of existential pain (e.g., suffering) in patients with advanced illness. All of these factors can influence the pharmacokinetics (absorption, distribution, metabolism, and excretion) and pharmacodynamics (pharmacologic effect) of the opioid, and they are largely unaccounted for in the Equianalgesic Opioid Dosing table.

Unidirectional Versus Bidirectional Equivalencies

In looking at the Equianalgesic Opioid Dosing table, we assume that the data are bidirectional. For example, we see that the oral morphine:hydromorphone ratio is approximately 5:1 (25-mg oral morphine is about equal to 5-mg oral hydromorphone), and we assume that ratio holds whether we are converting from morphine to hydromorphone or from hydromorphone to morphine. However, well-crafted cross-over trials have shown the oral morphine:hydromorphone ratio is actually 5-8:1, while the oral hydromorphone:morphine ratio is 1:3-4.[14] I'm sure you're holding your head in your hands right now, thinking "What do I do about this?" We'll discuss this later in the chapter, but basically you do the best you can, and you *monitor* your patient closely!

Bottom Line It for Me

Pereira and colleagues wrestled with the equianalgesia issue almost 20 years ago, reviewing opioid conversion literature from 1966 to 1999. They had six conclusions based on this review (which are still true today).

1. There exists a general paucity of data related to long-term dosing, and studies are heterogeneous in nature.
2. The ratios exhibit extremely wide ranges.
3. Methadone is more heterogeneous in nature.
4. The ratios related to methadone are highly correlated with the dose of the previous opioid.
5. The ratio may change according to the direction of the opioid switch.
6. Discrepancies exist with respect to both oxycodone and fentanyl.[50]

Their proposals for updating the equianalgesic dosing table (using prominent footnoting per their recommendation) are as follows:

1. Differentiate between single-dose conversion data versus steady-state data. Steady-state data are preferable when available.
2. Remember that an equianalgesic dosing table is a *guideline*; it's not set in concrete. No equianalgesic table accounts for the wide variation between individuals, the influence of repetitive opioid dosing, and varying opioid responsiveness. This is why smartphone apps that perform opioid conversion calculations are of limited usefulness.
3. When using equianalgesic dosing guidance, pay close attention to opioid titration and monitoring to ensure the patient is achieving pain relief as quickly as possible, while doing so in a safe fashion.
4. Recognize the lack of complete cross-tolerance between opioids; conversions should take into consideration factors such as available equianalgesic data (and are they steady-state data?), clinical factors, concerns for patient safety, and incomplete cross-tolerance. When switching from one opioid to a different opioid, dose reduction is advised.
5. Use extra caution when the patient has renal impairment. Fentanyl and methadone are less likely to be problematic in this situation, but opioids such as morphine and hydromorphone may result in neurotoxicity.[50]

As my good friend Dr. Mellar P. Davis says, "Opioid equianalgesia equivalencies are ranges with large variation, thanks to the heterogeneous populations from which this data are derived, and applied. Numbers in an equianalgesia table get you to the ballpark to play ball. Hitting a home run is dependent on the interactions between the pitcher and batter. Sometimes you strike out; sometimes there are base hits. You cannot make it neater than reality" (personal communication, February 2018).[51] Yeah, what he said!

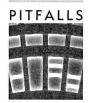

PITFALLS **Be Careful Which Rule You Slide On**

Many pharmaceutical manufacturers of opioid products will provide a conversion calculator for ease of converting to *their* product. In general, the guidelines they provide are fairly conservative for switching from other opioids to *their* product. Therefore, it is imperative that practitioners *not* use these conversion calculators to convert *from* the manufacturer's opioid to other opioids, or between other opioids. Obviously, if the conversion calculator is *conservative* going to the manufacturer's opioid, when used erroneously, it would be too *aggressive* when converting from their opioid.

INTRODUCTION TO THE PROCESS OF OPIOID CONVERSION CALCULATIONS

We will discuss opioid conversion calculations (OCC) at length in subsequent chapters, but it is important to recognize that there is a *process* to doing these calculations. This discussion includes the "art" as well as the "science" in OCC. Gammaitoni and colleagues recommended a five-step approach to OCC, which is shown in Table 1-2.[51] This five-step process illustrates the importance of calculating not only an effective dose, but even more important, a safe dose. As shown in Figure 1-1, your best option would be to calculate a safe *and* effective dose (top right quadrant). Barring that, a less effective but safer dose is your next best goal. When calculating a new opioid regimen, it is perfectly acceptable to be conservative with the scheduled, or long-acting, opioid dose. However, if you are being conservative (which is a good thing), the patient must have adequate rescue rapid- or short-acting analgesics available for breakthrough pain.

Safer	Most safe dose, but not as effective as it could be. **This is an Acceptable Quadrant.** Have a rescue plan in place (e.g., rapid- or short-acting opioid).	Most effective and most safe dose. **This is the Preferred Quadrant.**
Less Safe	Dose not safe or effective; clearly a place you do NOT want to be! **This is your Least Acceptable Quadrant!**	Most effective dose, but not as safe as it could be. **This is *Not* an Acceptable Quadrant.**
	Less Effective	More Effective

Figure 1-1. Opioid conversion calculations should be as safe *and* effective as possible.

Table 1-2

Five-Step Approach to Opioid Conversion

• **Step 1**—Globally assess the patient (i.e., PQRSTU, or another method) to determine if the uncontrolled pain is secondary to worsening of existing pain or development of a new type of pain.
• **Step 2**—Determine the total daily usage of the current opioid. This should include all long-acting and breakthrough opioid doses.
• **Step 3**—Decide which opioid analgesic will be used for the new agent and consult the established conversion tables to arrive at the proper dose of the new opioid, recognizing the limitations of the data.
• **Step 4**—Individualize the dosage based on assessment information gathered in Step 1 and ensure adequate access to breakthrough medication.
• **Step 5**—Patient follow-up and continual reassessment, especially during the first 7–14 days, to fine-tune the total daily dose (long-acting + short-acting) and increase or decrease the around the clock long-acting dosage accordingly.

Source: Reprinted with permission from: Gammaitoni AR, Fine P, Alvarez N, et al. Clinical application of opioid equianalgesic data. *Clin J Pain.* 2003;19:286-297.

Let's look at the five-step approach to opioid conversions.

Step 1

Lack of effectiveness is probably one of the most common reasons we switch to a new opioid. Before jumping in with your calculator, however, it is important to assess the pain. This will help the healthcare practitioner determine if continuing opioid therapy (including possibly switching to a new opioid) is the best course of action, versus adding a co-analgesic.

There are many proposed methods to assess a report of pain, but one of the most common is the *PQRSTU method.* The letters represent elements of symptom analysis that help the patient characterize the pain, and include

- ***P***—*precipitating and palliating:* What brings on or worsens the pain? What relieves the pain (nonpharmacologic and pharmacologic)? If pharmacologic, ask what the patient has taken (including breakthrough analgesics), what the response was, and if any side effects developed.

- ***Q***—*quality:* Can you describe the pain in your own words? You're looking for words such as *stabbing, shooting, throbbing, aching, gnawing,* etc.

- ***R***—*region and radiation:* Where is the pain? Does the pain move anywhere else? Is the pain deep inside or more superficial?

- ***S***—*severity:* There are many severity rating scales. For example, if *0* is no pain, and *10* is the worst pain you can imagine, how would you rate your pain right now? What is the *best* the pain is over the course of a day? The worst? The average? One hour after taking your rapid- or short-acting pain medication? You may need to consider nonverbal indicators of pain for patients who cannot describe it for you.

- ***T***—*temporal:* Is the pain constant or does it come and go? If it comes and goes, how many times per day does it occur? How long does it last? Is it increasing in frequency or duration over the past few days/weeks?

- ***U***—*you:* How is the pain affecting your life? How has the pain affected your ability to sleep, your appetite, your ability to ambulate, your mood, etc.?

This information, along with physical inspection of the painful areas will help you determine if this is the same pain the patient originally complained of, or if this is a new pain.

Step 2

Part of effective medication reconciliation is to get a complete and accurate list of all medications the patient is taking. You know what analgesics were *prescribed* for the patient, but this does not guarantee that's the way the patient has been taking these medications. Be sure to include both the long-acting and rapid- or short-acting analgesics the patient has been taking when determining the total daily dose of opioid. Of course, you will also ask about nonprescription, complementary, and alternative product use. The perceptive practitioner will also ask the patient about use of illicit substances such as heroin and will consider this in the total daily opioid consumption (good luck with that!).

Do You Know What I Know (About Your Medications)?

FAST FACTS 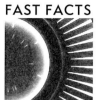 Unsurprisingly, patients frequently lack basic knowledge about their analgesics; this can often be a barrier to good pain management. When performing medication reconciliation, you can use this time to assess the patient's knowledge of his or her medications as well as ask how he or she is actually taking the medication (which may or may not reflect what is typed on the medication label). Taking it one medication at a time, show the patient the medication and say "Tell me how and when you take this medication." You can also ask if the patient knows the purpose, administration precautions, and potential adverse effects of the medications. This information will help you make clinical decisions (the "art") about the calculation.

PEARLS 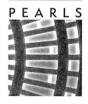 *I Spy With My Little Eye . . . Patients tend to forget to tell you about medications taken by the nonoral route of administration. This includes inhaled medications (e.g., metered dose inhalers or nebulized medications), injected medications (e.g., insulin), and topical products (e.g., ointments, creams, and transdermal medications). Detection of any transdermal opioids is critical when performing OCC. It is not uncommon for a patient to be admitted to the hospital or to hospice care and not tell the admitting nurse that he or she is wearing a transdermal fentanyl patch. If the nurse does not physically inspect the patient, this important piece of information may be missed. The healthcare team is often left scratching their heads wondering why the patient's pain control deteriorates 1 or 2 days later.*

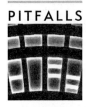

PITFALLS

The Whole Truth and Nothing But the Truth

It is critically important to ask the patient about *all* doses of rapid- or short-acting analgesics he or she is taking. Frequently, patients want to impress the healthcare provider with how severe the pain has been, so when asked, they claim "Doc, I've been taking that liquid medicine every 2 hours, just like it says on the label." This is a red flag—is the patient really, truly taking the rapid- or short-acting opioid *every* 2 hours around the clock? Literally, 12 doses on average over a 24-hour period? Patients are generally referring to the hours they are awake. If you take the "every 2 hours around the clock" report at face value and base your OCC calculation on that, you may be calculating too aggressive a dose and put the patient at risk for toxicity. Encourage use of a pain diary so the patient or caregiver records all doses of rapid- or short-acting opioids taken for breakthrough pain. Then you can average their use over 24 hours.

Step 3

Decide which opioid to switch to by using your knowledge of drug therapy selection. This decision may be influenced by the patient's ability to swallow medications or apply a transdermal system, renal function (drugs with pharmacologically active metabolites, such as morphine, are not the best choice in patients with end-stage renal disease), or the nature of the pain (perhaps you want to choose methadone because there is anecdotal evidence suggesting it is more effective for neuropathic or mixed nociceptive-neuropathic pain than other opioids). The decision may be driven by the availability of dosage formulations that are best suited to your patient's needs (e.g., oral concentrated solution, parenteral infusion). The potential for drug interactions (e.g., methadone can interact with many medications) and the patient's previous history of response to various opioids should be considered. Last, the decision may be influenced by formulary or financial limitations, or safety concerns (e.g., children in the home, risk of drug abuse and diversion).

Once you have decided which opioid you are switching to, consult the Equianalgesic Opioid Dosing table, and calculate the equianalgesic dose of the new opioid (this will be discussed at length in subsequent chapters). As stated earlier, using the Equianalgesic Opioid Dosing table is a ballpark estimate of the opioid dose to which you are switching. Let's take the ballpark analogy and run with it. Buying a ticket to the ballgame held in a stadium that seats 70,000 people is equivalent to consulting the Equianalgesic Opioid Dosing table and doing your calculation. Now you have your new opioid dose, but what do you do with it? It's like arriving at the ballpark with your ticket in hand. Now what? You have to consult your ticket to see what section you're in, which row, and which seat. How quickly you get to your seat depends on how quickly the game is going to start. You may have to get to your seat immediately, maybe even run and increase your risk of falling if you want to catch the early action. On the other hand, if you're early, you can probably score a hotdog and popcorn as you meander to your seat. Similarly, if the patient is in pain crisis, you will want to act immediately, be a bit more aggressive, and monitor him or her extremely closely. If you are switching to a new opioid for a less urgent reason, you can be more conservative and methodical. Integrating the art and science of OCC will help you hit this one out of the ballpark!

Step 4

Once you do your calculation, you will need to individualize the dose for the patient. Using the information you gathered in Step 1, you basically have three choices. You can use the dose you calculated, you can increase it, or you can decrease it. When converting from one opioid to another because of unacceptable adverse effects (where pain control was not an issue), it would be advisable to reduce the newly calculated dose by 25% to 50%. Patients likely develop some degree of **tolerance** to the therapeutic effects of an opioid, but when they convert to a new opioid, they will not show the same degree of tolerance. *Tolerance* is defined as a phenomenon where continued exposure to a drug reduces its effectiveness, occasionally necessitating a dosage increase. The increased opioid sensitivity seen with switching is known as *incomplete cross-tolerance*. Therefore, if you calculate an equivalent dose, but don't reduce it, the patient may experience an enhanced and possibly toxic effect from the new opioid. Another reason for reducing the dose of the new opioid has to do with the "ballpark" nature of the equivalency values in the Equianalgesic Opioid Dosing table (Table 1-1) discussed previously.

If you are switching the patient because his or her pain was not controlled on the original opioid, you may consider *not* reducing a full 25% to 50% of the calculated dose. The patient will experience a greater sensitivity to the new opioid, but this is a welcome effect, because the patient's pain was not controlled. It would be an extremely rare circumstance where you would calculate a new opioid regimen *and* increase the dose.

Fine and Portenoy established a "best practices" for opioid rotations based on consensus from an expert panel.[52] Their guidelines are as follows:

- Calculate the equianalgesic dose of the opioid to which you are switching.
- Reduce the calculated dose by 25% to 50% (this excludes methadone and fentanyl, which are seriously different—see Chapters 5 and 6).
  - The clinical situation will determine reduction by 25% versus 50%.
  - If switching from a high opioid dose, consider a larger reduction (e.g., 50%). Also consider this larger reduction if the patient is not Caucasian or is elderly or medically frail.
  - Less reduction (e.g., a 25% reduction or less) may be appropriate if the patient is switching from one route to another of the same opioid.
- Consider a 15% to 30% dosage adjustment (increase or decrease in dose) based on patient response to the initial dose. Always provide a rescue analgesic, and carefully assess the patient.[14]

So how do you decide how much to reduce the calculated dose? Here's where the art comes in (as in "art and science!"). We know that one size really *doesn't* fit all; therefore, you must consider your patient and his or her specific situation, and the data that supports this decision. Is the opioid conversion data you're using from single-dose studies or steady-state data? Is the patient at home? In the hospital? In a long-term care facility or assisted living? Is there a competent caregiver present or adequate nursing staff to assess for opioid-related adverse effects? How acute is the need to make this switch? How severe is the pain? Is the patient a 42-year-old man or a 94-year-old woman? Trust your gut!

- Once you've decided on the optimal total daily dose of the new opioid, you need to divide the 24-hour dose as appropriate for the new dosing interval (e.g., by the number of times the new medication will be administered in a 24-hour period). For example, if you're switching to an hourly infusion, you would calculate the dose to be delivered per hour by dividing the total daily dose by 24. If you will be advising the patient to take his or her opioid every 4 hours, you need to divide the total daily dose by 6.

- The individual dosage amount you calculate will then need to be rounded up or down to be a reasonable number: It must be "doable" with commercially available tablets, capsules, oral solution, or whatever dosage formulation you are going to use. You can be Albert Einstein and do complicated conversion calculations all day long, but there's no way in the world you can accurately give 12.75 mg of oxycodone every 4 hours with a tablet or capsule!

- The last step in individualization (and a very important step) is to account for residual drug in the patient's system (if any) during the conversion process. This is especially important when converting *from* long-acting oral opioids or transdermal patches. Starting the new drug, particularly a regularly scheduled, long-acting opioid (known as the **basal dose**), should be delayed if significant residual drug is in the body. In the meantime, the patient can use his or her rapid- or short-acting opioid should the pain recur. This will become clearer as you work through the problems included in this book.

Step 5

OK, you've done the deed! You've assessed the patient, picked the best opioid, sharpened your pencil, calculated a dose, adjusted it, and implemented your plan. But, your work is NOT done! This is where the real skill comes in: monitoring the patient for several days to 2 weeks after a medication change (duration of vigilant monitoring depends on time to achieve steady-state serum drug levels). Because the Equianalgesic Opioid Dosing table is not set in concrete, you may have been a bit over- or underaggressive with your dosing. You need to monitor the subjective and objective monitoring parameters for both therapeutic effectiveness (pain control) and potential toxicity from the opioid. Every patient's situation is different. Figure 1-2 is an example of a monitoring plan.

Armed with this information, you can fine-tune the opioid regimen over the ensuing hours and days. You may also adjust both the long- and short-acting opioid in the regimen as you monitor the patient's response. It is important to share your monitoring and titration plan with the patient, family, and caregiver; you are more likely to experience success if you explain the transition from one opioid to another, the importance of the rescue medications, and so forth.

	Subjective Parameters	Objective Parameters
Monitoring for therapeutic effectiveness	• Pain rating • Patient subjectively states he or she is better able to perform ADLs (e.g., personal care), sleep, ambulate, etc.	• Patient objectively reports he or she sleeps longer and does not awaken in pain. • Patient can objectively ambulate further without pain. • Limited use of rescue opioid
Monitoring for potential toxicity from an opioid	• Complaints of constipation, nausea, sedation, dizziness, confusion, itching, hallucinations, vomiting, dry mouth, urinary retention, sweating, rash, or hives	• Level of arousal/sedation • Unstimulated respiratory rate; pattern and depth of respiration • Pinpoint pupils • Bowel movement frequency • Episodes of emesis • Mini-mental state exam • Hours spent sleeping • Signs of excoriation

Figure 1-2. Example of a patient monitoring plan.

ADLs = activities of daily living

CONCLUSION

In this chapter, we have introduced the idea of opioid conversion calculations. There are many clinical situations where OCC is an appropriate intervention. It is important to use a systematic process when switching a patient from one opioid to another, and strongly consider patient variables when instituting a new regimen. Follow-up is critical to patient success. We will discuss numerous specific examples of opioid conversions in upcoming chapters.

Could I Get That to Go, Please? Bottom Line It for Me . . .

▶ Opioids are an important tool in the management of moderate-to-severe pain, but clinicians often need to switch from one opioid or dosage formulation, to another. This may be prompted by poor response, development of adverse effects, change in patient status, or other reasons.

▶ Based on the concepts of potency and bioavailability, Table 1-1, Equianalgesic Opioid Dosing, has been developed. Based on the best data available, doses of two different opioids (or routes of administration) would be considered equianalgesic when calculated using the ratios in the table.

▶ There are many limitations when using the Equianalgesic Opioid Dosing table such as design flaws in the research that produced the data and lack of consideration of patient-specific variables.

▶ A five-step process is recommended when doing an opioid conversion.

  ▶ Step 1—Assess the pain complaint carefully to determine if conversion is appropriate.

  ▶ Step 2—Determine patient's total daily consumption of opioid (prolonged-release opioid and average immediate-release opioid use).

  ▶ Step 3—Set up ratio using data from Equianalgesic Opioid Dosing table and calculate total daily dose of opioid regimen to which you are switching.

  ▶ Step 4—Modify the calculated dose, generally reducing by 25% to 50%, guided by the patient-specific situation. Determine the new opioid regimen (e.g., specific dose, dosing interval, breakthrough analgesia).

  ▶ Step 5—Implement recommendation and monitor patient's response carefully; adjust regimen further as clinically indicated.

▶ In conclusion, practitioners should strive to calculate the most *effective* dose for the patient, while valuing a *safe* dose above all. Liberal use of breakthrough analgesia should be available to minimize pain.

REFERENCES

1. Indelicato RA, Portenoy RK. Opioid rotation in the management of refractory cancer pain. *J Clin Oncol.* 2002;20:348-352.

2. Muller-Busch HC, Lindena G, Tietze K, et al. Opioid switch in palliative care, opioid choice by clinical need and opioid availability. *Eur J Pain.* 2005;9:571-579.

3. Dowell D, Haegerich TM, Chou R. CCD guideline for prescribing opioids for chronic pain—United States, 2016. *MMWR Recomm Rep.* 2016;65(No. RR-1):1-49.

4. Rennick A, Atkinson T, Cimino NM, et al. Variability in opioid equivalence calculations. *Pain Med.* 2015 Sep 9. Epub ahead of print.

5. Riley J, Ross JR, Rutter D, et al. No pain relief from morphine? Individual variation in sensitivity to morphine and the need to switch to an alternative opioid in cancer patients. *Support Care Cancer.* 2006;14:56-64.

6. Quigley C. Opioid switching to improve pain relief and drug tolerability. *The Cochrane Library.* 2004. http://onlinelibrary.wiley.com/doi/10.1002/14651858.CD004847/abstract. Accessed December 25, 2017.

7. Dale O, Moksnes K, Kaasa S. European Palliative Care Research Collaborative pain guidelines: Opioid switching to improve analgesia or reduce side effects. A systematic review. *Palliat Med.* 2010;25(5):494-503.

8. Mercadante S, Bruera E. Opioid switching in cancer pain: From the beginning to nowadays. *Crit Rev Oncol Hematol.* 2016;99:241-248.

9. Gatti A, Reale C, Luzi M, et al. Effects of opioid rotation in chronic pain patients: ORTIBARN study. *Clin Drug Investig.* 2010;30(suppl 2):39-47.

10. Mercadante S, Valle A, Porzio G, et al. Opioid switching in patients with advanced cancer followed at home. A retrospective analysis. *J Pain Symptom Manage.* 2013;45(2):298-304.

11. Gonzalez-Barboteo J, Alentorn XG, Manuel FA, et al. Effectiveness of opioid rotation in the control of cancer pain: the ROTODOL study. *J Opioid Manage.* 2014;10(6):395-403.

12. Mercadante S, Portenoy RK. Opioid poorly-responsive cancer pain. Part 1: Clinical considerations. *J Pain Symptom Manage.* 2001;21:144-150.

13. Ferrante FM. Principles of opioid pharmacotherapy: practical implications of basic mechanisms. *J Pain Symptom Manage.* 1996;11:265-273.

14. Patanwala AE, Duby J, Waters D, Erstad BL. Opioid conversions in acute care. *Ann Pharmacother.* 2007;41:255-267.

15. Carr DB, Jacox AK, Chapman CR, et al. *Acute Pain Management: Operative or Medical Procedures and Trauma. Clinical Practice Guideline No. 1.* AHCPR Pub. No. 92-0032. Rockville, MD: Agency for Health Care Policy and Research, Public Health Service, U.S. Department of Health and Human Services; 1992.

16. Jacox A, Carr DB, Payne R, et al. *Management of Cancer Pain. Clinical Practice Guideline No. 9,* AHCPR Publication No. 94-0592. Rockville, MD. Agency for Health Care Policy and Research, U.S. Department of Health and Human Services, Public Health Service; 1994.

17. Eastern Metropolitan Region Palliative Care Consortium. Opioid Conversion Ratios Guide to Palliative Care Practice 2016. Eastern Metropolitan Region Palliative Care Consortium; March 5, 2016. http://www.emrpcc.org.au/wp-content/uploads/2016/05/Opioid-Conversions-May-3-2016-final.pdf. Accessed August 28, 2017.

18. Syrmis W, Good P, Wootton J, et al. Opioid conversion ratios used in palliative care: Is there an Australian consensus? *Int Med J.* 2014;44(5):483-489.

19. American Pain Society. *Principles of Analgesic Use.* 7th ed. Chicago, IL: American Pain Society; 2016.

20. Inturrisi C. Clinical pharmacology of opioids for pain. *Clin J Pain.* 2002;18:S3-S13.

21. Kalso E, Vainio A. Morphine and oxycodone hydrochloride in the management of cancer pain. *Clin Pharmacol Ther.* 1990;47:639-646.

22. Reddy SK, Agloria M. Pain management. In: *The M.D. Anderson Supportive and Palliative Care Handbook.* 3rd ed. The University of Texas MD Anderson Cancer Center; 2008:19-43.

23. Westerling D, Lindahl S, Andersson KE, et al. Absorption and bioavailability of rectally administered morphine in women. *Eur J Clin Pharmacol.* 1982;23(1):59-64.

24. Brook-Williams P. Morphine suppositories for intractable pain. *Can Med Assoc J.* 1982;126:14.

25. Donner B, Zenz M, Tryba M, et al. Direct conversion from oral morphine to transdermal fentanyl: a multicenter study in patients with cancer pain. *Pain.* 1996;64:527-534.

26. Lawlor P, Pereira J, Bruera E. Dose ratios among different opioids: Underlying issues and an update on the use of the equianalgesic table. In: *Topics in Palliative Care.* Vol 5. New York, NY: Oxford University Press; 2001:247-276.

27. Nomura M, Inoue K, Matsushita S, et al. Serum concentration of fentanyl during conversion from intravenous to transdermal administration to patients with chronic cancer pain. *Clin J Pain.* 2013;29(6):487-491.

28. Solassol I, Caumette L, Bressolle F, et al. Inter- and intra-individual variability in transdermal fentanyl absorption in cancer pain patients. *Oncol Rep.* 2005;14(4):1029-1036.

29. Mather LE. Clinical pharmacokinetics of fentanyl and its newer derivatives. *Clin Pharmacokinet.* 1983;8:422-446.

30. Samala RV, Bloise R, Davis MP. Efficacy and safety of a six-hour continuous overlap method for converting intravenous to transdermal fentanyl in cancer pain. *J Pain Symptom Manage.* 2014;48(1):132-136.

31. Oosten AW, Abrantes JA, Jonsson S, et al. Treatment with subcutaneous and transdermal fentanyl: results from a population pharmacokinetic study in cancer patients. *Eur J Clin Pharmacol.* 2016;72:459-467.

32. Breitbart W, Chandler S, Eagel B, et al. An alternative algorithm for dosing transdermal fentanyl for cancer-related pain. *Oncology.* 2000;14:695-705.

33. Reddy A, Yennurajalingam S, Reddy S, et al. The opioid rotation ratio from transdermal fentanyl to "strong" opioid in patients with cancer pain. *J Pain Symptom Manage.* 2016;51(6):1040-1045.

34. Hallenbeck JL. *Palliative Care Perspectives.* New York, NY: Oxford University Press; 2003:71.

35. Reddy A, Yennurajalingam S, Desai H, et al. The opioid rotation ratio of hydrocodone to strong opioids in cancer patients. *Oncologist.* 2014;19:1186-1193.

36. Vallner JJ, Stewart JT, Kotzan JA, et al. Pharmacokinetics and bioavailability of hydromorphone following intravenous and oral administration to human subjects. *J Clin Pharmacol.* 1981;21:152-156.

37. Ritschel WA, Parab PV, Denson DD, et al. Absolute bioavailability of hydromorphone after per-oral and rectal administration in humans: saliva/plasma ratio and clinical effects. *J Clin Pharmacol.* 1987;27:647-653.

38. Parab PV, Ritschel WA, Coyle DE, et al. Pharmacokinetics of hydromorphone after intravenous, peroral and rectal administration to human subjects. *Biopharm Drug Dispos.* 1988;9:187-199.

39. Reddy A, Vidal M, Stephen S, et al. The conversion ratio from intravenous hydromorphone to oral opioids in cancer patients. *J Pain Symptom Manage.* 2017;54(3):280-288.

40. Lawlor P, Turner K, Hanson J, et al. Dose ratio between morphine and hydromorphone in patients with cancer pain: a retrospective study. *Pain.* 1997;72:79-85.

41. Anderson R, Saiers JH, Abram S, et al. Accuracy in equianalgesic dosing: conversion dilemmas. *J Pain Symptom Manage.* 2001;21:397-406.

42. Pöyhiä R, Seppälä T, Olkkola KT, et al. The pharmacokinetics and metabolism of oxycodone after intramuscular and oral administration to healthy subjects. *Br J Clin Pharmacol.* 1992;33:617-621.

43. New Zealand Medicines and Medical Devices Safety Authority. Oxynorm (solution for injection or infusion). Medsafe. Published June 29, 2017. http://www.medsafe.govt.nz/profs/datasheet/o/oxynorminj.pdf. Accessed August 30, 2017.

44. Sloan P, Slatkin N, Ahdieh H. Effectiveness and safety of oral extended-release oxymorphone for the treatment of cancer pain: a pilot study. *Support Care Cancer.* 2005;13:57-65.

45. Mercadante S, Porzio G, Aielli GPF, et al. Opioid switching from and to tapentadol extended release in cancer patients: conversion ratio with other opioids. *Curr Med Res Opin.* 2013;29(6):661-666.

46. Wilder-Smith CH, Hill L, Wilkins J, et al. Effects of morphine and tramadol on somatic and visceral sensory function and gastrointestinal motility after abdominal surgery. *Anesthesiology.* 1999;91:639-647.

47. Grond S, Sablotzki A. Clinical pharmacology of tramadol. *Clin Pharmacokinet.* 2004;31:879-923.

48. Grond S, Radbruch L, Meuser T, et al. High-dose tramadol in comparison to low-dose morphine for cancer pain relief. *J Pain Symptom Manage.* 1999;18:174–179.

49. Christoph T, Kogel B, Strassburger W, et al. Tramadol has a better potency ratio relative to morphine in neuropathic than in nociceptive pain models. *Drugs R D.* 2007;8:51-57.

50. Pereira J, Lawlor P, Vigano A, et al. Equianalgesic dose ratios for opioids: A critical review and proposals for long-term dosing. *J Pain Symptom Manage.* 2001;22(2):672-687.

51. Gammaitoni AR, Fine P, Alvarez N, et al. Clinical application of opioid equianalgesic data. *Clin J Pain.* 2003;19:286-297.

52. Fine PG, Portenoy RK. Establishing "best practices" for opioid rotation: conclusions of an expert panel. *J Pain Symptom Manage.* 2009;38(3):418-425.

CHAPTER 2

Converting Among Routes and Formulations of the Same Opioid

INTRODUCTION

In Chapter 1, we discussed the reasons why a patient may need to be switched from one opioid to another. Frequently, a patient's pain is controlled on his or her current opioid, but he or she requires, or would benefit from, a different dosage formulation or route of administration. For example, approximately 70% of patients with advanced illness will require a nonoral route of administration prior to death due to difficulty swallowing.[1] Conversely, patients who receive parenteral opioid therapy postprocedure or to control a pain crisis would likely prefer the convenience of oral opioid therapy as soon as possible. The purpose of this chapter is to learn how to switch a patient between routes of administration or dosage formulations using the same opioid.

OBJECTIVES

After reading this chapter and completing all practice problems, the participant will be able to:

1. List the advantages and disadvantages of potential routes of administration for opioid analgesics.

2. Define *bioavailability* and explain factors that influence medication bioavailability such as the first-pass effect, solubility, gastrointestinal (GI) influences, and drug formulation considerations.

3. Given an actual or simulated patient with a complaint of pain, convert between dosage formulations and routes of administration for the same opioid (e.g., morphine, hydromorphone, oxycodone, and oxymorphone).

ROUTES OF ADMINISTRATION

As you can see from Table 2-1, most opioids are commercially available in a variety of dosage formulations, giving us flexibility in opioid administration. Morphine, for example, can be given by the oral route (immediate-release tablets, capsules, and oral solution, and prolonged-release tablets and capsules), rectal route (rectal suppositories and rectal insertion of long-acting tablets [not an FDA-approved route of administration]), parenterally (intravenous [IV], subcutaneous [sub-Q], or intramuscular [IM]), or via the neuroaxis (epidural or intrathecal routes; to be discussed in Chapter 7). Many short- and long-acting opioid tablets and capsules are formulated as abuse-deterrent formulations. ***Let's consider route of administration and formulation-specific issues that guide dosing equivalency considerations.***

Oral

Oral dosage formulations are preferred when feasible and effective, particularly for the management of chronic pain. Oral medications are usually cost effective, convenient,

Table 2-1
Opioid Formulations

Opioid	IR Oral Tablet or Capsule	CR Tablet or Capsule	Abuse Deterrent IR or CR Tablet or Capsule	Oral Solution, Suspension, or Elixir	Sublingual Tablet or Solution	Rectal Suppository	Injectable	Transdermal	Transmucosal*	Other
Buprenorphine					X		X	X	X	X**
Codeine	X			X						
Codeine plus nonopioid	X			X						
Fentanyl					X		X	X	X	
Hydrocodone		X	X							
Hydrocodone plus nonopioid	X			X						
Hydromorphone	X		X	X		X	X			
Methadone	X			X			X			
Morphine	X	X	X	X		X	X			
Oxycodone	X		X	X			X***			
Oxycodone plus nonopioid	X			X						
Oxymorphone	X	X					X			
Tapentadol	X	X								
Tramadol	X	X		X			X***			

*Transmucosal includes buccal, sublingual, and intranasal administration.

**Probuphine subcutaneous implant.

***Not available in the U.S.

IR = immediate-release; CR = controlled-release.

portable, flexible, reliable, result in relatively steady blood levels, and are less associated with the stigma of being sick.

Most opioids are short acting (immediate release), requiring frequent dosing (e.g., every 4 hours). Some practitioners may purposely choose to use a short-acting opioid to begin opioid therapy, and will titrate to adequate pain relief, then switch the patient to a long-acting (prolonged-release) oral opioid formulation. At present, morphine, hydromorphone, hydrocodone, oxycodone, oxymorphone, tapentadol, and tramadol are available in a variety of long-acting, modified-release oral formulations. Methadone is inherently a long-lasting opioid (e.g., 8–12 hours) and will be discussed in Chapter 6. Fentanyl is available in transdermal, transmucosal, and parenteral formulations and will be discussed in Chapters 4 and 5.

For patients who have difficulty swallowing tablets or capsules, they can be switched to a liquid opioid formulation. Alternately, long-acting morphine capsules such as Kadian may be opened, and the contents sprinkled on soft food such as applesauce. Kadian is also approved for administration through a 16-French gastrostomy tube:

- Flush tube with water to ensure it is wet.
- Sprinkle Kadian pellets into 10 mL of water.
- Swirl to pour pellets and water into gastrostomy tube through a funnel.
- Rinse beaker.
- Pour into funnel until no pellets remain in beaker.

Importantly, neither long-acting tablets nor the long-acting particles inside Kadian or generic morphine capsules should ever be crushed, chewed, or allowed to dissolve. Doing so would render a dose of opioid intended to be delivered over 12 to 24 hours to be immediately available. The patient would likely be *really* comfortable, but this will probably cause adverse effects that may be fatal (patients hate that side effect!).[2]

Xtampza ER is an extended-release (ER) capsule of oxycodone that must be taken with food, but may be swallowed whole, opened and sprinkled on soft food (e.g., one tablespoon of applesauce, pudding, yogurt, ice cream or jam), sprinkled into a cup and then directly into the patient's mouth, or administered via enteral (gastric/

Timing of Long-Acting Opioid Administration

FAST FACTS Researchers have long recognized that pain exhibits a diurnal variation, or circadian rhythm, although it is likely variable among patients and disease states. One recent study evaluated the impact of administering a once-daily oral morphine first thing in the morning versus at bedtime to patients with opioid-responsive advanced cancer pain. The results showed no difference in overall pain control, pain during the day, pain disturbing sleep, or use of breakthrough medications. The researchers concluded that any differences between AM and PM administration of this once-daily oral morphine product to advanced cancer patients were small, and unlikely to be clinically significant for most people. These data allow us to dose once-daily oral morphine products when it is most convenient for the patient or family.[4]

nasogastric [G/NG]) tube. The mouth or enteral tube should be rinsed or flushed after drug administration. Even though Xtampza ER capsules contain individual abuse-deterrent microspheres of oxycodone, let's not tempt fate by allowing the patient to crunch down on the little beads![3]

The primary disadvantage to oral dosage formulations, particularly opioids, is reduced **bioavailability** (see sidebar "Bioavailability"). **Bioavailability** is defined as "the rate and extent to which the active ingredient or active **moiety** [the active part of the drug molecule] is absorbed from a drug product and becomes available at the site of action."[5] In simpler terms, the bioavailability of a drug refers to the percentage of drug that eventually ends up in the systemic circulation. IV injection of a drug (where you *put* the drug in the systemic circulation) is considered to have 100% bioavailability. The bioavailability of other dosage formulations is determined by administering the same dose in a different formulation and determining how much of the dose ends up in the systemic circulation. The average bioavailability of oral morphine is approximately 30% to 40% but may be quite variable (e.g., 16% to 68%).[6] Oral hydromorphone has approximately 50% to 60% bioavailability (range 29% to 95%), while oral oxycodone is about 80% and oral oxymorphone is about 10%.[7-9] This means that you must give considerably more opioid by the oral route than by IV injection to get the same amount into the systemic circulation and a similar therapeutic effect. As shown in our Equianalgesic Opioid Dosing table (Table 1-1), the dose equivalency ratio between parenteral and oral morphine is 10:25—we must give two-and-a-half times as much morphine by tablet or capsule as we do by IV injection to achieve an equivalent blood level, and by inference, a similar level of analgesia. Things get a bit more complicated when we consider the role of morphine metabolites with chronic dosing, however. In single-dose studies, the ratio of IV to oral morphine is closer to 10:60. Accumulation of morphine-6-glucuronide (M6G) with repeated morphine dosing (especially oral) contributes to the analgesic activity of morphine; therefore, a true comparison of oral and IV morphine includes consideration of M6G.

- *For patients with normal kidney function*, and consequently adequate clearance of M6G, a 10:30 IV:oral ratio holds up under conditions of repeated dosing.

- *In patients with compromised renal function*, a more correct conversion would be 10:20 when going from IV to oral morphine, and conversely 20:10 when going from oral to IV morphine.[10]

Many variables affect the extent of drug absorption. One major influence on oral medication administration is the **first-pass effect**. When a medication is administered orally, after being absorbed from the GI tract, it first goes through the liver (see Figure 2-1). During transit through the GI tract, and the first pass through the liver, the GI enzymes and microsomal (P450) or glucuronide enzymes in the liver can metabolize a considerable portion of the administered dose to pharmacologically inactive metabolites. Other variables that may impact bioavailability include altered hepatic blood flow (reduced with aging), gastric pH, or GI motility; quantitative variance in metabolic enzymes; and drug recirculation. Individuals with liver disease may display greater medication bioavailability (sometimes approaching 100%) due to liver shunting and reduced liver metabolism. Other factors that affect bioavailability are discussed in the sidebar.

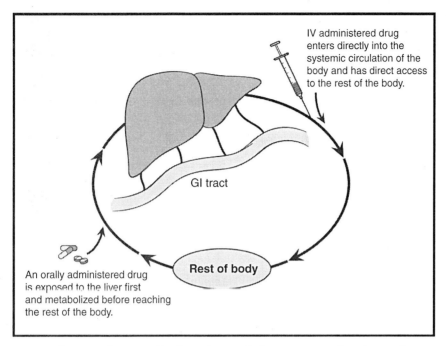

IV administered drug enters directly into the systemic circulation of the body and has direct access to the rest of the body.

GI tract

Rest of body

An orally administered drug is exposed to the liver first and metabolized before reaching the rest of the body.

Figure 2-1. Medications administered by the oral route of administration may be subject to first-pass metabolism by hepatic enzymes, reducing the amount of administered drug that reaches the systemic circulation.
GI = gastrointestinal; IV = intravenous

Buccal, Sublingual, and Transmucosal, Oh My!

Occasionally we need to administer opioids in the buccal or sublingual cavity. Fentanyl is now available as several transmucosal formulations intended for sublingual, buccal, or intranasal administration. Highly concentrated oral opioid solutions are frequently instilled in the buccal or sublingual cavity. A small, but variable portion of the oral solution is actually absorbed transmucosally, but the portion that gets absorbed through the mucosal membranes in the mouth bypasses the liver; therefore, it is not subject to a first-pass effect. The variability in transmucosal absorption reflects the lipophilicity of the opioid. Buprenorphine, fentanyl, and methadone are more lipophilic, and a larger percentage of the transmucosally administered dose is absorbed directly from the site of administration. Transmucosally absorbed opioids have a rapid onset of action due to the good blood supply to the area of absorption. The rest of the medication is swallowed and absorbed, subject to the first-pass effect.

Disadvantages to buccal and sublingual opioid administration include the inconvenience of holding the dosage formulation in the mouth and the relatively poor transmucosal absorption of morphine and oxycodone.

Rapid-acting fentanyl products will be discussed in detail in Chapter 4, and they have a much higher degree of transmucosal absorption than morphine or oxycodone solution.

Rectal

Medications administered by the rectal route are commonly suppositories or enemas. Morphine and hydromorphone are commercially available as rectal suppositories. Opioid suppositories inserted just past the rectal sphincter avoid first-pass hepatic metabolism, although suppositories inserted higher into the rectal vault are absorbed into the superior rectal vein that empties into the hepatic circulation, resulting in first-pass metabolism. Morphine rectal suppositories are approximately bioequivalent to oral morphine (1:1 dosing conversion), and are usually dosed every 4 hours.[11] There are fewer data on the bioequivalence of rectal hydromorphone; however, most practitioners would consider hydromorphone suppositories bioequivalent to oral hydromorphone due to similar pharmacokinetics as morphine. Rectal hydromorphone seems to have a longer duration of action possibly due to reduced first-pass metabolism or slower absorption, so the Food and Drug Administration (FDA)-approved dosing interval is every 6 hours. Rectal methadone is not commercially available; however, evidence shows it is approximately bioequivalent to oral methadone.

Although not FDA approved, controlled-release oral morphine tablets introduced many years ago to the market have been administered rectally to cancer patients (every 12 hours) and provided as good or better absorption than when administered orally. Generally, practitioners use a 1:1 ratio for oral:controlled-release morphine tablets administered rectally, although the rectal dose may require dosage reduction due to increased sedation from better absorption.[12,13] When the original controlled-release formulation of oxycodone tablets was administered by rectum, a significantly higher "area under the curve" (39% increase) and a higher maximum concentration (9%)

BIOAVAILABILITY

As discussed in the text, **bioavailability** is defined as "the rate and extent to which the active ingredient or active moiety [the active part of the drug molecule] is absorbed from a drug product and becomes available at the site of action."[5] Put more simply, bioavailability is expressed as a percent and represents the fraction of administered drug that eventually reaches the systemic circulation. For example, if 30 mg of oral morphine were administered by mouth, and 10 mg of the drug was absorbed unchanged, the bioavailability would be 1/3, or 33%.

You learned how the first-pass effect can dramatically affect bioavailability, as is the case with drugs such as fentanyl (metabolized to inactive metabolites by the P450 system), morphine (metabolized to active and potentially toxic metabolites via glucuronidation), lidocaine, and nitroglycerin. We can minimize this effect by giving nitroglycerin by the sublingual route, bypassing the liver prior to absorption, or administering lidocaine topically (Lidoderm topical patch) or intravenously.

Another factor that influences the bioavailability of a drug is its **solubility**. Medications that are either extremely water-soluble (hydrophilic) or extremely lipid-soluble (hydrophobic or lipophilic) are poorly absorbed either because they cannot cross the lipid-rich cell membranes or they cannot dissolve into solution. For optimal drug absorption, the medication must be primarily lipophilic, but also be sufficiently soluble in aqueous solutions.

Some medications are unstable in the pH of gastric contents, such as penicillin G. Enzymes in the GI tract degrade other medications, such as insulin.

Last, the nature of the **drug formulation** (e.g., tablet or capsule) can influence the bioavailability. This includes factors such as drug particle size, salt form, crystal polymorphism, and the presence of various excipients. **Excipient** is a fancy word for all the stuff aside from the drug itself in the tablet or capsule. Examples include the following:

- Lubricants
- Granulating agent
- Filler (to bulk up tablet or capsule so it's not too small)
- Wetting agent (to assist with penetration of water into the tablet)
- Disintegration agent (helps the tablet break apart)

Excipients can enhance tablet or capsule dissolution and, therefore, alter the rate and extent of absorption.

due to enhanced drug absorption were observed.[14] Of note, the rectal administration of oral tablets or capsules is not recommended (particularly modified-release formulations); absorption can be quite erratic.

The rectal route of administration is not appropriate for all patients. First, patients tend not to like this route, and it makes for uncomfortable family dynamics when a 60-year-old man has to administer a rectal suppository to his 85-year-old mother. In addition to emotional discomfort, rectal products can be physically uncomfortable for patients with advanced illnesses. Dehydrated patients may have insufficient fluid in the rectal vault to absorb medications delivered by this route. Rectal drug products should not be administered into surgically created openings, and are less helpful in patients with diarrhea, colostomy, hemorrhoids, anal fissures, or in neutropenic patients.[12]

Last, it is important to recognize that there is a high degree of interindividual absorption variability in rectally administered medications. Even though the rectal administration of oral prolonged-release opioids is tempting, it is important to remember that this is not an FDA-approved route of administration, and is probably not a good long-term drug administration strategy. Rectal doses can be expelled before they are fully absorbed, and, if the lower rectum is filled with stool, absorption will also be limited. This can only be proven by performing a rectal examination, and for obvious reasons, this creates an additional burden for the patient and caregiver.

Parenteral

When we speak of parenteral drug administration we are generally referring to IV, sub-Q, and IM administration, which are injected into the vein, subcutaneous tissue, or a muscle respectively (Figure 2-2). As discussed previously, medications administered by the IV route are 100% bioavailable. Drugs can be injected into a peripheral vein over several minutes, or administered by an intermittent or continuous infusion. The IV route allows the fastest onset of drug action.

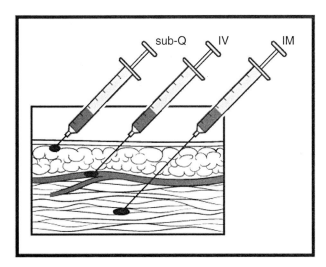

Figure 2-2. Commonly used parenteral injections include subcutaneous (sub-Q), intravenous (IV), and intramuscular (IM).

Disadvantages to the IV route of administration include the need to find a suitable vein, which in turn requires trained personnel and more expensive equipment to administer the drug. Patients are also frequently fearful of more invasive or painful medications given by injection.

Sub-Q administration of a medication involves much less equipment and may be administered by the patient or a family member. Although absorption is slower than an IV injection, it is usually complete. Opioids may be administered by intermittent sub-Q injections or continuous sub-Q infusion.

Disadvantages to the sub-Q route of administration include potential discomfort, local tissue irritation, and probably most important, the need to limit the volume injected (because the subcutaneous tissue has a limited capacity to absorb fluid). Some references cite a maximum of 2 mL per injection, or 1 to 2 mL/hr of continuous sub-Q infusion.

What do plastic silverware, jumbo shrimp, and an IM opioid all have in common? They are all oxymorons! An IM injection is painful, which is kind of a kick in the pants when we're administering an analgesic! The American Pain Society recommends that the IM route of administration be abandoned for this reason, as well as wide fluctuations in absorption from the site of injection, a 30- to 60-minute lag time to peak analgesic effect, and rapid falloff of action when compared to oral administration. Chronic use of IM injections can also lead to nerve injury with persistent neuropathic pain, sterile abscess formation, and muscle and soft tissue fibrosis.[15]

As you can see in the Equianalgesic Opioid Dosing table (Table 1-1), there is no differentiation between IV, sub-Q, and IM dosing in the "parenteral" column. Therefore, this implies a 1:1:1 ratio in dosing. If only life were that straightforward! Because we have already voted IM opioids off the island, let's focus on IV and sub-Q comparisons. Pharmacokinetic studies comparing sub-Q versus IV continuous infusions of identical doses of both morphine and hydromorphone have shown comparable plasma concentrations. Further, the sub-Q and IV routes provided equivalent analgesia and adverse effects.[16] The sub-Q route is preferred for the reasons described above, particularly for a patient at home without established IV access. With high doses, however, absorption may be more variable with sub-Q injections or infusion and may require dosage adjustment. Some literature suggests that the relative potency ratio of sub-Q to oral morphine is between 1:2 and 1:3 with doses in excess of 10 mg/hr (our table states it is 1:2.5 regardless of the parenteral route of administration, but these data bear consideration), while IV to oral morphine is predictably closer to the 1:3 ratio.[11]

Well, I'm sure that discussion left you holding your head in your hands! Let's jump into some calculations to clear the water! You can start by wearing your life vest and you'll be swimming with the sharks by the end of the chapter!

Remember the steps outlined in Chapter 1, Table 1-2, that summarize the five steps in opioid conversion calculations. Table 2-2 in this chapter shows you four possible conversion calculation methods—*What a deal!* You can do a simple ratio in your head (not recommended) or on paper (A), a mathematical proportion using cross-multiplication (B and C), or a mathematical proportion using ratios (D). We'll use methods B and D primarily, but method A is a good way to check yourself!

Table 2-2
Calculating the New Opioid Dose

Just as there are several ways to pluck a chicken, there are several ways you can use the Equianalgesic Opioid Dosing table data to calculate the dose of the opioid to which you are switching.

Several examples are as follows:

- Simple ratio (method A)
  - Oral morphine to oral morphine is a 1:1 conversion (or 25 mg:25 mg conversion). There is no dividing or multiplying to be done; oral morphine is oral morphine!
  - Oral morphine to parenteral morphine is a 2.5:1 conversion (or 25 mg:10 mg conversion).
  - You can apply the simple ratio practically in your head (not recommended) by dividing or multiplying by 2.5.
  - Even when switching from one opioid to another you can do a simple ratio. For example, oral hydromorphone to oral morphine is a 1:5 ratio (or 5-mg oral hydromorphone:25-mg oral morphine conversion). If the patient were getting 8 mg of oral hydromorphone per day, this would be approximately 40 mg of oral morphine per day.

- Mathematical proportion using cross-multiplication (methods B and C)
  - Set up a simple mathematical proportion using ratios. *This can be done several ways, but the important thing is that the ratios on both sides of the equation are parallel.* Here are two examples (reminder: TDD = total daily dose):

  - Method B:

    Actual Drug Doses: Equianalgesic Data from Chart:

    $$\frac{\text{"X" mg TDD new opioid}}{\text{mg TDD current opioid}} = \frac{\text{equianalgesic factor of new opioid}}{\text{equianalgesic factor of current opioid}}$$

  - Method C:

    New Opioid   Current Opioid

    $$\frac{\text{"X" mg TDD new opioid}}{\text{equianalgesic factor of new opioid}} = \frac{\text{mg TDD current opioid equianalgesic}}{\text{factors of current opioid}}$$

- Mathematical proportion using ratio (method D)
  - Instead of cross-multiplying, you can directly apply the ratio to the current total daily dose, and end up with the new opioid total daily dose as follows:

    $$\text{TDD current opioid} \times \frac{\text{equianalgesic factor of new opioid}}{\text{equianalgesic factor of current opioid}} = \text{TDD new opioid}$$

Wow! So many possible equations, so little time! I suggest you stick with method B or D, and keep method A as your "does that LOOK right?" method. Alternatively, use method B, and use method D to check yourself! *Whatever you pick, be consistent!*

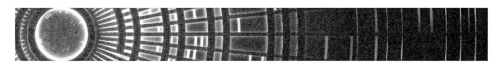

CASE 2.1

Same Opioid, Same Route of Administration (Oral), Different Formulation

HW is an 84-year-old man in a long-term care facility with general debility. He has moderate pain from spinal stenosis and other general aches and pains. HW has been having transient ischemic attacks (TIAs), and he has had increasing difficulty swallowing solid food and medications. Up to this point, his pain was well controlled on Percocet (5-mg oxycodone/325-mg acetaminophen per tablet), six tablets daily. To accommodate his difficulty swallowing, HW just had a feeding tube placed, and his physician asked that you convert HW to a liquid formulation to provide an equivalent degree of pain relief. HW tells you that the six Percocet tablets per day did a good job controlling his pain. You decide to switch HW to the Roxicet Oral Solution, which contains 5-mg oxycodone and 325-mg acetaminophen per 5 mL. What would be the correct regimen to recommend to HW's physician?

Let's look at our five-step opioid conversion calculation process:

STEP 1—HW's pain is well controlled on six Percocet tablets per day. When he was able to take the tablets, he was able to do his limited activities of daily living, and he reported he was comfortable. There appears to be no reason to suspect he should be switched to a different opioid, or have any co-analgesics added.

STEP 2—HW has been consistently taking six Percocet tablets (5-mg oxycodone/325-mg acetaminophen per tablet) per day, giving a total daily dose (TDD) of oxycodone of 30 mg. The acetaminophen dose is less important, but should always be less than 4 g per day (and lower in some patients).

STEP 3—We have already chosen our new formulation (Roxicet Oral Solution, 5-mg oxycodone/325-mg acetaminophen per 5 mL). This conversion is very straight forward! Oral oxycodone is oral oxycodone, and the amount of oxycodone (5 mg) in one tablet HW was taking happens to be the same as the amount of oxycodone (5 mg) in 5 mL of the solution. This makes your life a bit easier, but don't get used to it—things won't always be this easy! *The bioavailability of oxycodone from the tablet formulation is very similar to that of the oral solution; therefore, the dose is the same:* 30-mg TDD oxycodone.

STEP 4—In this step, we individualize the dose for the patient. There is no need to increase the dose because HW's pain was well controlled on 30-mg oxycodone per day, and there is no need to decrease the dose due to increased sensitivity to the new opioid (because we're not *switching* opioids—we're going from oxycodone to oxycodone—same drug!). Therefore, HW's new regimen is the same TDD (30-mg oxycodone), given as Roxicet Oral Solution, 5-mg oxycodone/325-mg acetaminophen (5 mL) every 4 hours by feeding tube. The last piece of business in individualizing the dose for HW is determining when to begin therapy with the new formulation. Because Percocet tablets only last approximately 4 hours, HW can begin the Roxicet Oral Solution anytime 4 or more hours after his last Percocet tablet.

STEP 5—HW begins therapy with the Roxicet Oral Solution. The nursing staff in the long-term care facility monitor HW closely. He has no complaints of sedation, confusion, nausea, or any other adverse effects. It has been 24 hours since his last Percocet tablet was administered (he received a very small dose of sub-Q morphine when the feeding tube was placed), but by the time HW had been receiving the Roxicet Oral Solution for 24 hours, he said the pain control was acceptable. You would continue to monitor HW and adjust his regimen as clinically indicated. Of course, if he continued to require more oxycodone, you would have to be cautious of the acetaminophen dose, and perhaps switch to a single ingredient oxycodone oral solution product.

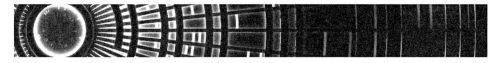

CASE 2.2
••
Same Opioid, Same Route of Administration (Oral), Different Formulation

RS is a 62-year-old man with a history of renal cancer, no metastatic disease noted. He has been experiencing visceral pain for the past several months, and his physician prescribed hydromorphone 2-mg tablets every 4 hours as needed for pain. He has been taking five or six tablets daily with good pain control. He rates his pain as a daily best of 3 (on a 0–10 scale; 0 = no pain, 10 = worst imaginable pain), a daily worst pain of 7, and an average of 4 or 5. He states that this level of pain control allows him to perform most of his activities of daily living, but he feels that the pain management could be improved. He does complain about having to either get up during the night to take another dose of hydromorphone, or of awakening in pain. What should be done?

STEP 1—You have carefully assessed RS's pain and have determined that he continues to experience nociceptive pain that is unlikely to be metastatic bone pain. You do not suspect neuropathic pain because the patient does not use any descriptors suggestive of neuro-pathic pain (stabbing, shooting, burning pain), and he has a normal neurologic exam. The pain has responded fairly well to five or six hydromorphone 2-mg tablets, but there is room for improvement.

STEP 2—We can calculate the TDD of hydromorphone RS is receiving as follows: five or six tablets of hydromorphone, 2 mg per tablet for a TDD of 10 to 12 mg oral hydromorphone. He is taking no other analgesic medications.

STEP 3—Hydromorphone is available as a sustained-release tablet (Exalgo), which is dosed every 24 hours. This would allow RS to sleep through the night without having to redose, and hopefully to not awaken in pain. Oral bioavailability is likely similar between the unmodified and the ER hydromorphone tablets; therefore, the equivalent TDD of ER hydro-morphone would be 10 to 12 mg.

STEP 4—Because RS's pain is likely visceral, he has shown good response to hydromor-phone and his pain is not quite controlled, a dosage increase would seem reasonable. Exalgo is available as 8-, 12-, 16- and 32-mg tablets. Because RS's pain wasn't quite at goal, it would be reasonable to select the 12-mg dose of Exalgo. RS could keep the hydro-morphone 2-mg tablets for additional or unanticipated pain. The Exalgo could be started approximately 4 hours after the last IR 2-mg hydromorphone tablet.

STEP 5—RS should be monitored clinically, and he should be encouraged to use a pain diary to record his pain ratings and his use of unmodified hydromorphone tablets. This will assist his healthcare team in titrating his long-acting oral opioid regimen.

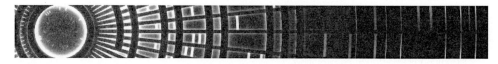

CASE 2.3

• •

Same Opioid, Same Route of Administration (Oral), Different Formulation

PL is an 82-year-old woman living in an assisted-living facility with lung cancer, with widespread metastatic disease, including bone involvement. PL also has end-stage Alzheimer disease. As her Alzheimer disease has worsened, her healthcare team has assessed her pain by observing her behavior, particularly during personal care. PL's pain was being managed with morphine sulfate IR tablets, 15 mg po (by mouth) every 4 hours until she began "pocketing" the tablets (between the cheek and the gum), which she later spit out. Her physician switched her to morphine sulfate oral solution at the same dose and dosing interval, but PL found it amusing to shoot the morphine solution out between her clenched teeth. PL's physician asks your help in treating this patient's pain.

STEP 1—On close observation, you determine that PL grimaces and moans loudly when receiving personal care. She seems to be guarding her right side, and is particularly disinclined to roll over on that side. Her physician agrees that it is likely that this behavior is due to painful metastatic bone disease. In response to this, you recommended adding a nonsteroidal anti-inflammatory drug such as naproxen, which PL takes with no commotion. She continues to spit out the morphine solution, and you aren't even sure how much she has been getting per day thanks to these antics. The naproxen has reduced but not eliminated behaviors that are thought to be related to pain; therefore, the decision has been made to continue PL on morphine, provided an acceptable regimen can be identified.

STEP 2—Had PL been taking all the morphine prescribed for her, this would be a TDD of 90 mg (15 mg by mouth every 4 hours = 15 × 6 times per day = 90 mg). The aides caring for PL estimate that she has been actually swallowing about 60% of her prescribed morphine per day since she started "acting out."

STEP 3—You decide to try Kadian, a once- or twice-a-day long-acting morphine capsule that can be swallowed whole or opened and the contents administered by a gastrostomy tube or sprinkled on soft food such as applesauce. Since PL adores applesauce, you decide to go with this option. Based on an estimated TDD of 54 mg of morphine from the morphine solution PL was taking (60% of 90 mg TDD), it would be the same TDD of Kadian.

STEP 4—So, should you keep the TDD of 54 mg, increase it, or decrease it? Because you don't know for sure how much morphine PL was getting, it would be prudent to go with a lower TDD of Kadian. You have also decided to go with an every 12-hour regimen so you can closely monitor PL's progress. Kadian is available as 10-, 20-, 30-, 40-, 50-, 60-, 70-, 80-, 100-, 130-, 150-, and 200-mg capsules. You decide to begin with Kadian 20 mg by mouth every 12 hours sprinkled on applesauce. The morphine oral solution is still available for additional breakthrough pain as needed (e.g., every 4 hours). Kadian therapy can begin at any time 4 hours after PL's last dose of oral morphine solution.

STEP 5—After instituting this plan, PL responded very well. Her pain seemed to be well controlled as evidenced by significantly less difficulty providing personal care. PL was happy to eat her applesauce twice daily (without crunching the morphine particles), with 20 mg of Kadian sprinkled on top. PL probably thought they were sprinkles—otherwise she probably would have pulled some other hijinks!

Long-Acting Opioid Capsules on Applesauce

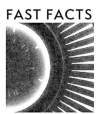

FAST FACTS *When opening a Kadian (morphine), or Xtampza ER capsule (oxyco-done), and sprin-kling the contents on applesauce,* **there are several important things to remember.**

▶ Do not use a large quantity of applesauce—this is not a meal, merely a drug delivery vehicle. A tablespoon should be sufficient.

▶ Never use a large quantity of applesauce with a higher strength capsule and attempt to give only a portion of the mixture. Use exactly the capsule strength prescribed *only*.

▶ Make sure the patient is able to swallow the morphine-applesauce mixture without crunching or chewing the beads, which are extended-release. Have the patient rinse his or her mouth and swallow after consuming the morphine-applesauce mixture to avoid having a little sustained-release snack hiding behind a molar.

▶ Do *not* heat the applesauce! Do not sprinkle cinnamon on the applesauce! Do not get out your Easy Bake Oven and whip up a batch of apple cinnamon morphine muffins! There are no data on the stability of the morphine should you heat this mixture, and other foodstuffs should not be added to the mixture!

Tapentadol

Tapentadol (Nucynta) is a novel analgesic that is classified as having *opioidergic* and *monoaminergic* mechanisms of action. It acts as a mu-opioid receptor agonist and a norepinephrine reuptake inhibitor. It also weakly inhibits serotonin reuptake but to a clinically insufficient degree to contribute to pain relief.[17] Tapentadol is indicated for the relief of pain severe enough to require daily, around-the-clock, long-term opioid treatment and for which alternative treatment options are inadequate.[18,19] The ER formulation also has an indication for diabetic peripheral neuropathy.[19] At present, there are three IR tablet formulations on the market in the United States: 50, 75, and 100 mg. Although dosing should be individualized to meet specific patient needs, the appropriate dose is 50, 75, or 100 mg every 4 to 6 hours. On the first day of dosing, if the first dose does not adequately relieve the pain, a second dose may be administered as soon as 1 hour after the first dose. Total daily doses in excess of 700 mg the first day or 600 mg on subsequent days have not been studied. The ER formulation (Nucynta ER) is available as 50-, 100-, 150-, 200-, and 250-mg tablets. The dose for opioid-naïve and opioid nontolerant patients is 50 mg by mouth every 12 hours.

When converting from the IR to the ER formulation of tapentadol, what do we have to take into consideration? You're switching from tapentadol to tapentadol, so the patient should not have any increase in sensitivity to the drug. The primary consideration is any difference in bioavailability. In other words, if you are switching to Nucynta ER and it had higher bioavailability, you would be overdosing the patient if you just gave the same TDD only as the twice-a-day ER formulation. Alternately, if Nucynta ER had LOWER bioavailability than Nucynta, giving the same TDD could leave the patient in pain. Interestingly, the oral bioavailability of both formulations is 32% (ha!! – why did I make you read all that?!).[18,19]

Per the package labeling, patients can be converted from Nucynta to Nucynta ER by dividing the tapentadol TDD in two, and administering at 12-hour intervals.[19]

What about Kadian or Xtampza ER by feeding tube?

FAST FACTS

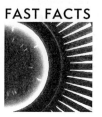

▶ Kadian pellets may be administered through a 16-French gastrostomy tube. Flush the gastrostomy tube with water to wet; sprinkle the Kadian dose into 10 mL of water. Swirl and pour the pellets and water into the gastrostomy tube through a funnel. Rinse the beaker with an additional 10 mL of water and pour this into the funnel. Kadian may not be administered by NG tube.

▶ Xtampza ER may be administered through a NG or gastrostomy tube. Flush the NG or gastrostomy tube with liquid (water, milk, or liquid nutritional supplement). Open an Xtampza ER capsule and carefully pour the contents of the capsule directly into the tube (do *not* premix the capsule contents with liquid). Administer 15 mL of liquid via syringe into the tube after administering capsule contents. Flush the tube two more times with 10 mL of liquid each time.

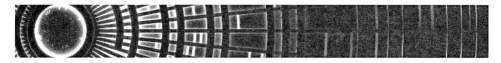

CASE 2.4

•••

Same Opioid, Same Route of Administration (Oral), Different Formulation

VA is a 62-year-old woman with severe osteoarthritis of both knees. Her orthopedic surgeon wants her to lose 100 more pounds before she will consider knee replacement surgery. VA has been taking Nucynta 100 mg when she awakens for severe knee pain, then three additional 50-mg Nucynta tablets spaced throughout the day (TDD 250 mg). This amount allows her to do most of her desired activities of daily living. She's working hard to lose the weight so she can have surgery, but she tells her prescriber she's tired of waking up in so much pain, and whenever she takes 100 mg she gets quite sleepy. She asks if there is a better regimen that she can use less often. What do you think?

STEP 1—You review VA's chart; her osteoarthritis is severe, and her pain is consistent with this presentation. She says when she takes the 250-mg Nucynta per day it gets the job done pretty well for her. Her concerns are noted above, however.

STEP 2—VA takes 100-mg Nucynta first thing in the morning, then three 50-mg tablets throughout the balance of the day, for a TDD of 250 mg.

STEP 3—We are switching from tapentatol to tapentadol, and the IR and ER formulation have equivalent bioavailability so the Nucynta ER dose calculates to 250 mg by mouth daily.

STEP 4—Because VA complains of drowsiness when she takes the 100-mg dose of Nucynta, we would be wise to reduce her TDD at this time. Nucynta ER is available as 50-, 100-, 150-, 200-, and 250-mg tablets. VA receives a prescription for Nucynta ER 100 mg by mouth, 1 tablet every 12 hours.

STEP 5—VA's prescriber checks in 1 week later, and VA states this regimen is holding her just fine. Now go get skinny woman!

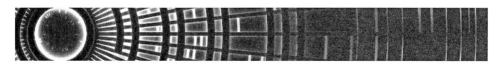

CASE 2.5

•••

Same Opioid, Same Route of Administration (Oral), Different Formulation

JN is a 37-year-old woman with a work-related back injury. She is receiving physical therapy (PT), but she states the pain is significant, particularly when undergoing PT. Her physician hopes for JN to have back surgery once PT has provided maximum benefit, which she believes is about 8 to 12 weeks in the future. To allow JN to tolerate PT and fully participate, her physician prescribed hydrocodone 7.5 mg/acetaminophen 300 mg, one tablet up to four times daily as needed (patient has been consistently using four tablets daily). JN tells you that this works quite well for her. Her favorite way to use this medication is to crush the tablet and sprinkle the powder into a cola (with crushed ice, naturally) because it "relaxes her" quite nicely. The patient has exhibited no other "red flags" of opioid misuse, and her response to therapy has allowed her to fully participate and make good progress. However, the prescriber is uncomfortable with JT altering the hydrocodone/acetaminophen tablets, and decides to switch JT to Zohydro ER, a 12-hour abuse-deterrent formulation of hydrocodone. The prescriber explains to JN that she cannot crush her medication, and the new formulation of hydrocodone is designed to withstand the "crushed with cola" treatment. However, what dose of Zohydro ER do you recommend?

Unless you've been off Earth for a decade or so, you have certainly heard of the opioid misuse, abuse, and overdose death epidemic we are currently experiencing. A variety of risk mitigation strategies has been implemented, and the use of **abuse-deterrent opioid formulations** is one such strategy. Although not *abuse-proof*, these tablets and capsules have been formulated to "target the known or expected routes of abuse, such as crushing in order to snort or dissolving in order to inject, for the specific opioid drug substance."[20] Examples of technology used to make an oral formulation abuse-deterrent include the following:[21]

- *Physical/chemical barrier*—prevents chewing, crushing, cutting, grating, or grinding the tablet or capsule

- *Agonist/antagonist combination*—adds a sequestered opioid antagonist that is only liberated on manipulation of the dosage formulation and counters the effect of the opioid

- *Aversion*—includes a substance that produces an unpleasant effect if the dosage formulation is manipulated or higher than recommended doses are ingested

- *Delivery system*—uses depot injections and implants that offer resistance to abuse

- *Prodrug*—uses a prodrug that is pharmacologically inactive prior to transformation in the GI tract (e.g., first-pass effect), rendering it unattractive for parenteral use

This sounds serious—I can put an OxyContin tablet in my driveway, ride over it with my SUV, and see the intact tablet in my rear-view mirror? So, does the opioid get *out* of the abuse-deterrent formulation to achieve a therapeutic serum level to provide pain relief? *Yes,* the manufacturer must show bioequivalence to traditional formulations.

So, how do we convert from unmodified opioids to these abuse-deterrent formulations, such as in the case of JN? Let's take a look at Table 2-3 for the scoop.

Meanwhile, back at the ranch, JN is patiently waiting for her prescription. Her pain is well controlled on hydrocodone 7.5 mg/acetaminophen 300 mg, four tablets daily. The prescriber is going to switch JN to Zohydro ER. Referring to Table 2-3, divide the patient's TDD of oral hydrocodone in half and administer as Zohydro ER every 12 hours. Note that we are ignoring any analgesia provided by acetaminophen; this can be administered separately if appropriate to continue.

JN is taking 30-mg hydrocodone per day; the order for Zohydro ER should be 15 mg by mouth, every 12 hours. Monitor the patient's response to therapy and adherence to *not* attempting to manipulate the dosage formulation.

Table 2-3
Abuse-Deterrent Opioid Formulations

Generic	Brand	Formulation	Abuse-Deterrent Mechanism	Equivalence to Unmodified Opioid Ingredient
Hydrocodone	HYSINGLA ER[22,23]	ER tablets	RESISTEC technology—confers tablet hardness (makes the tablet difficult to crush, break, or dissolve); imparts viscosity when dissolved in aqueous solutions.	Administer total daily dose of hydrocodone as Hysingla ER once daily (every 24 hours).
Hydrocodone	VANTRELA ER[24]	ER tablets	Physiochemical properties to make tablet more difficult to manipulate for misuse and abuse.	Divide the patient's total daily oral hydrocodone dose in half and administer as VANTRELA ER every 12 hours.
Hydrocodone	ZOHYDRO ER[25,26]	ER capsule	BeadTek technology—a combination of hydrocodone beads and inactive PEO beads. When crushed and dissolved in liquids or solvents, the PEO beads are designed to immediately form a viscous gel.	Divide the patient's total daily oral hydrocodone dose in half and administer as ZOHYDRO ER every 12 hours.
Hydromorphone	EXALGO[28,29]	ER tablet	Uses tamper-resistant OROS technology—tablet is difficult to crush or extract for injection. OROS is a push-pull osmotic system that releases hydromorphone at a controlled rate.	Administer TDD of immediate-release hydromorphone as a single Exalgo dose once daily (every 24 hours).
Morphine	ARYMO ER[30,31]	ER tablet	Guardian technology—provides resistance to manipulation (cutting, crushing, grinding, or breaking) or chemical extraction. Has physical and chemical properties that are expected to make abuse by injection difficult.	Divide the patient's total daily oral morphine dose in half and administer as Arymo ER every 12 hours, or divide the patient's total daily oral morphine dose in thirds and administer as Arymo ER every 8 hours.
Morphine	MORPHABOND ER[32]	ER tablets	Increased resistance to cutting, crushing, or breaking. Forms a viscous material when subjected to a liquid environment.	Divide the patient's total daily oral morphine dose in half and administer as MORPHABONDER every 12 hours.
Morphine/ naltrexone	EMBEDA[27,33]	ER capsule	Embeda contains ER morphine pellets that contain a sequestered core of the opioid-antagonist naltrexone. If the pellets are swallowed, the naltrexone core passes through the gut intact. If pellets are crushed, chewed, or dissolved, naltrexone is released and blocks morphine-induced euphoria.	Divide the patient's total daily oral morphine dose in half and administer as Embeda every 12 hours, or administer the total daily dose of oral morphine as Embeda once every 24 hours.

(continued)

Table 2-3
Abuse-Deterrent Opioid Formulations *(continued)*

Generic	Brand	Formulation	Abuse-Deterrent Mechanism	Equivalence to Unmodified Opioid Ingredient
Oxycodone	OXAYDO[34,35]	IR tablets	AVERSION technology—includes sodium lauryl sulfate, which causes nasal burning and throat irritation when snorted. If dissolved for IV injection, forms gelatinous mixture, trapping oxycodone inside.	Available as a 5- and 7.5-mg IR tablets.
Oxycodone	OXYCONTIN[36]	ER tablets	INTAC technology—employs physiochemical barrier to impede chewing, crushing, snorting, and injecting. Also contains PEO, which forms a viscous gel matrix that traps oxycodone inside when tablet dissolved.	Divide the patient's total daily oral oxycodone dose in half and administer as OxyContin every 12 hours.
Oxycodone	ROXYBOND[38,39]	IR tablets	Tablet is more difficult to manipulate, with increased resistance to cutting, crushing, grinding, or breaking. When exposed to a liquid environment, forms a viscous material.	Convert from IR oxycodone to ROXY-BOND at same dose and dosing interval.
Oxycodone	XTAMPZA ER[40,41]	ER capsules	DETERx microsphere technology—resists manipulation including cutting, crushing, grinding, melting, chewing, or dissolving.	Xtampza ER contains oxycodone base (capsule is approximately 90% of oxycodone hydrochloride formulation). Divide the patient's total daily oral oxycodone dose in half and administer as Xtampza ER every 12 hours.

ER = extended release; IV = intravenous; OROS = osmotic extended-release oral delivery system; PEO = polyethylene oxide

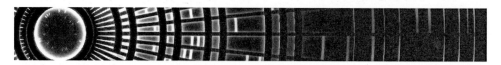

CASE 2.6
••

Same Opioid, Different Formulation and Route of Administration (Oral to Rectal)

KT is a 72-year-old woman with advanced stage pancreatic cancer. She had recently been in the hospital receiving a low-dose morphine IV infusion for pain control, and was converted to oral morphine solution for discharge home when she decided not to pursue any additional chemotherapy. KT's pain was well controlled on morphine 10-mg oral solution, but she started throwing up after most doses, and her pain has returned. KT's physician has prescribed haloperidol for the nausea and vomiting, but it has had little impact. KT is likely to die within the next 48 hours. What do you recommend?

STEP 1—KT is very weak but she states that the pain is exactly the type and intensity she had in the hospital, which responded very well to the morphine infusion. She tells you the oral morphine solution worked well also when she was able to keep it down. She does not have complaints or physical findings that are suggestive of metastatic bone pain or neuropathy; therefore, it seems appropriate to continue the morphine.

STEP 2—KT achieved good pain relief with a TDD of 60-mg oral morphine when she was able to take the oral morphine solution.

STEP 3—Because morphine worked well for KT, she is close to death, and she has a strong family support system and caregivers in place, you decide to switch her to rectal morphine suppositories. As you know, oral:rectal morphine is 1:1 and the dosing interval is the same for IR oral morphine and rectal morphine suppositories (every 4 hours).

You can obviously figure this out in your head (morphine 10 mg pr every 4 hours), or you can set up a mathematical proportion by ratio (method D) as follows:

$$\text{TDD current opioid} \times \frac{\text{equianalgesic factor of new opioid}}{\text{equianalgesic factor of current opioid}} = \text{TDD new opioid}$$

$$\text{TDD 60 mg oral morphine} \times \frac{30 \text{ mg rectal morphine}}{30 \text{ mg oral morphine}} = \text{TDD mg pr morphine}$$

Cancel out like units as shown below:

$$\text{TDD 60 } \cancel{\text{mg oral morphine}} \times \frac{30 \text{ mg rectal morphine}}{30 \; \cancel{\text{mg oral morphine}}} = \text{TDD mg pr morphine}$$

Solve for TDD mg pr morphine: $60 \times 30/30 = 60$

The TDD pr morphine is 60 mg.

STEP 4—We have no reason to increase the TDD morphine dose because her pain was well controlled on this regimen previously. We have no reason to reduce the TDD because we are not switching opioids (going from morphine to morphine), so the only thing left to consider is *can we do morphine by rectal suppository 10 mg every 4 hours? By golly, we can*—morphine rectal suppositories are available as 5-, 10-, 20-, and 30-mg suppositories. You definitely don't want to get into the business of carving up commercially available suppositories to create new strengths. If you really feel the need for a different strength rectal suppository, talk to a pharmacist who can compound (these people are angels of mercy) and they can whip you up a batch. Fortunately, we can rock and roll with an order for "morphine 10 mg by rectal suppository every 4 hours." Because the patient threw up her last dose of oral morphine, you can start the rectal morphine suppositories as soon as they are delivered.

STEP 5—You would monitor KT's response as she uses the morphine suppositories for both therapeutic effect (pain relief) and potential toxicity, particularly nausea. An important point to mention is that as KT declines, she may lose consciousness. Sometimes family members, caregivers, and even other healthcare providers question the continued need for the opioid once a patient becomes obtunded. If the patient is free from physical signs of opioid overdose (e.g., reduced respirations, pinpoint pupils), there is no reason to suspect the pain magically went away, so you should continue the opioid throughout the duration of the patient's life. However, if the patient becomes oliguric, leading you to suspect reduced renal clearance, the dosing interval may be extended. Each case must be assessed independently, because physiologic functions, especially at life's end, are variable among patients.

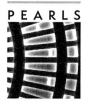

P E A R L S

In the case of KT (Case 2.6), if she had been receiving MS Contin 30 mg by mouth every 12 hours and experienced nausea and vomiting, what could you have done? Certainly, you could have calculated her TDD of oral morphine to be 60 mg, and again gone with the morphine 10-mg rectal suppository every 4 hours. Alternately, if KT lived far from the pharmacy, or was even closer to death, you could insert an MS Contin 30-mg tablet rectally every 12 hours. As discussed in the text, the tablet would have fairly equivalent bioavailability and should keep KT comfortable. I generally do not order a large quantity (e.g., a month's worth) of long-acting morphine tablets with the idea of giving them rectally for as long as needed, but for a patient who is very close to death, or in a situation where you are unable to get the dosage formulation you'd prefer, this is an acceptable option. <u>Remember,</u> this is <u>not</u> an FDA-approved route of administration for these tablets.

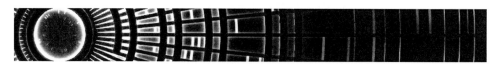

CASE 2.7

Same Opioid, Different Formulation and Route of Administration (Oral to Parenteral)

WP is a 62-year-old man with multiple myeloma and diffuse bony metastasis admitted to hospice several weeks ago. His analgesic regimen has been increased since admission to his current regimen of ER morphine 30 mg by mouth every 12 hours, plus IR morphine oral solution 10 mg every 2 hours as needed for breakthrough pain. WP is also receiving dexamethasone 4 mg by mouth twice daily for bone pain, senna twice daily to prevent constipation, temazepam 15 mg by mouth at bedtime, and lorazepam 1 mg by mouth every 4 hours as needed for anxiety. Over the past few days WP's wife tells you the patient has been taking the IR morphine approximately six times during a 24-hour period. When you visit the patient, you review the pain diary and confirm that WP really has been taking five to six doses of the IR morphine over a 24-hour period for the previous 3 days. Despite this, WP is complaining of pain that he rates as 5 to 7 (on a 0–10 scale; 0 = no pain, 10 = worst imaginable pain). WP has also been taking the lorazepam around the clock due to extreme agitation and worry about the pain, and he claims the bedtime temazepam is marginally effective. WP accepts your offer of inpatient admission to switch to parenteral morphine for more rapid titration.

STEP 1—WP and his wife are obviously distressed over WP's pain situation. He is fearful of the meaning of the pain (disease progression, approaching death, etc.). WP is especially terrified that the pain will never get under control and that he will die a painful, undignified death. WP's physician feels that increasing the dexamethasone is unlikely to provide significantly more relief, and that IV morphine is the best way to go. WP does not describe the pain such that the physician suspects neuropathic pain, nor are there physical findings to suggest such.

STEP 2—As described in the case above, WP was receiving ER morphine tablets, 30 mg by mouth every 12 hours plus five to six daily doses of IR morphine 10-mg oral solution.

WP's TDD of morphine is calculated as follows: 30 mg by mouth every 12 hours = 30 × 2 = 60 mg, plus 10 mg by mouth every 2 hours prn × 5 doses a day = 10 × 5 = 50 mg, for a grand TDD of 110 mg oral morphine (prn = as needed).

STEP 3—WP's physician has asked that you calculate an appropriate starting dose of IV morphine for the patient. An IV line was started, and the plan is to dose WP every 4 hours with morphine and increase the dose as clinically indicated. The first step is to determine how much IV morphine would replace a TDD of 110-mg oral morphine.

We can calculate this using the mathematical proportion by ratio (method D) as follows:

$$\text{TDD current opioid} \times \frac{\text{equianalgesic factor of new opioid}}{\text{equianalgesic factor of current opioid}} = \text{TDD new opioid}$$

$$\text{TDD 110 mg oral morphine} \times \frac{\text{10 mg IV morphine}}{\text{25 mg oral morphine}} = \text{TDD mg IV morphine}$$

Cancel out like units as shown below:

$$\text{TDD 110} \; \cancel{\text{mg oral morphine}} \times \frac{\text{10 mg IV morphine}}{\text{25} \; \cancel{\text{mg oral morphine}}} = \text{TDD mg IV morphine}$$

Solve for TDD mg IV morphine: 110 × 10/25 = 44

The TDD IV morphine is 44 mg.

STEP 4—At this point, we need to decide whether to go with the 44-mg TDD IV morphine, to increase the dose, or decrease the dose.

First the easy one. We would be unlikely to decrease the dose due to incomplete cross-tolerance because we are not switching opioids (we're going from morphine to morphine). We could go with the 44 mg, divide by 6 to get our every 4-hour dose, and increase from there, but we already *know* the patient is in pain. We also know the pain is opioid-responsive; we just need to give *more* morphine. Therefore, it would be clinically appropriate to increase the TDD of morphine at this time.

You will learn more about opioid titration in Chapter 4, but for now accept that a 25% to 50% increase would be appropriate. A 25% increase of 44 mg per day would be 55 mg per day. A 50% increase would be an additional 22 mg per day, or a TDD of 66-mg parenteral morphine. Let's split the difference and go with morphine 10 mg IV every 4 hours (TDD of

60-mg IV morphine). This is in keeping with the admonition to use caution when switching, even though we are not switching *between* opioids.

When should he start this new regimen? The last dose of ER morphine was administered about 7 hours ago, with two doses of the IR morphine given since the last one given 3 hours ago. WP is complaining of considerable pain now, thanks to the ambulance ride and all the transfer maneuvers. It would be appropriate to give WP his first IV injection of 10 mg morphine now.

STEP 5—After giving an IV injection of morphine, WP's pain level should be assessed within 20 to 60 minutes. The onset of action of IV morphine is 2 to 4 minutes, with approximate time to peak of 15 to 20 minutes. It will take 12 to 24 hours to achieve steady state with this dosage increase, but WP should be getting more pain relief from this increased dose, starting with the very first dose. If he does *not* achieve pain relief with the first injection, it would be appropriate to consider a modest increase in the next injection (about 25% to 50%), such as 12.5- or 15-mg morphine IV. Continued use of the original or this higher dose requires continuous monitoring for sedation and other potential toxicities of morphine.

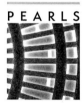

PEARLS **Monitoring for Oversedation**

One method used frequently to monitor the "sleepiness" index from opioid therapy is referred to as the Modified Ramsay Scale for rating sedation. Originally published in 1974, Figure 2-3 is an adapted version.

Indication	Score
• Patient is anxious, agitated, restless.	1
• Patient is awake, cooperative, oriented, tranquil.	2
• Patient is semi-asleep, responds to commands only.	3
• Patient is asleep but responds briskly to glabellar tap, loud auditory stimulus, or gentle shaking.	4
• Patient is asleep with sluggish or decreased response to glabellar tap, loud auditory stimulus, or other noxious stimuli.	5
• Patient does not respond to firm nailbed pressure or other noxious stimuli.	6

Figure 2-3. Modified Ramsay Scale.

Source: Adapted from Ramsay MA, Savege TM, Simpson BR, et al. Controlled sedation with alphaxalone-alphadolone. Br Med J. 1974;2(920):656-659; Blanchard AR. Sedation and analgesia in intensive care. Postgrad Med. 2002;111(2):59-74.

The goal would be a level of arousal rated as a 2; 3 or 4 is acceptable but warrants close monitoring; 5 is not a good look; and 6 is really bad news. If the patient is oversedated, you would need to hold the next dose of opioid, and perhaps lower the dose and/or extend the dosing interval. Rarely do you need to resort to using an opioid antagonist such as naloxone.

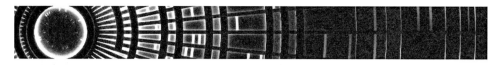

CASE 2.8
• •

Same Opioid, Different Formulation and Route of Administration (Parenteral to Oral)

Let's look at the reverse of the previous case. But, before we fire up the calculator, let's consider some important data from Reddy and colleagues.[44]

Can We Be Steadies?

*Let's stop and consider evidence from crossover, **steady-state** trials of opioid conversions. These data are more robust than data based on single-dose crossover trials using an experimental pain model or based on bioavailability.*

Reddy and colleagues evaluated the conversion ratio from IV hydromorphone to oral hydromorphone (see Chapter 1), oral morphine, and oxycodone.[44]

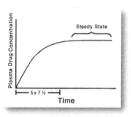

Their results were as follows:

▶ The median conversion ratio from IV hydromorphone to oral hydromorphone was 2.5 (1-mg IV hydromorphone converted to 2.5-mg oral hydromorphone) in patients receiving <30-mg IV hydromorphone/day.

▶ The median conversion ratio from IV hydromorphone to oral hydromorphone was 2.1 (1-mg IV hydromorphone converted to 2.1-mg oral hydromorphone) in patients receiving ≥30-mg IV hydromorphone/day.

▶ The median conversion ratio from IV hydromorphone to oral morphine was 11.54 (1-mg IV hydromorphone converted to 11.54-mg oral morphine) in patients receiving <30-mg IV hydromorphone/day.

▶ The median conversion from IV hydromorphone to oral morphine was 9.86 (1-mg IV hydromorphone converted to 9.86-mg oral morphine) in patients receiving ≥30-mg IV hydromorphone/day.

▶ The median conversion from IV hydromorphone to oral oxycodone was 8.06 (1-mg IV hydromorphone converted to 8.06-mg oral oxycodone).

BOTTOM LINE RECOMMENDATION: From IV hydromorphone to oral hydromorphone

▶ 1:2.5 (IV hydromorphone → oral hydromorphone)

BOTTOM LINE RECOMMENDATION: From IV hydromorphone to oral morphine

▶ 1:10 (IV hydromorphone → oral morphine)

BOTTOM LINE: From IV hydromorphone to oral oxycodone

▶ 1:8 (IV hydromorphone → oral oxycodone)

VF is a 62-year-old man recently diagnosed with colon cancer, who was admitted for surgical resection of the lesion. Post-operatively he was given hydromorphone 2 mg IV every 4 hours as needed for pain control. On post-operative day 1, he used 12 mg of IV hydromorphone, post-operative day 2 he used 10 mg, and post-operative day 3 he used 8 mg. This is the morning of day 4, and he is preparing for discharge. VF has a history of itching when taking oxycodone; therefore, the physician does not want to transition the patient to Percocet as is her usual habit. Instead, she wants to discharge the patient with oral hydromorphone and asks your advice on dosing. What do you recommend?

STEP 1—On reviewing VF's chart, you see that he has used less and less hydromorphone each day, and he reports good pain control. His last dose of hydromorphone was 3 hours ago, and he is rating his pain as a 2 or 3 (on a 0–10 scale; 0 = no pain, 10 = worst imaginable pain). His pain is entirely consistent with a normal post-operative course, and there does not seem to be any reason to consider adding a co-analgesic at this time.

STEP 2—Over the 24-hour period of day 3, VF used 8 mg of sub-Q hydromorphone (TDD).

STEP 3—The physician has already stated that she would like to transition VF to oral hydromorphone because hydromorphone has worked very well for this patient, and it is less likely to cause itching (which is a "pseudoallergic" reaction to opioids, probably related to histamine release).

Consulting our Equianalgesic Opioid Dosing table, we see that 2-mg parenteral hydromorphone is approximately equivalent to 5-mg oral hydromorphone. If we use a simple ratio, this is a 2.5-fold difference. Therefore, we can do a simple ratio and determine that this would be 2.5 times the 8-mg TDD sub-Q hydromorphone, or 20-mg TDD oral hydromorphone.

Alternately, we could use the mathematical proportion using the cross-multiplication method:

Actual Drug Doses: **Equianalgesic Data from Chart:**

$$\frac{\text{"X" mg TDD new opioid}}{\text{mg TDD current opioid}} = \frac{\text{equianalgesic factor of new opioid}}{\text{equianalgesic factor of current opioid}}$$

Filling in the numbers we find:

$$\frac{\text{"X" mg TDD new opioid}}{\text{8 mg TDD sub-Q hydromorphone}} = \frac{\text{5 mg oral hydromorphone}}{\text{2 mg parenteral hydromorphone}}$$

We cross multiply:

$(8) \times (5) = (X) \times (2)$

$40 = X \times 2$

$X = 20$

This method also shows the TDD oral hydromorphone would be 20 mg.

Let's do the calculation using the mathematical proportion by ratio (method D) just for grins, as follows:

$$\text{TDD current opioid} \times \frac{\text{equianalgesic factor of new opioid}}{\text{equianalgesic factor of current opioid}} = \text{TDD new opioid}$$

$$\text{TDD 8 mg sub-Q hydromorphone} \times \frac{\text{5 mg oral hydromorphone}}{\text{2 mg sub-Q hydromorphone}} = \text{TDD mg oral hydromorphone}$$

Cancel out like units as shown below:

$$\text{TDD 8 } \cancel{\text{mg sub-Q hydromorphone}} \times \frac{\text{5 mg oral hydromorphone}}{\text{hydromorphone 2 } \cancel{\text{mg sub-Q hydromorphone}}} = \text{TDD mg oral}$$

Doing the math shows us: $8 \times 5/2 = 8 \times 2.5 = 20$ mg.

Confirming for the third time that the TDD of oral hydromorphone is 20 mg. Eureka! I'm convinced! Hold up there, cowboy! Don't reach for the party hat just yet.

STEP 4—Working from an equivalent TDD of oral hydromorphone is 20 mg, we must decide if we should increase the dose, decrease the dose, or run with the 20 mg. Because VF's pain is well controlled at this time, there's no need to increase the dose. Further, VF has been using less and less IV hydromorphone every day since surgery—his pain is getting better on its own. Therefore, it would be reasonable to expect he would continue to improve, and we can reduce this dose for discharge.

If we look at the oral equivalent of VF's post-operative daily use of hydromorphone since surgery, it would be 30 mg, 25 mg, and then 20 mg. As we think ahead to discharge, hydromorphone is available as 2-, 4-, and 8-mg tablets. VF is able to swallow tablets; therefore, this makes the most sense. We generally dose hydromorphone every 4 hours. If we recommend 2-mg oral hydromorphone every 4 hours, that's a potential TDD of 12-mg oral hydromorphone. If we recommend 4-mg oral hydromorphone every 4 hours, that's a potential TDD of 24-mg oral hydromorphone. VF probably will not need 24-mg of oral hydromorphone per day, but 12-mg per day may be insufficient. Let's hope for the best but plan for the worst and order the following: hydromorphone 2 mg by mouth every 4 hours as needed for pain rated 6 or less; or 4 mg by mouth for pain rated 7 or higher. The surgeon anticipates VF will only need hydromorphone for 3 to 4 days after discharge, so we order 28, 2-mg tablets. We will also encourage VF to maintain a pain diary over the next few days. We could even anticipate his opioid requirements declining further over the next few days and recommend the physician prescribe the 2-mg tablet, allowing the patient to self-taper off opioids (e.g., use one or two 2-mg tablets every 4 hours initially for a day or two, then reduce to one 2-mg tablet every 4 hours for a day or two, then halve the tablets or discontinue therapy).

STEP 5—As discussed above, we will ask VF to maintain a pain diary, recording his pain ratings and use of hydromorphone. We will also do a phone follow-up to ask about his ability to perform activities of daily living and his ability to sleep and ambulate. We will ask VF's wife to monitor his level of arousal/sedation to make sure he doesn't become too sedated, and we will encourage VF to use a bowel regimen if necessary and ask about constipation.

Wow! We've talked about several situations where we need to switch from one formulation or route of administration to another using the same opioid. You have learned about several methods to calculate the dose you are switching to, and have seen how all roads really do lead to Rome!

- It's a good idea to use one method for your calculation, and another method to check yourself.

- *Always* use common sense.

- When you are switching from a parenteral to a nonparenteral route, the dose will *always* be higher.

- When you are switching from a nonparenteral to a parenteral route, the TDD will *always* be lower.

On to the practice problems—your ears aren't ringing enough yet!

PRACTICE PROBLEMS

P2.1. Same Opioid, Same Route of Administration (Oral to Oral/Buccal), Different Formulation

JM is an 86-year-old woman with dementia and uterine cancer. She is very confused and has difficulty swallowing tablets, so her prescriber put her on Kadian (once-daily ER morphine capsule), and titrated her to 60 mg once daily, sprinkled on applesauce. She is close to death at this point, and eating applesauce is not an option. Because JM is in a long-term care facility, the prescriber would like to avoid starting parenteral morphine. You suggested switching JM to a morphine oral concentrated solution and instilling it in the buccal cavity. The prescriber thinks that's a fabulous idea and asks you to determine an equivalent dosage regimen to Kadian 60 mg by mouth every day.

P2.2. Same Opioid, Different Formulation and Route of Administration (Oral to Rectal)

HZ is a 92-year-old man who lives at home, diagnosed with lung cancer. His pain has been well controlled on hydromorphone 2 mg, one to two tablets every 4 hours as needed. His average TDD over the past few days is 14 to 16 mg. At this time, he is unable to swallow either hydromorphone tablets or oral solution, and you decide to switch him to hydromorphone rectal suppositories. What dose and regimen do you recommend and when should it start?

P2.3. Same Opioid, Same Route of Administration (Oral), Different Formulation

LK is a 42-year-old man who injured his back several years ago while unloading a truck. He has had three back surgeries since his initial injury and is no longer a surgical candidate. At present, LK complains of pain in his sacral area, which he rates as a best of 2 and a worst of 4 on average per day (on a 0–10 scale; 0 = no pain, 10 = worst imaginable pain) while taking his pain medications. At present, LK is taking the following analgesic regimen:

- Percocet (10-mg oxycodone/325-mg acetaminophen per tablet), two tablets every 6 hours
- Gabapentin 900 mg by mouth every 8 hours
- Desipramine 75 mg by mouth at bedtime

LK states he is content with his level of pain control and that it allows him to perform his desired activities of daily living. He enjoys the little "kick" he gets when he takes his two Percocet tablets every 6 hours.

As his prescriber, however, you are not as amused by the Percocet "kick." You are also concerned about the amount of acetaminophen LK is getting per day (325 mg × 8 tablets = 2.6 g per day), since LK enjoys an alcoholic beverage or three on the weekends (alcohol use increases risk of acetaminophen toxicity and is never a good idea with concurrent opioid therapy). You decide to switch his Percocet to OxyContin. What dosage regimen do you recommend? When can it be initiated? What educational tips should you give LK about his analgesics?

P2.4. Same Opioid, Same Route of Administration (Oral), Different Formulation

DM is a 48-year-old man diagnosed with non-small cell lung cancer. His disease has progressed, and he is now using hydromorphone 2 mg by mouth every 4 hours, including during the night. This regimen helps his pain, but he is not at goal. He rates his pain on average as a 6 or 7 (on a 0–10 scale; 0 = no pain, 10 = worst imaginable pain), and he finds the frequent redosing distressing and would like a longer-acting opioid. His prescriber has optimized adjunctive analgesic therapy. What dose of Exalgo would you recommend?

P2.5: Same Opioid, Different Formulation and Route of Administration (Parenteral to Oral)

BC is a 48-year-old woman who injured her back in a motor vehicle accident recently, for which she required immediate surgical repair. Post-operatively she was started on intermittent sub-Q injections of morphine every 4 hours. It has been 5 days since surgery, and BC has been stabilized on a TDD of 15-mg sub-Q morphine. BC is ready for transfer to a rehabilitation facility, and it is anticipated that she will require chronic opioid therapy for the near future. What dosage regimen of long-acting oral morphine would you recommend and why? What dose of oral morphine should be made available to the patient for breakthrough or incident pain?

P2.6: Same Opioid, Different Formulation and Route of Administration (Parenteral to Oral)

MV is a 62-year-old woman with stage IV breast cancer. She has been experiencing significant pain and was maintained on oral long-acting morphine at home. Unfortunately, she has experienced a pain crisis and is admitted to hospice for pain control. Her pain is controlled within a few days on IV hydromorphone 0.4 mg per hour, with only occasional bolus dose of 0.2 mg. She is anxious to go home so she can be with her family, but still have this same level of pain control. What do you recommend?

Could I Get That to Go, Please? Bottom Line It for Me . . .

▸ In this chapter, we discussed how to switch from one dosage formulation and/or route of administration to another using the same opioid.

▸ Staying with the same opioid alleviates the need to worry about tolerance and potency concerns; switching between routes of administration is more a concern of bioavailability. Timing in these switches is also an important consideration.

▸ If pain is not controlled when switching, do not reduce the newly calculated dose; depending on the clinical scenario, you may round up to the next appropriate dosage strength.

▸ If pain is controlled when switching, you can either use the calculated dose or round down to the next appropriate dosage strength.

▸ Consider the timing of switches when switching to or from prolonged-release dosage formulations.

REFERENCES

1. Mercadente S. Opioid rotation for cancer pain: rationale and clinical aspects. *Cancer.* 1999;86:1856-1866.

2. Kadian Prescribing Information. https://www.allergan.com/assets/pdf/kadian_pi. Published December 2016. Accessed February 10, 2017.

3. Xtampza ER Prescribing Information. http://www.xtampzaer.com/hcp/assets/pdf/xtampza-pi.pdf. Published December 2016. Accessed February 10, 2018.

4. Currow DC, Plummer JL, Cooney NJ, et al. A randomized, double-blind, multi-site, crossover, placebo-controlled equivalence study of morning versus evening once-daily sustained-release morphine sulfate in people with pain from advanced cancer. *J Pain Symptom Manage.* 2007;34:17-23.

5. U.S. Department of Health and Human Services, Food and Drug Administration, Center for Drug Evaluation and Research (CDER). Guidance for Industry: Bioavailability and Bioequivalence Studies for Orally Administered Drug Products – General Considerations; March 2003; p. 6. https://www.fda.gov/ohrms/dockets/ac/03/briefing/3995B1_07_GFI-BioAvail-BioEquiv.pdf. Accessed February 10, 2018.

6. Lugo RA, Kern SE. Clinical pharmacokinetics of morphine. *J Pain Palliat Care Pharmacother.* 2002;16(4):5-18.

7. Vallner JJ, Stewart JT, Kotzan JA, et al. Pharmacokinetics and bioavailability of hydromorphone following intravenous and oral administration to human subjects. *J Clin Pharmacol.* 1981;21:152-156.

8. Parab PV, Ritschel WA, Coyle DE, et al. Pharmacokinetics of hydromorphone after intravenous, peroral and rectal administration to human subjects. *Biopharm Drug Dispos.* 1988;9:187-199.

9. Amabile CM, Bowman CJ. Overview of oral modified-release opioid products for the management of chronic pain. *Ann Pharmacother.* 2006;40:1327-1335.

10. Patanwala AE, Duby J, Waters D, et al. Opioid conversions in acute care. *Ann Pharmacother.* 2007;41:255-267.

11. Hanks GW, DeConno F, Ripamonti C, et al. Expert Working Group of the European Association for Palliative Care. Morphine in cancer pain: modes of administration. *Br Med J.* 1996;312:823-826.

12. Mercadante SG. When oral morphine fails in cancer pain: the role of the alternative route. *Am J Hosp Palliat Care.* 1998;15:333-342.

13. Walsh D, Tropiano P. Long-term rectal administration of high-dose sustained release morphine tablets. *Support Care Cancer.* 2002:10:653-655.

14. American Pain Society. *Principles of Analgesic Use in the Treatment of Acute Pain and Cancer Pain.* 5th ed. Glenview, IL: American Pain Society; 2003.

15. Moulin DE, Kfreedt JH, Murray-Parsons N, et al. Comparison of continuous subcutaneous hydromorphone infusions for management of cancer pain. *Lancet.* 1991;337:465-468.

16. Waldman CS, Eason JR, Rambohul E, et al. Serum morphine levels: a comparison between continuous subcutaneous infusion and continuous intravenous infusion in post-operative patients. *Anesthesia.* 1984;39:768-771.

17. Frampton JE. Tapentadol immediate release: A review of its use in the treatment of moderate to severe acute pain. *Drugs.* 2010;70(13):1719-1743.

18. Nucynta Prescribing Information. https://www.nucynta.com/sites/default/files/pdf/nucynta-pi_0.pdf. Accessed February 10, 2018.

19. Nucynta ER Prescribing Information. https://www.nucynta.com/sites/default/files/pdf/nucyntaer-pi_0.pdf. Accessed February 10, 2018.

20. Food and Drug Administration. Opioids. https://www.fda.gov/Drugs/DrugSafety/InformationbyDrugClass/ucm337066.htm. Accessed February 10, 2018.

21. MPR. Opioids with abuse deterrent properties. http://www.empr.com/opioids-with-abuse-deterrent-properties/slideshow/1279/. Accessed February 10, 2018.

22. Hysingla ER Prescribing Information. http://app.purduepharma.com/xmlpublishing/pi.aspx?id=h. Accessed February 10, 2018.

23. Hysingla ER. https://hysinglaer.com/. Accessed February 10, 2018.

24. Vantrela ER Prescribing Information. https://www.accessdata.fda.gov/drugsatfda_docs/label/2017/207975s000lbl.pdf. Accessed February 10, 2018.

25. Zohydro ER Prescribing Information. http://www.zohydroer.com/downloads/ZOHYDROERFullPrescribingInformation.pdf. Accessed February 10, 2018.

26. What Is Zohydro ER with BeadTek? http://zohydroer.com/how-beadtek-works.php. Accessed February 10, 2018.

27. Abuse-Deterrent Opioid Formulations. *The Medical Letter* 2015;1476. https://secure.medicalletter.org/w1476a. Accessed February 10, 2018.

28. Exalgo Prescribing Information. https://www.accessdata.fda.gov/drugsatfda_docs/label/2010/021217lbl.pdf. Accessed February 10, 2018.

29. Moorman-Li R, Motycka CA, Inge LD, et al. A review of abuse-deterrent opioids for chronic nonmalignant pain. *P&T.* 2012;37(7):412-421.

30. Arymo ER. https://www.arymoer.com/. Accessed February 10, 2018.

31. Arymo ER Prescribing Information. https://dailymed.nlm.nih.gov/dailymed/drugInfo.cfm?setid=e60552c9-06ce-4790-95e7-aadd4df12b2a. Accessed February 10, 2018.

32. MORPHABOND ER Prescribing Information. http://dsi.com/prescribing-information-portlet/getDocument?product=MB&inline=true. Accessed February 10, 2018.

33. Embeda Prescribing Information. http://labeling.pfizer.com/ShowLabeling.aspx?id=694. Accessed February 10, 2018.

34. Oxaydo. http://www.oxaydo.com/hcp/why-oxaydo/. Accessed February 10, 2018.

35. Oxaydo Prescribing Information. https://dailymed.nlm.nih.gov/dailymed/drugInfo.cfm?setid=cff0c64a-63f5-4b3c-909a-cdecf6755cbe. Accessed February 10, 2018.

36. Bulloch M. Abuse-deterrent opioids: A primer for pharmacists. *Pharmacy Times.* 2015. http://www.pharmacytimes.com/print.php?url=/contributor/marilyn-bulloch-pharmd-bcps/2015/10/abuse-deterrent-opioids-a-primer-for-pharmacists. Accessed February 10, 2018.

37. MORPHABOND ER Prescribing Information. http://dsi.com/prescribing-information-portlet/getDocument?product=MB&inline=true. Accessed February 10, 2018.

38. ROXYBOND Prescribing Information. https://www.accessdata.fda.gov/drugsatfda_docs/label/2017/209777lbl.pdf. Accessed February 10, 2018.

39. Inspirion Delivery Sciences receives FDA approval for RoxyBond™ (oxycodone hydrochloride) tablets CII, the first and only immediate release opioid analgesic with abuse-deterrent label claims [news release]. Basking Ridge, NJ: Inspirion Delivery Sciences, LLC; April 26, 2017. http://www.prnewswire.com/news-releases/inspirion-delivery-sciences-receives-fda-approval-for-roxybond-oxycodone-hydrochloride-tablets-cii-the-first-and-only-immediate-release-opioid-analgesic-with-abuse-deterrent-label-claims-300445964.html. Accessed February 10, 2018.

40. Xtampza ER. http://www.xtampzaer.com/hcp/deterx-technology.html#tab-2. Accessed February 10, 2018.

41. Xtampza ER Prescribing Information. http://www.xtampzaer.com/hcp/assets/pdf/xtampza-pi.pdf. Accessed February 10, 2018.

42. Ramsay MA, Savege TM, Simpson BR, et al. Controlled sedation with alphaxalone-alphadolone. *Br Med J.* 1974;2(920):656-659.

43. Blanchard AR. Sedation and analgesia in intensive care. *Postgrad Med.* 2002;111(2):59-74.

44. Reddy A, Vidal M, Stephen S, et al. The conversion ratio from intravenous hydromorphone to oral opioids in cancer patients. *J Pain Symptom Manage.* 2017;54:280-288.

SOLUTIONS TO PRACTICE PROBLEMS

P2.1

STEP 1—Per the prescriber, JM's pain is well controlled.

STEP 2—JM is receiving Kadian 60 mg once daily, so her TDD of oral morphine is 60 mg.

STEP 3—The prescriber has already accepted the idea of switching JM to an oral morphine concentrated solution. Because we're switching from oral morphine to oral morphine, the TDD remains the same, 60-mg oral morphine.

STEP 4—The patient's pain was controlled; therefore, an increase in dose is not necessary. We're not switching opioids, so a decrease is not necessary. Oral morphine concentrated solution is dosed every 4 hours, or six doses per day. This gives us a regimen of oral morphine solution 20 mg/mL, 10 mg (0.5 mL) every 4 hours, instilled in the buccal cavity.

STEP 5—JM's upper body should be propped up 30 degrees before instilling the morphine in her buccal cavity and monitored to ensure she does not aspirate the morphine solution. She should also be monitored for pain control and any potential toxicity.

P2.2

STEP 1—HZ's pain is well controlled, and he is doing well on his current regimen (aside from the inability to swallow).

STEP 2—HZ's TDD of oral hydromorphone is between 14 and 16 mg.

STEP 3—We have already decided to switch HZ to rectal hydromorphone suppositories. The data on the bioequivalence of rectal hydromorphone suppositories are not as strong as they are for oral:rectal morphine, but most practitioners consider the ratio to be 1:1 for hydromorphone as well.

STEP 4—Some data suggest that hydromorphone may be a bit more potent when given as a rectal suppository, and it seems to last 6 hours, as opposed to 4 hours with oral hydromorphone. For this reason, it would be prudent to switch to hydromorphone 3 mg by rectum every 6 hours, which is a TDD of 12 mg (slightly less than the oral regimen).

STEP 5—Monitor HZ for adverse effects to the hydromorphone, including rectal irritation and pain control.

P2.3

STEP 1—You have assessed LK's complaint of pain and believe you have maximized his analgesic regimen at this point. More important, LK feels his current analgesic regimen has met his goals for pain management.

STEP 2—Focusing just on the Percocet, LK's TDD of oral oxycodone is 80 mg (two Percocet tablets every 6 hours = 20-mg oxycodone × 4 = 80 mg).

STEP 3—LK admits to enjoying one or more alcoholic beverages on the weekend. Based on the tendency for individuals to underreport the amount of alcohol they consume and FDA recommendations, you have already decided to switch LK to OxyContin and not to replace the acetaminophen. In addition, opioids and alcohol are not a great idea; LK needs to promise to stop consuming alcohol or his opioid regimen should be tapered down and discontinued. Assuming he's agreeable to that plan, we can move forward with the opioid conversion. Oxycodone is equally bioavailable in Percocet and

OxyContin; therefore, the TDD of OxyContin would be 80 mg before any TDD dose change considerations.

STEP 4—As stated earlier, LK is content with his current level of pain control. Therefore, a TDD of 80-mg OxyContin should give equivalent pain relief, while only requiring twice-daily dosing. A regimen of OxyContin 40 mg by mouth every 12 hours would be appropriate. There is no need either to increase the TDD or to decrease it. The OxyContin should be started probably at a convenient time in the evening or morning, at least 4 hours after his last dose of Percocet. Should the patient's pain not be controlled on this new regimen, it may be due to eliminating the acetaminophen. If this is the case, you can add acetaminophen back to the regimen separately (if he is agreeable to discontinue drinking alcohol), adjust his co-analgesic regimen, or increase the opioid dose a bit.

STEP 5—LK should be monitored for therapeutic effectiveness including pain rating and performance of activities of daily living and parameters that would indicate toxicity. Alcohol consumption (or hopefully discontinuation) should be monitored as well.

Educational points for LK include the following:

- We would rather you not appreciate the "kick" from your opioid. The opioid is to control your pain and to allow you to perform your activities of daily living, not for your entertainment pleasure. OxyContin will give you 12 hours of steady pain relief; there will be no "kick."

- It is very important to tell LK that he should take his OxyContin tablets every 12 hours—don't say "take twice a day." To many patients, "take twice a day," means take with breakfast and dinner!

- You should advise LK to discontinue drinking alcohol. He is taking a potent medication, along with two co-analgesics, and alcohol doesn't play well in the sandbox with the others. He should avoid taking acetaminophen on top of this regimen, especially if he does not give up alcohol. If he does not give up alcohol, consider tapering down and stopping the opioid.

P2.4

STEP 1—DM's pain is not well controlled at this time, and his prescriber has maximized adjunctive therapy. The patient's pain is opioid-responsive, but he probably needs a dosage increase.

STEP 2—DM is taking hydromorphone 2 mg by mouth every 4 hours (6 doses) for a TDD of 12 mg.

STEP 3—Exalgo is a once-a-day prolonged-release hydromorphone tablet available as 8, 12, 16, and 32 mg. The conversion from oral immediate-release hydromorphone to Exalgo is 1:1; therefore, Exalgo 12 mg a day would provide DM the same degree of pain relief as he's experiencing at this time.

STEP 4—Technically, you could increase to 16 mg, but it may be worth trying the 12-mg tablet for several days to see how smoothing things out would work.

STEP 5—After 4 days on Exalgo 12 mg po every day, the patient tells you his pain is a 5 on average (on a 0–10 scale; 0 = no pain, 10 = worst imaginable pain), but he is needing two to three doses of the IR hydromorphone per day. At this point, you elect to increase Exalgo to 16 mg po every day and continue IR hydromorphone for breakthrough pain. You will continue to monitor the patient's response to therapy.

P2.5

STEP 1—BC's pain is stable on her current sub-Q morphine regimen and does not require the addition of any co-analgesics at this time.

STEP 2—BC's TDD of parenteral morphine is 15 mg.

STEP 3—The prescriber has already requested that BC be converted to oral morphine, using ER tablets for her baseline sub-Q analgesia, and to have an IR morphine tablet available for breakthrough or incident pain.

In comparison to IV morphine, oral morphine is approximately 35% bioavailable. A simple ratio tells us that we must multiply the parenteral TDD of morphine by 2.5 to determine the TDD of oral morphine, or in this case, 37.5 mg.

Or, you can directly apply the ratio to the current total daily dose and end up with the new opioid total daily dose as follows:

$$15 \text{ mg TDD } \cancel{\text{parenteral morphine}} \times \frac{25 \text{ mg oral morphine}}{10 \text{ mg } \cancel{\text{parenteral morphine}}} = 37.5 \text{ mg TDD oral morphine}$$

STEP 4—There is no reason to increase the amount of morphine the patient is receiving per day because her pain is controlled. We do not need to reduce her TDD due to incomplete cross-tolerance since we are converting from morphine to morphine. We will work with the TDD of 37.5-mg oral morphine to determine her exact regimen.

Our formulation options include generic long-acting morphine (every 8 or 12 hours) or Kadian (every 12 or 24 hours).

Possible recommendations include

- Generic long-acting morphine 15 mg by mouth every 12 hours
- Kadian 20 mg by mouth every 12 hours
- Kadian 40 mg by mouth every 24 hours

For breakthrough pain (which you will learn all about in Chapter 4), we generally offer 10% to 15% of the total daily dose of scheduled opioid, every 2 hours as needed. In this case, it would be about 5-mg oral morphine. This dose may be offered 1 hour before events known to produce pain (e.g., PT in the rehabilitation center) or when the pain increases to an unexpectedly higher level. BC's pain should continue to resolve as days and weeks go on.

STEP 5—We should monitor the medication administration record from the rehabilitation facility to determine how many doses of short-acting morphine the patient requires per day on top of her scheduled long-acting morphine. If she is consistently requiring four additional doses of IR morphine, we could consider increasing the long-acting morphine. Importantly, we will also monitor BC's ability to participate in PT, and for any potential signs of opioid toxicity.

P2.6

STEP 1—MV states she has acceptable pain control on her current regimen; therefore, it is unlikely we would need to add a co-analgesic at this time.

STEP 2—MV's TDD of IV hydromorphone is 9.6 mg (0.4 mg/hr = $0.4 \times 24 = 9.6$ mg).

STEP 3—We decide to switch MV to oral hydromorphone.

Consulting our Equianalgesic Opioid Dosing table, we see that 2-mg parenteral hydromorphone is approximately equivalent to 5-mg oral hydromorphone (a factor of 2.5). Using this method, an equivalent TDD of oral hydromorphone would be about 24 mg.

STEP 4—As we've discussed, the work by Reddy[44] illustrates that the median dose of oral hydromorphone when switching from IV hydromorphone in cancer patients is closer to 1:2.5 (IV to oral hydromorphone), which would give us 24-mg oral hydromorphone per day (9.6-mg TDD IV hydromorphone × 2.5 = 24 mg). Let's recommend oral hydromorphone 4 mg every 4 hours, with an extra 2-mg oral hydromorphone every 2 hours as needed for additional pain.

STEP 5—We will ask MV to maintain a pain diary when she goes home, and track how often she uses the breakthrough dose of oral hydromorphone. If we aimed too low, we can increase the dose of hydromorphone very quickly. A few days after MV gets home and we determine her optimal total daily oral hydromorphone dose, we could even consider switching her to Exalgo, the once-daily oral hydromorphone formulation. *Strong work everyone!*

CHAPTER 3

Converting Among Routes and Formulations of Different Opioids

INTRODUCTION

You learned all about why we switch opioids in Chapter 1, and how to switch from one route of administration or dosage formulation to a different one using the same opioid in Chapter 2. Sometimes in clinical practice, we need to switch from one opioid to an entirely different opioid. Consider the case of PJ, a 22-year-old man who had all four impacted wisdom teeth extracted during one procedure. The dentist realized this would cause PJ moderate pain post-operatively, and she prescribed Percocet (5-mg oxycodone/325-mg acetaminophen per tablet), one to two tablets every 4 hours as needed. When PJ recovered from anesthesia at home, he felt dreadful and took two Percocet tablets. Within 1 hour, PJ was itching and scratching all over like nobody's business. The dentist realized that the pruritus PJ was experiencing was due to the oxycodone (probably due to histamine release, not a true allergy), and switched him to Vicodin (5-mg hydrocodone/300-mg acetaminophen per tablet). PJ took the Vicodin with good success and his pain resolved over the next few days. Conversion calculations weren't really necessary in this case because PJ was opioid naïve, and received a starting dose for both the Percocet and Vicodin prescriptions.

As discussed in Chapter 1, the development of adverse effects is only one reason why we might switch opioids. Additional reasons include lack of therapeutic response, change in the patient's clinical condition (e.g., inability to use original dosage formulation), and a myriad of other reasons such as opioid product availability; formulary restriction; and patient, caregiver, or prescriber health beliefs. In Chapter 2, we discussed how to switch between routes of administration and formulations of the *same* opioid; in this chapter, we will make the leap *between* opioids (potentially changing the route of administration and formulation as well!). We will hold our discussions of switching to and from methadone and fentanyl until later in the book—they have very specific dosing considerations and deserve devoted discussion. We will also hold discussions of conversions to and from continuous intravenous (IV) or subcutaneous (sub-Q) opioid infusions for a later chapter.

As you may recall, the concepts of **potency** (the intensity of analgesic effect for a given dose), **equianalgesia** (doses of two different opioids that provide the same

OBJECTIVES

After reading this chapter and completing all practice problems, the participant will be able to:

1. List reasons why a healthcare professional may need to switch a patient from one opioid to a different opioid.

2. Given an actual or simulated case of a patient in pain, calculate an equivalent regimen of a different opioid, both by the same route of administration, as well as alternate routes of administration.

degree of pain relief), and **bioavailability** (the percentage of drug that is detected in the systemic circulation after its administration) were discussed in Chapter 1. These concepts were considered, along with the limited primary literature we have available, to craft an Equianalgesic Opioid Dosing table (see Chapter 1, Table 1-1). Remember the doses shown in Table 1-1 are *equivalent* doses, not actual doses.

Again referring to Chapter 1, tables such as Table 1-1 constitute rough estimates of dose equivalencies—most of the data used to determine these equivalencies are from single-dose cross-over studies, usually in acute pain patients, do not take into consideration patient-specific variables (e.g., age, body mass index [BMI], frailty, comorbidities, duration of exposure to opioids, concurrent use of other medications), and may be unidirectional. This is why we include a step in the opioid conversion calculation process where we carefully consider whether we should reduce the calculated dose (which is usually the case), use the calculated dose, or (rarely) increase the dose from that calculated. Where available, conversion ratios derived from switches done at steady state are introduced in this edition of *Demystifying*. Maybe by the fifth edition we'll have all solid data for our equianalgesic table! As a reminder, the five steps we use in opioid conversion calculations are shown in Chapter 1, Table 1-2. Enough talking already, let's jump into some calculations—you scream, I scream, we all scream for morphine (calculations!).

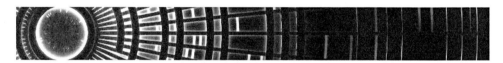

CASE 3.1
. . . .

Switching from Oral Acetaminophen/Oxycodone to Oral Extended-Release Morphine

PA is a 44-year-old man with chronic low back pain, a consequence of a work-related injury in construction. He has undergone surgery several times, and his healthcare team doesn't believe his pain will improve with further surgical interventions. He has completed numerous physical therapy sessions and is adherent to his exercise plan. PA's current analgesic regimen consists of Percocet (10-mg oxycodone/325-mg acetaminophen per tablet), one to two tablets every 6 hours as needed, and pregabalin (Lyrica) 100 mg three times a day. PA tells you, his community pharmacist, that taking the Percocet every 6 hours means he always awakens in pain, and he would really prefer to take medications less often. He's tried cutting back, but that causes his pain to get much worse.

STEP 1—When you ask PA about the pain, he tells you that it is an achy, occasionally "grabbing" pain localized in the lumbosacral area (he points to the small of his back, down into his buttocks). Lifting anything greater than 15 or 20 pounds increases the pain, he can only stand about 30 minutes before his back starts to hurt, and his left leg tingles and eventually becomes numb. Rest, the analgesics, and the application of heat relieve the pain. When he tries to go without the Percocet, or when he awakens 4 to 6 hours after taking a dose, he rates the pain as a 7 or 8 (on a 0–10 scale; 0 = no pain, 10 = worst imaginable pain). When he takes eight Percocet tablets per day, his average pain rating is a 3 or 4 (on a 0–10 scale), which he finds acceptable. He also tells you that the Lyrica has reduced the tingling and numbness in his leg, and it is tolerable at this point. This analgesic regimen allows him to perform the majority of his activities of daily living and sleep fairly well (aside from awakening in pain). He denies incontinence of bowel or bladder, fever, weight loss, or other constitutional symptoms.

STEP 2—PA is consistently taking eight Percocet tablets a day, along with pregabalin (Lyrica) 100 mg three times daily. You want PA to sleep through the night without awakening in pain. You check PA's prescription drug coverage and discover that extended-release (ER) oxycodone is not on the formulary; however, morphine ER is. PA has no history of morphine intolerance, and his renal function is normal for his age. You consult with the prescriber who agrees with your plan to switch PA's Percocet to morphine ER, and she asks you to calculate an equivalent dose. *Yikes—what do we do first?*

Clearly, what you must do now is calculate the total daily dose (TDD) of oxycodone PA is receiving. He tells you he's taking two tablets every 6 hours around the clock. Therefore, we determine the TDD as follows:

2 tablets every 6 hours means PA is taking two tablets four times daily, which means PA's total daily dose of oxycodone is 80 mg.

$$\frac{8 \text{ tablets}}{\text{day}} \times \frac{10 \text{ mg oxycodone}}{\text{tablet}} = \frac{8 \text{ \cancel{tablets}}}{\text{day}} \times \frac{10 \text{ mg oxycodone}}{\text{\cancel{tablet}}} = \frac{80 \text{ mg oxycodone}}{\text{day}}$$

Therefore, PA's TDD of oral oxycodone = 80 mg.

Please note that we are ignoring the acetaminophen component at this point. If necessary, the patient can take acetaminophen separately (up to 4,000 mg/day). The contribution of acetaminophen to the patient's overall analgesia should not be underestimated or forgotten.

STEP 3—Now we need to convert the 80-mg TDD oxycodone to a TDD of morphine.

Let's use the mathematical proportion method using cross-multiplication (method B) as follows:

$$\frac{\text{"X" mg TDD new opioid}}{\text{mg TDD current opioid}} = \frac{\text{equianalgesic factor of new opioid}}{\text{equianalgesic factor of current opioid}}$$

As you recall from Chapter 1 and consulting our Equianalgesic Opioid Dosing table (Table 1-1), the doses listed *across* a row for a given opioid show equipotent doses. Also, doses for different opioids in a *column* are also equipotent. We can also use this chart to look at equivalent doses between opioids and routes of administration. Therefore, looking at the table, we can fill in the appropriate data as follows:

$$\frac{\text{"X" mg TDD new opioid (morphine)}}{80 \text{ mg TDD oral oxycodone}} = \frac{25 \text{ mg oral morphine}}{20 \text{ mg oral oxycodone}}$$

Cross-multiplication gives us:

$(80) \times (25) = (X) \times 20$

$2,000 = 20X$

$X = 100$

Using this method, we see a TDD of 100 mg oral morphine is approximately equipotent to 80-mg TDD of oxycodone.

Before we move on to Step 4, let's consider the answer we calculated. *Does it LOOK right?* Fire up those synapses and think it through. If 20-mg oral oxycodone is approximately equivalent to 25-mg oral morphine, then 80-mg oral oxycodone (which is 4 times 20) must be about equivalent to 100-mg morphine (which is 4 times 25). *Yep—checks out using common sense.* It takes about 25% more milligrams of oral morphine as it does oral oxycodone to get the same job done (20-mg oral oxycodone ≈ 25-mg oral morphine; therefore, 80-mg oral oxycodone ≈ 100-mg oral morphine). *Excellent, let's press on.*

STEP 4—As you read in Chapter 1, once you do your mathematical computation, you will need to individualize the dose for the patient. We can go with a TDD of 100-mg oral morphine per day, reduce the morphine TDD dose, or increase the TDD (rare and very unlikely). Because there are discrete differences in the way different opioids bind and/or activate receptors, there is no complete "cross-tolerance" among opioids. In other words, PA will be more sensitive to the pharmacologic effects of morphine; therefore, giving him 100 mg per day of morphine would cause a greater pharmacologic effect than the 80 mg of oral oxycodone per day despite the fact that they are approximately equipotent. This would be a good plan (e.g., no dose adjustment) if we were switching because his pain was not controlled on the oxycodone, but that's not the case. Therefore, it would be prudent to reduce his TDD oral morphine by 25% to 50%. Reducing a 100-mg TDD oral morphine by 25% to 50% leaves us with about 50- to 75-mg TDD oral morphine. Let's go with 60 mg a day oral morphine.

We already discussed that we want to recommend an morphine ER tablet or capsule. Our options include the following:

- MS Contin, Arymo ER, or a similar generic 30 mg by mouth every 12 hours

- Kadian 60 mg once every 24 hours

- Kadian 30 mg once every 12 hours

To be conservative, let's go with MS Contin 30 mg by mouth once every 12 hours. We can continue to use the Percocet for breakthrough pain, particularly during the next few days as we titrate to effectiveness. Alternately, you could use oxycodone (without the acetaminophen) or morphine for breakthrough pain.

STEP 5—Once the prescriber agrees with the recommendation, the pharmacist can counsel the patient about how to transition from Percocet to the ER morphine product. Percocet is a short-acting product, and modified-release morphine products take several hours to reach therapeutic levels after the first dose. Therefore, the ER morphine could be started the very next morning, and at *most* one additional dose of Percocet could be taken within the first 4 hours after starting morphine, if pain is not sufficiently controlled and there is no appreciable sedation, nausea, or other untoward central nervous system (CNS) effects from the morphine. The patient should maintain a pain diary and note pain intensity, relationship to activity, and any adverse effects experienced, if any. The pharmacist will follow up with a phone call to ask if the patient is able to sleep through the night without awakening in pain and assess his continued ability to perform activities of daily living. The pharmacist will also ask about adverse effects (e.g., constipation, sedation, confusion, pruritus). If you chose to use oxycodone (instead of Percocet) or a different opioid for breakthrough pain, you could still offer acetaminophen separately, not to exceed 4 grams a day.

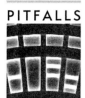

PITFALLS Double-Check Those Dosing Intervals!

Always stop yourself and make SURE you are CLEAR on how many doses the patient is actually taking per day. A common mistake is to hear "every 6 hours" and think "six" doses—or "every 4 hours" and think "four" doses per day.

Remember to divide the hourly dosing interval into 24 (hours per day)—obviously "every 6 hours" means four doses per day (24 hours divided by 6-hour intervals) and "every 4 hours" means six doses per day (24 hours divided by 4-hour intervals). *This common mathematical error could result in overdosage or undertreatment of pain.*

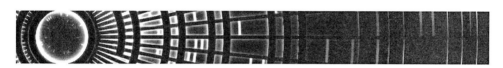

CASE 3.2

Switching from Oral Oxymorphone to Oral Oxycodone

ZH is a 68-year-old woman who is being discharged from a rehabilitation center after left total knee replacement. She has received extensive physical therapy, which caused some discomfort. Her physiatrist wants the patient to continue opioid therapy at home (plus she still needs her right knee replaced and it's quite painful). The patient's pain has been well controlled on oxymorphone ER 10 mg by mouth every 12 hours, and oxymorphone immediate release (IR) 5 mg every 4 hours as needed (takes about two doses per day). The surgeon is poised to discharge ZH home on this regimen, only to learn that ER oxymorphone is hard to readily obtain from a community pharmacy, since the Food and Drug Administration (FDA) requested Opana ER be removed from the market.[1] The surgeon has asked that you switch ZH to OxyContin. When you point out that there are other long-acting generic oxymorphone formulations on the market (which would be a simple 1:1 conversion from Opana ER), the surgeon declines. "No, those aren't abuse-deterrent, so I sure don't want to do this dance again." Ok, OxyContin it is! Cleary and colleagues provide an excellent discussion on considerations when rotating from Opana ER.[2]

STEP 1—ZH describes her pain as well-localized in her left knee and also present in her right knee. She says the physical therapy exacerbates the left knee pain, and rest, ice, and the opioid regimen relieve the pain. She describes the pain as achy and sometimes throbbing immediately after physical therapy. On her current analgesic regimen, she rates the pain as 1 or 2 (on a 0–10 scale; 0 = no pain, 10 = worst imaginable pain) at rest, 4 with normal movement, and 6 or 7 toward the end of a physical therapy session; she finds this level of pain control acceptable. She states the opioid regimen is necessary to allow her to continue physical therapy, which she will continue on an outpatient basis. ZH denies any burning, tingling, or numbness. The pain does not prevent her from sleeping, although her limited mobility at this time prevents her from several activities of daily living (e.g., housecleaning, grocery shopping) and hobbies (gardening, walking for exercise).

STEP 2—ZH is currently receiving oxymorphone ER 10 mg by mouth every 12 hours, and oxymorphone IR 5 mg by mouth every 4 hours as needed for breakthrough pain. She usually takes two of the 5-mg short-acting tablets per day, for a TDD of oral oxymorphone of 30 mg.

STEP 3—When we consult the Equianalgesic Opioid Dosing table (Table 1-1), we see the following data (abstracted from the table):

	Equianalgesic Doses (mg)	
Drug	Parenteral	Oral
Morphine	10	25
Oxycodone	10*	20
Oxymorphone	1	10

*Not available in the United States.

We are switching from oxymorphone to oxycodone—can we do this in one jump, or do we need to switch from oxymorphone to morphine, then from morphine to oxycodone? Some practitioners feel that it should be a two-step process (the latter scenario), but whether you do it in one step or two, you end up with the same answer. This being the case, it seems much easier just to make the leap. *But, for all you Doubting Thomases out there, let's do it both ways, so we can put this to bed!*

Let's use method B and go from oxymorphone to morphine, then morphine to oxycodone.

$$\frac{\text{"X" mg TDD oral morphine}}{30 \text{ mg TDD oral oxymorphone}} = \frac{25 \text{ mg equianalgesic factor of oral morphine}}{10 \text{ mg equianalgesic factor of oral oxymorphone}}$$

Cross-multiply:

(X)(10) = (30)(25)

10X = 750

X = 75

This calculation shows a TDD of 75-mg oral morphine is approximately equivalent to a TDD of 30-mg oral oxymorphone.

OK, now let's take this morphine dose and convert to oxycodone.

$$\frac{\text{"X" mg TDD oral oxycodone}}{75 \text{ mg TDD oral morphine}} = \frac{20 \text{ mg equianalgesic factor of oral oxycodone}}{25 \text{ mg equianalgesic factor of oral morphine}}$$

Cross multiply:

(X)(25) = (20)(75)

25X = 1,500

X = 60

This calculation shows a TDD of 60-mg oral oxycodone is approximately equivalent to a TDD of 75-mg oral morphine.

<u>So, doing the two steps (via morphine) takes us from:</u>

Oral oxymorphone 30-mg TDD → oral morphine 75-mg TDD → oral oxycodone 60-mg TDD

Gee, I wonder how this would work if we just switched right from oral oxymorphone to oral oxycodone? I can't stand the suspense, how about you? Let's do it by golly!

$$\frac{\text{"X" mg TDD oral oxycodone}}{\text{30 mg TDD oral oxymorphone}} = \frac{\text{20 mg equianalgesic factor of oral oxycodone}}{\text{10 mg equianalgesic factor of oral oxymorphone}}$$

Cross-multiply:

(X)(10) = (20)(30)

10X = 600

X = 60

This calculation (going straight from oral oxymorphone to oral oxycodone) shows a TDD of 60-mg oral oxycodone is approximately equivalent to a TDD of 30-mg oral oxymorphone.

Whether you feel obligated to go to morphine first and then to your opioid of choice, or take the short cut and go directly to your opioid of choice, you get the same answer. Actually, doing it both ways is a good check of your math.

Just for laughs, let's do the direct conversion (oxymorphone to oxycodone) using method D.

As you recall, method D is as follows:

$$\text{TDD current opioid} \times \frac{\text{equianalgesic factor of new opioid}}{\text{equianalgesic factor of current opioid}} = \text{TDD new opioid}$$

Let's plug and chug:

$$\text{30 mg TDD oral oxymorphone} \times \frac{\text{20 mg equianalgesic factor of oral oxycodone}}{\text{10 mg equianalgesic factor of oral oxymorphone}}$$

$$= \text{30 mg TDD } \cancel{\text{oral oxymorphone}} \times \frac{\text{20 mg equianalgesic factor of oral oxycodone}}{\text{10 mg equianalgesic factor of } \cancel{\text{oral oxymorphone}}}$$

$$= 30 \times 20/10 = 30 \times 2 = \textbf{60-mg TDD oral oxycodone}$$

By gosh, I think we have a winner! Before we individualize the dose for this patient, we have conclusively shown that a TDD of 30-mg oral oxymorphone is approximately equivalent to a TDD of 60-mg oral oxycodone.

STEP 4—Because ZH has acceptable pain control on her current opioid regimen, and we know she will probably be more sensitive to the oxycodone due to incomplete cross-tolerance, it would be prudent to reduce our TDD of oral oxycodone. Using the one-third rule, this reduces the TDD oral oxycodone to 40 mg.

Extended-release (ER) oxycodone tablets are available as 10-, 15-, 20-, 30-, 40-, 60-, and 80-mg tablets. An appropriate order would be for 20 mg oxycodone ER by mouth every 12 hours. The surgeon could write the order for 20-mg tablets, or if he suspects the patient's pain will be improving fairly quickly, he may want to write for 10-mg tablets and instruct the patient to take two 10-mg tablets by mouth every 12 hours, then reduce the dose to one tablet (10 mg) by mouth every 12 hours at some point later. In addition, the surgeon should write a prescription for 5-mg oxycodone short-acting tablets, one tablet every 4 hours as needed for breakthrough pain. ZH can begin the oxycodone ER 12 hours after her last dose of oxymorphone ER.

STEP 5—It would be optimal for the surgeon to switch ZH to the new regimen while she is still in the rehabilitation hospital to observe her response. In any case, ZH should keep a pain diary, and self-monitor her therapeutic response and signs of toxicity. The nursing and physical therapy staff should assist in monitoring ZH's response to the oxycodone regimen if she is switched while still in the facility. If, for example, the patient finds that her pain has increased substantially after the switch, and she is requiring four to six doses of the short-acting oxycodone per day (e.g., 20 to 30 mg per day), it may be necessary to increase the oxycodone ER to 30 mg by mouth every 12 hours and continue monitoring the patient.

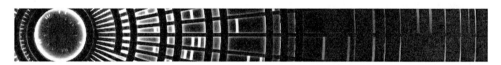

CASE 3.3
• •
Switching from Oral Morphine to Parenteral Hydromorphone

BL is a 74-year-old woman with a diagnosis of end-stage breast cancer, with diffuse bony metastasis, admitted to hospice several weeks ago. At the time of admission, the patient was clinically stable and receiving oral morphine ER 60 mg every 8 hours and oral naproxen 500 mg every 12 hours. Over the past 72 hours, the patient has deteriorated rapidly; she has difficulty swallowing her tablets, her pain is increasing significantly, and she has become quite weepy with all that's transpired. BL is very clear that she does not want to die at home, and the hospice team feels that her time is near; therefore, a decision is made to transfer her to the hospice's high-acuity inpatient facility.

STEP 1—The hospice nurse made an unscheduled visit, at which time the decision was made to transfer BL to the inpatient hospice unit. When the nurse asks BL about the pain, she moans while crying and says "it's just awful, please make it stop." The patient is unable to describe precipitating and palliating factors. She says the pain is constant and everywhere, and she describes it as throbbing, aching, and piercing. The patient is unable to rate the pain, but it is clear from observing her that it is severe.

STEP 2—The family states that BL was able to get down her last scheduled doses of morphine and naproxen, although with significant difficulty.

STEP 3—Upon arrival at the hospice facility, the attending advanced practice registered nurse (APRN) decides to switch BL to sub-Q injections of hydromorphone every 4 hours. *Let's help the APRN do this calculation.*

Assuming BL did not miss any doses of oral morphine, her TDD was 180 mg (60 mg every 8 hours).

Using method B, we can set up the following ratio:

$$\frac{\text{"X" mg TDD new opioid}}{\text{mg TDD current opioid}} = \frac{\text{equianalgesic factor of new opioid}}{\text{equianalgesic factor of current opioid}}$$

$$\frac{\text{"X" mg TDD sub–Q hydromorphone}}{\text{180 mg TDD oral morphine}} = \frac{\text{2 mg parenteral hydromorphone}}{\text{25 mg oral morphine}}$$

Cross-multiply:

(X)(25) = (2)(180)

25X = 360

X = 14.4

This method shows the TDD parenteral (sub-Q) hydromorphone is 14.4 mg.

STEP 4—We now need to decide whether to go with 14.4-mg sub-Q hydromorphone per day, to reduce it for incomplete cross-tolerance, or to increase the TDD. Because BL is in severe pain, it would be reasonable to go at least no lower than 14.4-mg TDD sub-Q hydromorphone. Hydromorphone is a relatively short-acting opioid, so it should be dosed at least every 4 hours (and perhaps even every 3 hours). If we give the TDD of 14.4 mg on an every 4 hour basis, this would be 2.4-mg sub-Q hydromorphone every 4 hours. Let's be bold and increase this to 2.5-mg sub-Q every 4 hours, and observe her response. The sub-Q hydromorphone can be started whenever clinically indicated; the last dose of ER oral morphine peaks about 3 to 4 hours after administration. If 3 to 4 hours have passed since BL took her last oral morphine ER tablet, and she is in pain, it would be appropriate to begin the sub-Q hydromorphone now. The patient may also require a further increase in hydromorphone if pain is not adequately controlled.

STEP 5—Parenterally administered hydromorphone peaks in about 30 minutes; therefore, BL should be closely monitored and given a repeat dose as clinically indicated. Alternately, BL could receive one or more IV or sub-Q injections of hydromorphone, and once made comfortable, switched to a continuous infusion of hydromorphone with a bolus option (discussed in Chapter 7).

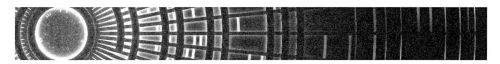

CASE 3.4

Switching from Oral Meperidine to Oral Oxycodone

CP is a 72-year-old obese woman with a long-standing history of osteoarthritis of the hips, knees, and lower lumbar vertebrae. She presents in the Medication Refill Clinic for routine follow-up and a new prescription for oral meperidine (Demerol) 100 mg, which she takes four times daily. You are a recent hire at this hospital, and you are taken aback to see this prescription. Meperidine is not recommended because it is short acting, and with repeat dosing, the metabolite normeperidine accumulates and can cause CNS excitation and possibly seizures. Meperidine should be especially avoided in patients with impaired renal function (because normeperidine is eliminated from the body by the kidneys), and you are keenly aware of the fact that renal function deteriorates as we age.

STEP 1—CP describes her pain as widely spread in the lumbar area, made worse with standing more than 5 minutes (e.g., doing the dishes) and with activities that require bending (e.g., vacuuming, laundry). She tells you the pain is dull and aching, and she rates it as a 7 or an 8 on average (on a 0–10 scale; 0 = no pain, 10 = worst imaginable pain) with no medication, and 4 or 5 with the meperidine. The pain does not affect her sleep (although she has more pain in the morning) or appetite, and although she is not happy about her pain status, she finds it bearable. CP has a past medical history of type 2 diabetes mellitus, hypertension, and peptic ulcer disease. She has tried maximum doses of acetaminophen without relief, and NSAID therapy is contraindicated due to a past history of duodenal ulcer. She has been taking meperidine for several years. Her most recent serum creatinine was 1.4 mg/dL.

STEP 2—CP does not take any extra doses of meperidine, nor does she miss any doses. She is very adherent to her regimen of 100-mg oral meperidine four times daily—with breakfast, lunch, dinner, and at bedtime.

STEP 3—Although CP has been fortunate not to have suffered adverse effects from meperidine, as time goes by, she is at high risk due to advancing age and reduced renal clearance (calculated creatinine clearance is approximately 36 mL/min; normal is 100 mL/min). Because morphine also has pharmacologically active metabolites that can cause toxicity, morphine is not a great choice for CP. A better choice would be oxycodone, hydromorphone, oxymorphone, methadone, or fentanyl. For educational purposes, let's choose oxycodone.

If you look at the Equianalgesic Opioid Dosing table (Table 1-1 and below), you will find meperidine listed. However, this does not imply that it is recommended patients be switched *to* meperidine—most contemporary pain management guidelines have eliminated meperidine from the list of recommended opioids due to its potential toxicity. Nevertheless, there are dose-equivalency studies with meperidine that can be used to develop an equianalgesic conversion *from* meperidine to another opioid. For purposes of saving CP from a potentially adverse outcome, let's look at the estimated equivalency data with meperidine:

Drug	Equianalgesic Doses (mg)	
	Parenteral	Oral
Morphine	10	25
Hydrocodone	NA	25
Hydromorphone	2	5
Oxycodone	10*	20
Oxymorphone	1	10
Meperidine	100	300

*Not available in the United States.

Let's use method C to switch the patient to oxycodone:

$$\frac{\text{"X" mg TDD new opioid}}{\text{equianalgesic factor of new opioid}} = \frac{\text{mg TDD current opioid}}{\text{equianalgesic factor of current opioid}}$$

$$\frac{\text{"X" mg TDD oral oxycodone}}{\text{20 mg oral oxycodone}} = \frac{\text{400 mg TDD oral meperidine}}{\text{300 mg oral meperidine}}$$

Cross-multiply:

(X)(300) = (400)(20)

300X = 8,000

X = 26.7 mg

This method shows an equivalent TDD of oral oxycodone would be 26.7 mg.

STEP 4—Because the patient was content with her current level of pain control, it would be prudent to reduce the TDD of oral oxycodone. Extended-release oxycodone tablets are available as 10 mg, so it would be reasonable to switch her to 10 mg by mouth every 12 hours (TDD 20-mg oral oxycodone). You could also prescribe short-acting oxycodone 5-mg tablets for breakthrough pain if desired. This regimen may be started 3 to 4 hours or greater after the last meperidine dose. Alternately, you could start with oxycodone 5 mg by mouth every 4 hours as needed, and after 48 hours, you'll have a better idea of the patient's 24-hour oxycodone requirement. At that point, you could switch to long-acting oxycodone.

STEP 5—CP should keep a pain diary, recording her pain ratings, use of short-acting oxycodone tablets (if prescribed), signs or symptoms of toxicity, and ability to perform activities of daily living.

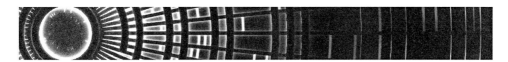

CASE 3.5

Switching from IV Hydromorphone to Oral Morphine or Oral Oxycodone

PR is a 58-year-old man with end-stage chronic obstructive pulmonary disease (COPD), receiving hospice care. He was admitted directly to the hospice inpatient unit with a complaint of uncontrolled pain. Over half of patients with advanced COPD experience pain, usually of musculoskeletal or pleuropulmonary origin.[3] PR is started on an IV infusion of hydromorphone at 0.2 mg/hr, which was titrated up over 4 days to 0.5 mg/hr with a bolus of 0.2 mg every 15 minutes as needed. PR is using the bolus about 4 times in a 24-hour period. It is time to discharge PR to home with hospice care, and you would like to switch him to either oral morphine or oral oxycodone to maintain this level of comfort. *What dosage regimen do you select?*

STEP 1—PR describes his pain as deep in his chest and extremely achy. He says all his ribs "feel tired," and it's exhausting and painful to draw breath. Physical assessment and imaging shows he does not have any broken ribs due to coughing, and pleural inflammation from infection has been ruled out as well. His average pain rating has declined from an average of 8 or 9 (on a 0–10 scale; 0 = no pain; 10 = worst imaginable pain) to a 3 on the current regimen. He is anxious to go home to his family and dogs.

STEP 2—PR is receiving IV hydromorphone 0.5 mg/hr every 24 hours, which totals 12 mg/day, plus four doses on average of the 0.2-mg bolus (0.8 mg), for a TDD of 12.8-mg IV hydromorphone.

STEP 3—*Decisions, decisions—should we convert to oral morphine or oral oxycodone? Why choose?—Let's do both!* Before we do, let's refresh our memory of where the equianalgesic ratios come from regarding IV hydromorphone.

Can We Be Steadies?

*Let's stop and consider evidence from crossover, **steady-state** trials of opioid conversions. These data are more robust than data based on single-dose crossover trials using an experimental pain model or based on bioavailability.*

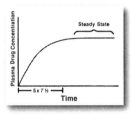

Reddy and colleagues evaluated the conversion ratio from IV hydromorphone to oral hydromorphone (see Chapter 2), oral morphine and oxycodone.[4]

Their results were as follows:

▸ The median conversion ratio from IV hydromorphone to oral hydromorphone was 2.5 (1-mg IV hydromorphone converted to 2.5-mg oral hydromorphone) in patients receiving <30-mg IV hydromorphone/day.

▸ The median conversion ratio from IV hydromorphone to oral hydromorphone was 2.1 (1-mg IV hydromorphone converted to 2.1-mg oral hydromorphone) in patients receiving ≥30-mg IV hydromorphone/day.

▸ The median conversion ratio from IV hydromorphone to oral morphine was 11.54 (1-mg IV hydromorphone converted to 11.54-mg oral morphine) in patients receiving <30-mg IV hydromorphone/day.

▸ The median conversion from IV hydromorphone to oral morphine was 9.86 (1-mg IV hydromorphone converted to 9.86-mg oral morphine) in patients receiving ≥30-mg IV hydromorphone/day.

▸ The median conversion from IV hydromorphone to oral oxycodone was 8.06 (1-mg IV hydromorphone converted to 8.06-mg oral oxycodone).

BOTTOM LINE RECOMMENDATION: From IV hydromorphone to oral hydromorphone

▸ 1:2.5 (IV hydromorphone → oral hydromorphone)

BOTTOM LINE RECOMMENDATION: From IV hydromorphone to oral morphine

▸ 1:10 (IV hydromorphone → oral morphine)

BOTTOM LINE: From IV hydromorphone to oral oxycodone

▸ 1:8 (IV hydromorphone → oral oxycodone)

Ok, back to business. Let's start with converting to oral morphine. Use method B to figure this out, as follows:

$$\frac{\text{"X" mg TDD new opioid (oral morphine)}}{\text{mg TDD current opioid (IV hydromorphone)}}$$

$$= \frac{\text{equianalgesic fact of new opioid (oral morphine)}}{\text{equianalgesic factor of current opioid (IV hydromorphone)}}$$

$$\frac{\text{"X" mg TDD new opioid (oral morphine)}}{\text{12.8 mg TDD IV hydromorphone}} = \frac{\text{25 mg oral morphine}}{\text{2 mg IV hydromorphone}}$$

Cross-multiply:

$(X)(2) = (25)(12.8)$

$2X = 320$

$X = 160$

The calculated TDD of oral morphine is 160.

Ok, so let's try converting to oral oxycodone instead. Our equation sets up as follows:

$$\frac{\text{"X" mg TDD new opioid (oral oxycodone)}}{\text{12.8 mg TDD IV hydromorphone}} = \frac{\text{20 mg oral oxycodone}}{\text{2 mg IV hydromorphone}}$$

Cross-multiply:

$(X)(2) = (20)(12.8)$

$2X = 256$

$X = 128$

The calculated TDD of oral oxycodone is 128. Just as a mental check—*does this LOOK right?* Remember that 20-mg oral oxycodone ≈ 25-mg oral morphine. So, does 128 mg (oral oxycodone) approximately equal 160-mg oral morphine? *Good golly Miss Molly, it does! We're cooking with gas now!*

STEP 4—*What to do with those calculated numbers?* PR's pain is well controlled on this regimen, and we are switching from one opioid to another (whether we end up with the oral morphine or the oral oxycodone), so dose reduction is what is wanted. In general, we reduce by 25% to 50% when switching from one opioid to a different opioid, particularly when the patient is not experiencing increased pain. However, the equianalgesic calculations are based on steady-state data.

If we reduce the total daily dose by 25%, it would be as follows:

- Oral morphine TDD of 160, reduce by 25% → 120-mg oral morphine TDD

- Oral oxycodone TDD of 128, reduce by 25% → 96-mg oral oxycodone TDD

Let's compare all this—PR was receiving 12.8-mg IV hydromorphone per day. Our columns include the calculated dose using the ratios provided in the Equianalgesic Opioid Dosing table, a 25% reduction for lack of complete cross-tolerance in the next column, and the dose using the conversion ratio from the Reddy recommendations.[4]

Switching from 12.8-mg IV Hydromorphone to:	Using Equianalgesic Dosing Table	Reduce Calculated Dose by 25%	Reddy Recommendation
Converting to oral morphine	Calculated 160-mg TDD	Reduced to 120-mg TDD	Using 1:10 ratio (IV hydromorphone to oral morphine) = 128-mg TDD
Converting to oral oxycodone	Calculated 128-mg TDD	Reduced to 96-mg TDD	Using a 1:8 ratio (IV hydromorphone to oral oxycodone) = 102-mg TDD

IV = intravenous; TDD = total daily dose.

Don't you love it when things work out?! Based on this approach, it would be reasonable to switch to oral morphine 120 mg a day (either as long-acting with short-acting morphine for breakthrough pain) or oral oxycodone 90 mg a day (long-acting or short-acting).

STEP 5—The hospice nursing staff will monitor PR's response to either regimen carefully, and adjust the dose as clinically appropriate.

TRAMADOL AND TAPENTADOL

Tramadol and tapentadol are classified as having *opioidergic* and *monoaminergic* mechanisms of action. They both act as mu-opioid receptor agonists and inhibit norepinephrine reuptake; tramadol also inhibits the reuptake of serotonin. Some would argue that tramadol and tapentadol shouldn't even be included in an equianalgesic opioid dosing table.[5]

Reasons include the following:

- The dual mechanisms of action (and a lack of clarity on the degree of analgesia provided by mu-opioid agonism versus other mechanisms of action)
- Polymorphism
- Partial agonism at the mu-receptor
- A changing dose response depending on the nature of the pain (neuropathic versus nociceptive)

The prescribing information for tapentadol does not provide any guidance for switching from IR tapentadol to ER tapentadol; the prescribing information for Nucynta ER states "There are no established conversion ratios for conversion from other opioids to Nucynta ER defined by clinical trials. Initiate dosing using Nucynta ER 50 mg orally every 12 hours."[6,7] *Are we going to take that lying down? Well, how about in a semi-recline position?*

Mercadante and colleagues investigated switching to and from tapentadol ER and other opioids in cancer patients.[8] Patients with cancer who presented to an acute inpatient palliative care unit and home care unit on an opioid, and were exhibiting an adverse effect, poor analgesic response, poor pain response, or those who chose to switch for convenience in dosing were included. The initial conversion ratio was based on a 1:3.3 (morphine:tapentadol) ratio in both directions. Results showed the conversion ratio when switching from tapentadol to morphine was 3.9:1 (tapentadol:morphine) (standard deviation [SD] 2.3). When switching from morphine to tapentadol, the conversion ratio was 1:4.5 (morphine:tapentadol) (SD 3.2). The authors considered their initial conversion ratio of 1:3.3 (morphine:tapentadol) to be a reasonable conversion strategy. Our Equianalgesic Opioid Dosing table shows 25 mg oral morphine ~ 100 mg oral tapentadol. *Let's take this conversion out for a spin, shall we?*

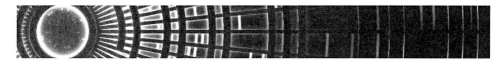

CASE 3.6
• •

Switching from Oral Morphine to Oral Tapentadol

JCM is a 72-year-old man with pain from spinal stenosis. He is taking gabapentin and Percocet (5-mg oxycodone/325-mg acetaminophen), one or two tablets four times a day. He is taking, on average, about six tablets per day. Unfortunately, this is not controlling his pain well; you think using a dual mechanism analgesic such as tapentadol may be beneficial. *Let's run this up the flagpole.*

STEP 1—The patient is experiencing a fair amount of neuropathic pain, rating his pain as an average of 6 or 7, best of 5, worst of 10 (on a 0–10 scale; 0 = no pain, 10 = worst imaginable pain). The pain keeps him from sleeping well; he just can't get comfortable.

STEP 2—His TDD of oral oxycodone is 30 mg.

STEP 3—Our first step is to switch the oral oxycodone TDD to oral morphine (this is how you calculate oral morphine equivalents). You've done enough of these calculations, so you know 30-mg oral oxycodone ≈ 37.5-mg oral morphine (using the 25:20 oral morphine:oral oxycodone ratio). Using our 1:3.3 (morphine:tapentadol) conversion ratio, 37.5-mg oral morphine would be about 124-mg oral tapentadol per day.

Using the data from our Equianalgesic Opioid Dosing table, when we convert from oral oxycodone to oral tapentadol (20:100), 30-mg oral oxycodone per day would be equivalent to 150-mg oral tapentadol. Because we are switching opioids, we would reduce by 25-50%, giving us somewhere between 75 and 112.5-mg tapentadol per day.

STEP 4—If we want to use Nucynta ER, we have several tablet strengths to choose from—50, 100, 150, 200, and 250 mg. Our only choice is to go with Nucynta ER 50 mg po every 12 hours, which is coincidentally what the prescribing information recommends. We could also use tapentadol IR 50 mg for breakthrough pain, or keep the Percocet he was receiving initially.

STEP 5—We will monitor JCM's response to Nucynta ER and his use of breakthrough analgesics. Nucynta ER prescribing information recommends increases of 50 mg no more than twice daily every 3 days.[7]

BUPRENORPHINE

Buprenorphine is a mu-opioid partial agonist administered via the parenteral route for moderate-to-severe acute pain and the oral route to treat opioid addiction. It is now available in the United States in two additional formulations for pain—transdermal buprenorphine (Butrans) and a buccal film formulation (Belbuca).[9,10] Both are indicated for the management of pain severe enough to require daily, around-the-clock, long-term opioid treatment and for which alternative treatment options are inadequate.

Davis provides an overview of why clinicians should consider buprenorphine as a frontline analgesic in management pain, including the following:

- Effectiveness in treating a variety of pain syndromes
- Less adverse effects (constipation, cognitive impairment, respiratory depression, immunosuppression, hypogonadism)
- A better safety profile in vulnerable populations (the elderly, those in renal failure and on dialysis)
- Fewer withdrawal symptoms[11]

Transdermal buprenorphine has been shown to be effective in treating a wide variety of moderately to severely painful conditions including chronic cancer and noncancer pain, ischemic pain, osteoarthritis pain, and neuropathic pain.[12] Butrans is meant to be worn for 7 days, after which time a new transdermal patch should be applied to a different location (wait a minimum of 3 weeks before reapplying to the same site). Recommended application sites include the upper outer arm, upper chest, upper back, or the side of the chest (eight possible application sites). This opioid delivery system is available in five strengths: 5, 7.5, 10, 15, and 20 mcg/hr.

Butrans therapy may be initiated in opioid-naïve patients with the 5-mcg/hr system. Because it takes 3 days to achieve steady-state serum levels of buprenorphine with the transdermal system, the dosage should not be increased for at least 72 hours, although many practitioners will wait a full week. The decision to move to the next higher Butrans strength should be based on the patient's need for supplemental short-acting opioid use, pain severity, and functional status. The maximum dose of Butrans is 20 mcg/hr (in the United States); higher doses (e.g., 40 mcg/hr) have resulted in prolongation of the QTc interval.

So what guidance do we have for switching an opioid-tolerant patient from his or her current opioid to Butrans? The manufacturer's guideline is as follows:[9]

- Oral morphine equivalent <30 mg a day → Butrans 5 mcg/hr
- Oral morphine equivalent 30 to 80 mg a day → Butrans 10 mcg/hr

The prescribing information advises that there is a potential for buprenorphine to precipitate withdrawal in patients who are already on opioids. The manufacturer recommends tapering the patient's current around-the-clock opioid, for up to 7 days, to no more than the equivalent of 30 mg of oral morphine before switching to Butrans. It is unclear if the rationale is concern that buprenorphine theoretically has a greater affinity for mu-opioid receptors than other opioids such as morphine, or acknowledgment that the recommended conversion ratio is low. The prescribing information further recommends using caution when prescribing Butrans to opioid-tolerant patients receiving >80 mg/day of morphine or its equivalent. The concern is that Butrans 20 mcg/hr may not provide adequate analgesia for patients receiving >80 mg/day of oral morphine or an equivalent.

An equipotency ratio of oral morphine to transdermal buprenorphine of 75:1 has been proposed; however, in recent years some data have suggested the ratio may range from 70:1 to 100:1.[12-15] As a reminder, an *equipotency ratio* is defined as the ratio of the doses of two opioids required to achieve the same degree of analgesia.

As discussed above, the oral morphine:transdermal buprenorphine equipotent ratio that has been proposed is 75:1, explained by the following mathematical equation:

- mg buprenorphine/day × 75 = mg oral morphine/day

For example, consider the Butrans 10 mcg/hr patch:

$$\frac{(\text{buprenorphine 10 mcg})}{\text{hr}} \times \frac{(24 \text{ hr})}{\text{day}} \times \frac{(1 \text{ mg})}{1{,}000 \text{ mcg}} = 0.24 \text{ mg buprenorphine/day}$$

0.24 mg buprenorphine/day × 75 = 18 mg oral morphine/day

Sittl and colleagues calculated an equipotency ratio of oral morphine to transdermal buprenorphine by comparing *identical-cohort* groups of patients with cancer and noncancer pain, using a drug utilization database.[14] Using this methodology, they determined an oral morphine to transdermal buprenorphine ratio of 110:1 or 115:1. However, their methodology was to use retrospective data from identical-cohort groups, not a methodology where patients served as their own control.

Mercadante and colleagues evaluated the equianalgesic ratio between oral morphine and transdermal buprenorphine in cancer patients receiving oral morphine ranging from 120 to 240 mg a day at stable doses for at least 6 days.[13] Patients served as their own controls and were switched from oral morphine to transdermal buprenorphine using a 70:1 ratio. Pain levels were assessed on days 3 and 6 post-switch. This was a small study (four patients), but all patients maintained good control of their pain and other symptoms, and the only clinical difference in switching to transdermal buprenorphine was an improvement in constipation. Their conclusion was that the proposed conversion ratio from oral morphine to transdermal buprenorphine of 70:1 was appropriate.[13]

If we believe Mercadante and colleagues that the oral morphine:transdermal buprenorphine ratio is 70:1, or if we accept Sittl and colleagues' conclusion that the ratio is 100:1 (or more), clearly the conversions recommended by the manufacturer of Butrans are low.

Look at the following table:

Buprenorphine TD Dose (using 70:1 ratio)		Equipotent Oral Morphine Dose (mg)	Buprenorphine TD Dose (using 100:1 ratio)		Butrans Recommended Conversion (mcg/hr)
mcg/hr	mg/day		mcg/hr	mg/day	
17.9	0.43	30 mg	12.5	0.3	5
47.6	1.14	80 mg	33.3	0.8	10

TD = transdermal

For example, if a patient was receiving 30 mg/day of oral morphine, using the 70:1 ratio, it calculates to a hypothetical equivalent potency of 17.9 mcg/hr transdermal buprenorphine. Using the 100:1 ratio, it would be 12.5 mcg/hr transdermal buprenorphine. However, the manufacturer of Butrans, in this example, would recommend starting with the 5-mcg/hr transdermal system. Similarly, for total daily oral morphine doses up to 80 mg a day, the manufacturer of Butrans recommends starting with a 10-mcg/hr patch. However, the data that support a 70:1 ratio would suggest a 47.6 mcg/hr patch, and the 100:1 ratio would suggest a 33.3 mcg/hr patch.

The bottom line from all this is that we should follow the prescribing guidelines, but know that the recommended Butrans dosage conversion is very conservative, and an analgesic for breakthrough pain should also be prescribed simultaneously.

Mercadente also considered the conversion of patients receiving transdermal fentanyl 50 to 100 mcg/hr to transdermal buprenorphine, using a transdermal fentanyl:transdermal buprenorphine ratio of 0.6:0.8.[16] Their methods were as follows:

Number of Patients	Current Therapy for at least 6 Days and Receiving No More than 2 Doses of Oral Morphine per Day for Breakthrough	Switched to for 3 Days	After 3 Days Switched Back to
16	TDF 25 mcg/hr	TDB 35 mcg/hr	TDF 25 mcg/hr
16	TDF 50 mcg/hr	TDB 50 mcg/hr	TDF 50 mcg/hr
6	TDB 35 mcg/hr	TDF 25 mcg/hr	TDB 35 mcg/hr
6	TDB 70 mcg/hr	TDF 50 mcg/hr	TDB 70 mcg/hr

TDF = transdermal fentanyl; TDB = transdermal buprenorphine.

Pain and other symptoms were evaluated at days 3 and 6, and no significant changes were noted (except improvement in reported constipation with transdermal buprenorphine). These findings are again considerably more aggressive than those from the manufacturer of Butrans.

The only other issue to consider is that of QTc prolongation associated with use of Butrans in excess of 20 mcg/hr. The risk associated with QTc prolongation is the development of torsades de pointes, a potentially fatal ventricular arrhythmia. According to the prescribing information, a Butrans dose of 40 mcg/hr (given as two 20-mcg/hr Butrans transdermal systems) prolonged the mean QTc by up to 9.2 ms across 13 assessment time points. For this reason, in the United States, Butrans is only approved for dosages up to 20 mcg/hr. However, higher concentration buprenorphine patches have been available in Europe for almost 10 years (Transtec 35 mcg/hr, Transtec 52.5 mcg/hr, and Transtec 70 mcg/hr).[17] According to the FDA, the threshold level for regulatory concern is "around 5 ms as evidenced by an upper bound of the 95% confidence interval around the mean effect on QTc of 10 ms."[18] Prescribers should be mindful of the other risk factors for the development of torsades or prolongation of the QTc when using Butrans in their patients.

BELBUCA is a newer formulation of buprenorphine, also indicated for opioid-requiring severe pain. It is a long-acting opioid that is formulated as a buccal film intended to be applied to the inner aspect of the cheek (buccal area) once, or if tolerated, twice daily.[19] The buccal film is available in strengths of 75, 150, 300, 450, 600, 750, and 900 mcg. The dose for opioid-naïve or opioid-nontolerant patients is a 75-mcg film once daily, or if tolerated, every 12 hours for at least 4 days, then increase dose to 150 mcg every 12 hours.[10]

When converting from other opioids, the manufacturer recommends discontinuing all other around-the-clock opioids when starting therapy with BELBUCA. Due to the risk of buprenorphine-induced withdrawal, the recommendations are to taper patients to no more than 30-mg oral morphine sulfate equivalents (MSE) per day before starting BELBUCA.

After tapering down to this level, the manufacturer recommends the following:[10]

Prior Daily Dose of Opioid Analgesic Before Taper to 30-mg Oral MSE	Initial BELBUCA Dose
Less than 30 mg	BELBUCA 75 mcg once daily or every 12 hours
30-mg to 89-mg oral MSE	BELBUCA 150 mcg every 12 hours
90-mg to 160-mg oral MSE	Belbuca 300 mcg every 12 hours
Greater than 160-mg oral MSE	Consider alternate analgesic

MSE = morphine sulfate equivalents.

The minimum titration interval of BELBUCA is 4 days, and the maximum daily dose of 900 mcg every 12 hours is due to the risk of QTc interval prolongation.[10]

Webster and colleagues investigated the feasibility of switching opioid-dependent patients with chronic pain directly to buccal buprenorphine without a taper (clearly they are rebels!).[20] Chronic pain patients receiving between 80- and 160-mg oral MSEs were switched to 300-mcg buccal buprenorphine (which represents a 50% reduction of the patient's original oral MSE dose, based on a conversion ratio of 100:1 for oral morphine to buprenorphine). Three of 35 patients experienced symptoms of opioid withdrawal of at least moderate intensity. Their conclusion was that patients receiving full mu-agonist therapy can be switched to buccal buprenorphine at 50% of the equivalent full mu-agonist dose without significantly increased risk of opioid withdrawal or loss of pain control.[20] Despite these findings, it is probably wise to follow the manufacturers' recommendation and titrate full mu-agonist therapy down to 30-mg oral MSE prior to beginning BELBUCA therapy.

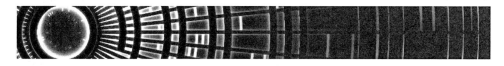

CASE 3.7

Switching from Oral Oxycodone to Transdermal Buprenorphine

BW is a 62-year-old woman with a history of severe osteoarthritis of both knees, for which she receives OxyContin 20 mg by mouth every 12 hours, and she has oxycodone 5 mg for breakthrough pain (which she uses at least once a day, rarely twice a day). She tells her prescriber that she hates taking medication all day long, saying, "it makes me feel like a druggie." The prescriber decides to switch her to transdermal buprenorphine, so the patient only has to re-dose every 7 days. *How would you recommend we make this transition?*

STEP 1—BW's pain is in both knees; her prescriber states that she has "bone-on-bone" disease, and due to her obesity, she is not a surgical candidate. BW states that her current opioid regimen controls her pain fairly well; she just doesn't like taking pain pills.

STEP 2—BW's total daily dose of oxycodone is 45 to 50 mg. This is approximately equivalent to 56- to 62-mg oral morphine per day (based on our 25:20 oral morphine:oral oxycodone equivalency).

STEP 3—Per the Butrans prescribing information, because the patient is receiving between 30- and 80-mg oral morphine equivalents per day, she will have to be tapered down to no more than 30-mg oral morphine per day prior to beginning Butrans. We will instruct the patient to reduce her OxyContin to 10 mg po every 12 hours for 5 to 7 days. She can supplement the OxyContin with a nonopioid analgesic such as acetaminophen or a nonsteroidal anti-inflammatory agent (if appropriate). After that time, we will instruct BW to discontinue OxyContin, begin Butrans 10 mcg/hr, and supplement with oxycodone 5 mg as needed every 4 hours for additional pain.

STEP 4—After 72 hours, if necessary, we can increase the Butrans to 15 mcg/hr.

STEP 5—We will monitor BW's pain ratings and her functional status to guide further dose adjustment or potential toxicity.

PRACTICE PROBLEMS

P3.1: Switching from Oral Acetaminophen/Hydrocodone to Oral Extended-Release Morphine

RD is a 48-year-old man who has residual pain from a motor vehicle accident. His pain is moderately controlled on Vicodin (10-mg hydrocodone and 300-mg acetaminophen), one tablet every 4 hours (he usually skips the middle-of-the-night dose). He also receives desipramine 50 mg by mouth at bedtime and gabapentin (Neurontin) 900 mg by mouth every 8 hours. RD rates his pain as 4 to 5 (on a 0–10 scale; 0 = no pain, 10 = worst imaginable pain) on average. RD is complaining about the need to take Vicodin every 4 hours, and that when he wakes up each morning, he is in pain. His pharmacy insurance plan covers generic ER morphine, and you are asked to recommend an appropriate dose.

P3.2: Switching from IV Hydromorphone to Oral Oxycodone

FA is a 62-year-old man with colon cancer who underwent tumor debulking 3 days ago. Over the past 24 hours, he has received 3 mg of IV hydromorphone. He has good pain control, and the attending physician would like to send him home on an equivalent regimen of long- and short-acting oxycodone. The physician anticipates FA will be able to taper down this dose significantly over the next few days.

P3.3: Switching from Oral Morphine to Oral Oxymorphone

SJ is an 84-year-old woman with general debility, significant renal impairment, and generalized aches and pains. She has been receiving ER morphine 30 mg by mouth every 12 hours for the past several months with good success. Over the past couple of weeks, she has developed delirium, with both visual and auditory hallucinations. Other reversible causes have been ruled out, and the prescriber is concerned that the active metabolites of morphine are accumulating given SJ's renal function, and causing or contributing to the delirium. The prescriber asks that you calculate an equivalent regimen using oxymorphone (generic long- and short-acting). *Just for fun, use all four methods to calculate the oxymorphone regimen. That should keep you out of trouble for a while!*

P3.4: Switching from Oral Acetaminophen/Codeine to Oral Morphine

KK is a 72-year-old opioid-naïve woman receiving rehabilitation services for a total hip replacement several weeks ago. KK had a stroke several years ago, and she has residual swallowing difficulties. She has an order for Tylenol with Codeine oral solution, 2 tablespoons every 4 hours as needed for pain (12-mg codeine phosphate and 120-mg acetaminophen per 5 mL). She has asked for the Tylenol with Codeine on several occasions, and it relieved the pain sufficiently, but she got so nauseated that she couldn't participate in therapy. You decide to switch her to oral morphine solution. *What would be the appropriate dose to give an equivalent therapy effect?*

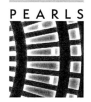

P E A R L S   What Do You Mean You're "Allergic" to It?

It is not uncommon for patients to say they are "allergic" to an opioid, when in fact they are referring to an adverse effect. Codeine is a perfect example—it seems that everyone and their mother can experience nausea from codeine, which can be quite severe (think Linda Blair, The Exorcist, pea soup). A patient may be given too high a dose of an opioid such as morphine and experience delirium. When a patient says he or she is "allergic" to any medication, it is important to ask what happened when the patient took the medication, and how the event was handled by the healthcare team (discontinue medication versus administer epinephrine). However, be careful if the patient really DOES have an allergic reaction to codeine. The patient could easily be cross allergic to any phenanthrene opioid, especially morphine, a metabolite of codeine. Make sure you adequately document your findings to increase patient safety and to inform better decisions for the next practitioner!

Could I Get That to Go, Please? Bottom Line It for Me . . .

▸ In this chapter, we discussed how to switch from one opioid to a different opioid, regardless of route of administration of dosage formulation.

▸ Clinicians should always use best evidence Equianalgesic Opioid Dosing data, but should reduce calculated doses to be safe. Always provide effective rescue analgesics during periods of conversion.

▸ Use conversion ratios derived from steady-state studies when available, such as the Reddy study that shows 1-mg IV hydromorphone ≈ 2.5-mg oral hydromorphone ≈ 10-mg oral morphine ≈ 8-mg oral oxycodone.[4]

▸ Tramadol and tapentadol have opioidergic and monoaminergic mechanisms of action and warrant conservative conversions.

▸ Buprenorphine is available as a transdermal delivery system and buccal film for severe chronic pain. Opioid-tolerant patients should be titrated down to 30-mg oral morphine equivalent per day (or less) prior to switching to Butrans or BELBUCA.

REFERENCES

1. FDA requests removal of Opana ER for risks related to abuse [news release]. Silver Spring, MD: US Food and Drug Administration; June 8, 2017. https://www.fda.gov/newsevents/newsroom/pressannouncements/ucm562401.htm. Accessed February 16, 2018.

2. Cleary J, Brennan M, Fudin J. Opioid rotation from Opana ER following FDA call for removal. *Pract Pain Manage.* 2017;July/August:50-57.

3. Spathis A, Booth S. End of life care in chronic obstructive pulmonary disease: In search of a good death. *Int J Chron Obstruct Pulmon Dis.* 2008;3(1):11-29.

4. Reddy A, Vidal M, Stephen S, et al. The conversion ratio from intravenous hydromorphone to oral opioids in cancer patients. *J Pain Symptom Manage.* 2017;54:280-288.

5. Fudin J, Raouf M, Wegrzyn E. Opioid Dosing Policy: Pharmacological considerations regarding equianalgesic dosing. A white paper from the Academy of Integrative Pain Medicine; September 2017. http://c.ymcdn.com/sites/www.integrativepainmanagement.org/resource/resmgr/docs/MEDD_White_Paper.pdf. Accessed February 16, 2018.

6. Nucynta Prescribing Information. https://www.nucynta.com/sites/default/files/pdf/nucynta-pi_0.pdf. Accessed February 16, 2018.

7. Nucynta ER Prescribing Information. https://www.nucynta.com/sites/default/files/pdf/nucyntaer-pi_0.pdf. Accessed February 16, 2018.

8. Mercadante S, Porzio G, Aielli F, et al. Opioid switching from and to tapentadol extended release in cancer patients: conversion ratio with other opioids. *Curr Med Res Opin.* 2013;29(6):661-666.

9. Butrans Prescribing Information. http://app.purduepharma.com/xmlpublishing/pi.aspx?id=b. Accessed February 16, 2018.

10. BELBUCA Prescribing Information. https://s3.amazonaws.com/belbuca/website/pdfs/belbuca-prescribing-info.pdf. Accessed February 16, 2018.

11. Davis MP. Twelve reasons for considering buprenorphine as a frontline analgesic in the management of pain. *J Support Oncol.* 2012;10(6):209-219.

12. Hans G, Robert D. Transdermal buprenorphine—a critical appraisal of its role in pain management. *J Pain Res.* 2009;2:117-134.

13. Mercadante S, Casuccio A, Tirelli W, Giarratano A. Equipotent doses to switch from high doses of opioids to transdermal buprenorphine. *Support Care Cancer.* 2009;17:715-718.

14. Sittl R, Likar R, Nautrup BP. Equipotent doses of transdermal fentanyl and transdermal buprenorphine in patients with cancer and noncancer pain: results of a retrospective cohort study. *Clin Ther.* 2005;27:225-237.

15. Skaer TL. Dosing considerations with transdermal formulations of fentanyl and buprenorphine for the treatment of cancer pain. *J Pain Res.* 2014;7:495-503.

16. Mercadante S, Porzio G, Fulfaro F, et al. Switching from transdermal drugs: an observational "N of 1" study of fentanyl and buprenorphine. *J Pain Symptom Manage.* 2007;34(5):532-538.

17. EMC. Transtec 35, 52.5 and 70 micrograms transdermal patch. https://www.medicines.org.uk/emc/medicine/8864. Accessed February 16, 2018.

18. US Department of Health and Human Services, Food and Drug Administration, Center for Drug Evaluation and Research (CDER), Center for Biologics Evaluation and Research (CBER), October 2005. Guidance for Industry: E14 Clinical Evaluation of QT/QTc Interval Prolongation and Proarrhythmic Potential for Non-Antiarrhythmic Drugs. https://www.fda.gov/downloads/Drugs/GuidanceCompliance RegulatoryInformation/Guidances/UCM073153.pdf. Accessed February 16, 2018.

19. BELBUCA Application. https://www.belbuca.com/hcp/belbuca-application-instructions/. Accessed February 16, 2018.

20. Webster L, Gruener D, Kirby T, et al. Evaluation of the tolerability of switching patients on chronic full μ-opioid agonist therapy to buccal buprenorphine. *Pain Med.* 2016;17:899-907.

SOLUTIONS TO PRACTICE PROBLEMS

P3.1

STEP 1—Per the patient, his pain is fairly well controlled, but could stand to be improved a bit. He would like to switch due to the inconvenience of Vicodin dosing, and the fact that the Vicodin doesn't last all night, causing him to awaken with pain.

STEP 2—Patient is taking 5 Vicodin tablets per 24-hour period, in addition to desipramine and gabapentin. This is a total of 50-mg oral hydrocodone.

STEP 3—RD would benefit from an ER opioid. His pharmacy insurance plan covers long-acting oral morphine. RD's TDD of hydrocodone is 50 mg (5 doses × 10 mg per tablet).

Using method D, we can determine the equivalent dose of morphine:

$$50 \text{ mg TDD oral hydrocodone} \times \frac{25 \text{ mg oral morphine}}{25 \text{ mg oral hydrocodone}}$$

$$50 \text{ mg TDD oral } \cancel{\text{hydrocodone}} \times \frac{25 \text{ mg oral morphine}}{25 \text{ mg oral } \cancel{\text{hydrocodone}}}$$

Completing the mathematics, we see the TDD oral morphine is also 50 mg. This is kind of a no-brainer since oral morphine and oral hydrocodone are equivalent on a mg:mg basis (25-mg oral morphine ≈ 25-mg oral hydrocodone). Unsurprisingly, 50-mg TDD oral hydrocodone ≈ 50-mg TDD oral morphine.

Remember, though, this "equivalency" is *not* based on solid evidence. We could be over- or underestimating the equivalent amount of morphine.

The ER morphine can be started 4 or more hours after the last Vicodin tablet is taken.

STEP 4—Given the 50-mg TDD oral morphine, we could use this number, increase, or decrease for lack of cross-tolerance. RD is not pleased with his level of pain control, so even though we are switching from one opioid to a different opioid, we probably only want a slight decrease in the calculated dose. We could consider Kadian 40 mg by mouth every 24 hours or MS Contin 15 mg by mouth every 8 hours.

STEP 5—The patient needs to be counseled to avoid driving or operating machinery until he knows how he will react to the new opioid regimen. He should maintain a pain diary and self-monitor his therapeutic and toxic response to the new regimen.

P3.2

STEP 1—Per the physician, the patient's pain is well controlled.

STEP 2—Patient's TDD IV hydromorphone is 3 mg.

STEP 3—The physician has already asked that you calculate an equivalent dose of long- and short-acting oral oxycodone.

Using method B, we can set up the following ratio:

$$\frac{\text{"X" mg TDD oral oxycodone}}{3 \text{ mg IV hydromorphone}} = \frac{20 \text{ mg oral oxycodone}}{2 \text{ mg parenteral hydromorphone}}$$

Cross multiply:

$(X)(2) = (20)(3)$

$2X = 60$

$X = 30$

This method shows that the TDD oral oxycodone would be 30 mg.

Remember the steady-state data from the Reddy trial in cancer patients?[4] In their trial, they found that a conversion ratio from IV hydromorphone to oral oxycodone was approximately 8. Because the patient's TDD of IV hydromorphone is 3 mg, this would be about 24-mg oral oxycodone per day.

STEP 4—Using the data from the Equianalgesic Opioid Dosing table, and calculating a TDD of oxycodone 30 mg, it would be prudent to reduce the TDD of oral oxycodone by 25% (for a new TDD of 22.5-mg per day), particularly because his pain was well controlled. The physician anticipates that the patient will be able to taper down the oxycodone dose significantly over the next few days, so we can be more conservative with the long-acting oral oxycodone, and more liberal with the short-acting. For example, it would be reasonable to recommend OxyContin 10 mg by mouth every 12 hours with oxycodone 5 mg by mouth every 4 hours as needed for additional pain. Alternatively, you could just go with oxycodone 5 mg every 4 hours as needed for pain. This is also consistent with the calculated dose based on the steady-state model described above.

STEP 5—The patient should maintain a pain diary, and the healthcare team should follow his therapeutic and toxic response to this regimen.

P3.3

STEP 1—SJ has had good pain control per her prescriber with her analgesic regimen.

STEP 2—SJ is receiving ER oral morphine 30 mg every 12 hours, for a TDD of 60-mg oral morphine.

STEP 3—The physician has asked that you calculate an equivalent dose of oxymorphone for SJ.

What does method A tell us (this is the eye-ball method)? Our Equianalgesic Opioid Dosing table shows that 25-mg oral morphine ≈ 10-mg oral oxymorphone. The 10-mg oxymorphone is a little less than half of the 25-mg morphine; therefore, an oxymorphone dose equivalent to 60 mg oral morphine should be a little less than 30 mg (50%). Let's press on.

Use methods B, C, and D to calculate your answer, and compare. Let's take a look:

Method B

$$\frac{\text{"X" mg TDD oral oxymorphone}}{60 \text{ mg TDD oral morphine}} = \frac{10 \text{ mg oral oxymorphone}}{25 \text{ mg oral morphine}}$$

Cross multiply:

$(X)(25) = (10)(60)$

$25X = 600$

$X = 24$

This method shows that the TDD oral oxymorphone would be 24 mg.

Method C

$$\frac{\text{"X" mg TDD oral oxymorphone}}{10 \text{ mg oral oxymorphone}} = \frac{60 \text{ mg TDD oral morphine}}{25 \text{ mg oral morphine}}$$

Cross-multiply:

$(X)(25) = (10)(60)$

$25X = 600$

$X = 24$

This method shows that the TDD oral oxymorphone would be 24 mg.

Method D

$$60 \text{ mg TDD oral morphine} \times \frac{10 \text{ mg oral oxymorphone}}{25 \text{ mg oral morphine}}$$

$$60 \text{ mg TDD oral } \cancel{\text{morphine}} \times \frac{10 \text{ mg oral oxymorphone}}{25 \text{ mg oral } \cancel{\text{morphine}}}$$

Multiplying through, we see 60 × 10/25 = 24.

This method shows that the TDD oral oxymorphone would be 24 mg.

As we can see, all three methods give us the same answer, a TDD of 24-mg oral oxymorphone. Outstanding; milk bones for everyone!

STEP 4—Now that everybody and their dog believes the TDD of oral oxymorphone should be 24 mg, we need to decide if we're going to go with this number, increase, or decrease. Because the patient had good pain control (and renal impairment), it's probably a good idea to reduce the dose. Generic ER oxymorphone comes in 5-, 7.5-, 10-, 15-, 20-, 30-, and 40-mg strengths, so we can recommend ER oxymorphone 7.5 mg po every 12 hours. We can also order IR oxymorphone, 5 mg by mouth as needed for breakthrough pain every 4 hours. If the patient consistently uses two or three doses per day of the short-acting oxymorphone, we can increase the ER to 15 mg by mouth every 12 hours.

STEP 5—Monitor the patient for subjective and objective signs of therapeutic effectiveness and toxicity. *Importantly, we should monitor the patient carefully for resolution of hallucinations.*

P3.4

STEP 1—Patient reports that the Tylenol with Codeine helped the pain, but she couldn't tolerate it (nausea).

STEP 2—KK only uses the analgesic as needed. She has tried the Tylenol with Codeine several times.

STEP 3—KK has not taken the Tylenol with Codeine consistently enough to calculate a TDD, but we can calculate an equivalent dose of a different opioid to be used "as needed" for pain. In this case, you have already decided to switch to morphine solution. *We need to calculate an equivalent dose.*

KK was prescribed 2 tablespoons (30 mL) of Tylenol with Codeine solution.

How much codeine is she getting with every dose?

$$\frac{12 \text{ mg codeine}}{5 \text{ mL}} \times 30 \text{ mL}$$

$$\frac{12 \text{ mg codeine}}{5 \text{ mL}} \times 30 \text{ mL} = 12 \text{ mg codeine} \times 6 = 72 \text{ mg codeine}$$

Now we need to calculate a dose of oral morphine that is equivalent to 72-mg codeine. Let's use method D.

$$\text{TDD } 72 \text{ mg oral codeine} \times \frac{25 \text{ mg oral morphine}}{200 \text{ mg oral codeine}}$$

$$\text{TDD } 72 \text{ mg oral codeine} \times \frac{25 \text{ mg oral morphine}}{200 \text{ mg oral codeine}}$$

$72 \times 25/200 = 9$

This method shows an equivalent dose of oral morphine is approximately 9 mg.

STEP 4—Now we need to individualize the dose for the patient. As explained in the case, KK was opioid-naïve (she had not received opioids for some period of time post-operatively, before beginning rehabilitation). For an older adult, morphine 9 mg is a high dose—this could have been part of the nausea problem with the Tylenol with Codeine. This fact, along with incomplete cross-tolerance would make a strong argument to recommend 5 mg of oral morphine as needed every 4 hours for pain, instead of 10 mg (rounding up from 9 mg).

STEP 5—The patient's pain level should be assessed prior to morphine administration and 1 hour later. Signs and symptoms of toxicity should also be monitored and documented, and the opioid regimen adjusted as indicated.

CHAPTER 4

Titrating Opioid Regimens: Around the Clock and to the Rescue!

INTRODUCTION

When crafting an opioid regimen for a patient with persistent pain, we generally have one opioid strategy for the baseline pain and a different opioid strategy for breakthrough pain. In most cases, the same opioid is used, although they may be different for various reasons. *In the face of increasing pain:*

- How does the astute healthcare practitioner know whether to increase the baseline opioid or the rescue opioid?

- How much and how quickly can we increase each opioid?

- How about the patient who needs to decrease his or her opioid dose due to the development of an adverse effect or implementation of an opioid-sparing intervention—how quickly can we decrease the dose and not cause opioid withdrawal symptoms?

OBJECTIVES

After reading this chapter and completing all practice problems, the participant will be able to:

1. Recommend and initiate opioid therapy for opioid-naïve patients with acute severe pain and transition to around-the-clock opioid dosing.

2. Describe different types of breakthrough pain and recommend and titrate an opioid regimen to treat these pains.

3. Determine an appropriate strategy to increase an opioid regimen, including both the regularly scheduled and rescue opioid for breakthrough pain.

4. Recommend a dosing strategy to wean or taper a patient from opioids when adverse effects occur or as other clinical situations dictate.

Even though this chapter is not specifically about *conversion* calculations, opioid titration is a critical calculation skill. We discussed the paradigm of safety and efficacy in Chapter 1—the same principles apply here. After reading this chapter, practitioners in the know will be able to calculate dosage increases (or decreases) that allow the patient to achieve pain relief as quickly as possible, while remembering "safety first!" Why does that sound like a Boy Scout doing drug math?

INITIATING OPIOID THERAPY

There are several excellent review articles and consensus guidelines that will be of assistance as we consider the calculations in this chapter.[1-6] In this section, we will discuss dose-finding strategies for patients moving from nonopioids, combination analgesics, or occasional opioid use to around-the-clock opioid therapy, as well as management of the opioid-naïve patients with acute, severe sudden-onset pain. Calculations specific to methadone, fentanyl, and continuous opioid infusions will be addressed in subsequent chapters.

Acute Severe Pain in the Opioid-Naïve Patient

Most patients transition to opioid therapy after nonopioid or co-analgesic therapy fails to adequately control pain. Occasionally, however, a patient who has not been taking opioids previously will experience acute-onset severe pain. Examples include patients who suffer a pathologic fracture or nerve compression.

The Cleveland Clinic guidelines for managing acute severe pain in opioid-naïve patients in a supervised inpatient setting (or very closely monitored outpatient setting) are as follows[1]:

- Morphine 1 mg intravenously (IV) every minute for 10 minutes, followed by a 5-minute respite, and repeated until pain is controlled. The healthcare practitioner (physician or licensed independent practitioner) should closely monitor (really closely, meaning park yourself by the bedside and don't leave!) sensorium and pain response. It is critically important to monitor level of arousal because sedation precedes respiratory depression. If the patient has not achieved pain relief after 30 mg of parenteral morphine has been administered, and/or the patient is sedated or respiratory rate is <10 breaths per minute, further investigation of the pain complaint should commence. Alternate opioids include fentanyl 20 micrograms (mcg) per minute or hydromorphone 0.2 mg per minute.

- If subcutaneous (sub-Q) dosing is preferred, morphine 2 mg every 5 minutes (or fentanyl 40 mcg or hydromorphone 0.4 mg) until pain is managed. Follow the monitoring and precautions discussed above.

- Using the oral route of administration, 5 mg of immediate-release (IR) morphine (or 1-mg hydromorphone or 5-mg oxycodone) is given every 30 minutes until pain recedes.

What Do You Mean "Until Pain Is Controlled?"

FAST FACTS 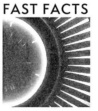 It is important to describe clearly what we mean by repeating doses of the opioid "until pain is controlled. *How do you know when the pain is "controlled?"* What you're looking for is an initial two to four point drop in the pain rating, not *complete* pain relief. Practitioners must recognize that using a strategy such as described above (morphine 1-mg IV every minute up to 10 doses) is *dose stacking* (because the peak effect of IV morphine is no sooner than 15 minutes). **If the practitioner continues to administer the opioid until complete pain relief is achieved, this may result in overadministration of the opioid when the entire drug administered achieves peak effect.**

Another guideline we can draw on comes from the National Comprehensive Cancer Network (NCCN) *Clinical Practice Guidelines in Oncology: Adult Cancer Pain.*[6] These guidelines state that opioid-naïve patients who experience moderate-to-severe pain should receive between 2 to 5 mg of IV morphine (or the equivalent with a different opioid) and reassess pain at 15 minutes. If the pain has increased or persists at 15 minutes, increase dose by 50% to 100% and reassess after 15 minutes. They advise considering an alternate strategy if the pain is not improved after two to three cycles (a *cycle* refers to administer opioid, then reassess pain in 15 minutes) as described. If the pain has decreased but is still inadequately controlled, repeat the same dose and continue monitoring patient response. If the pain is improved and adequately controlled, the guidelines recommend continuing at the current effective dose as needed over the initial 24 hours at an appropriate dosing interval and continue monitoring patient response.

The NCCN guidelines also provide guidance using oral opioids. For moderate-to-severe pain in an opioid-naïve patient, the guidelines recommend the following:

- Administer an initial dose of 5 to 15 mg of oral short-acting morphine or equivalent opioid.
- Reassess efficacy and adverse effects at 60 minutes.
- If pain is unchanged or increased, increase morphine dose by 50% to 100%.
- After two to three cycles, consider switching to IV opioid therapy for subsequent management.
- If after 60 minutes the pain has decreased but is still inadequately controlled, the guidelines recommend repeating the same oral dose and continue monitoring.[6]

It is critically important to recognize that the guidelines listed above pertain to patients in a *very closely monitored* environment, such as a hospital. In other words, an opioid antagonist such as naloxone (Narcan) is standing by if needed. These protocols would *not* be used for a home-based patient. For one thing, it would be unlikely that a home-based patient would have a parenteral opioid sitting around "just in case." However, patients admitted to hospice care may very well have a starter kit or emergency kit that contains a few doses of the most commonly used rescue medications, including an oral opioid. If this were the case, it would be appropriate for the prescriber to order the visiting nurse (*not* the patient or family of their own volition) to administer 5 mg of IR morphine (e.g., oral morphine solution) every 30 to 60 minutes up to a total of 20 or 30 mg for an acute pain crisis. This may, in fact, be a stopgap intervention pending inpatient admission to determine the cause of this sudden-onset severe pain. *Let's look at a case of an opioid-naïve patient who experiences sudden-onset acute pain.*

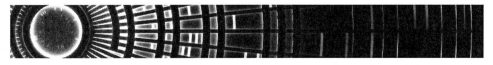

CASE 4.1
• •
Acute Pain Management in an Opioid-Naïve Patient

HY is a 72-year-old man diagnosed with colon cancer 8 years ago, subsequently diagnosed with prostate cancer 2 years ago, who is currently on hormone therapy for the prostate cancer. HY presents to the emergency department (ED) today complaining of sudden-onset severe pain of the right proximal femur. He describes the pain as agonizing and rates it as a 10 (on a 0–10 scale; 0 = no pain, 10 = worst imaginable pain). HY takes only naproxen 500 mg by mouth twice daily for pain; he has not taken an opioid since his prostate surgery 2 years ago. Before beginning diagnostic proceedings, it is imperative that HY's pain be treated. HY has no contraindications to opioid therapy (including any history of morphine allergy), and IV access is quickly established. The ED physician sits bedside and administers 1-mg IV morphine every minute for 10 minutes (total dose 10 mg). During this time, HY's respiratory rate decreases from 38 breaths per minute to 22 breaths per minute. He rates his pain as a 9 after the tenth injection. The ED physician waits 5 minutes, at which point the patient says his pain is now an 8; respiratory rate is 20 breaths per minute and patient is very much awake with a clear sensorium. The ED physician administers an additional milligram of IV morphine every minute for the next 5 minutes at which point, the patient reports the pain is less than 6 and tolerable. The respiratory rate is now 16 breaths per minute, and the patient has relaxed considerably. With 15 mg of morphine on board, the patient can tolerate an x-ray, which confirms a fractured right femur, and a chest x-ray shows a solid mass in the hilum of his right lung. HY's fractured right femur was thought to be due to primary pulmonary cancer and his fracture was surgically repaired.

Acute/Uncontrolled Moderate-to-Severe Pain in the Opioid-Tolerant Patient

The NCCN guidelines also provide direction for opioid-tolerant patients experiencing moderate-to-severe pain.[6]

- If administering the opioid by the IV route of administration, the recommendation is to administer the IV (or sub-Q) opioid dose equivalent to 10% to 20% of the total opioid taken in the previous 24 hours (does not include transmucosal fentanyl doses).

- Reassess efficacy and adverse effects in 15 minutes. If the pain is unchanged or increased, administer another dose, 50% to 100% higher than the initial dose.

- Repeat for two to three cycles; if pain is not improving, consider a consult from pain management or palliative care service, or the need for interventional strategies.

- If the pain is decreased but still inadequately controlled, repeat the initial dose.

- If pain improved and was adequately controlled, continue at current (last administered) effective dose, at an appropriate dosing interval, as needed over initial 24 hours.

If using the oral route of administration, the guidelines recommend the following:

- Administer the oral opioid dose equivalent to 10% to 20% of the total opioid taken in the previous 24 hours.

- Reassess efficacy and adverse effects at 60 minutes; if pain is unchanged or increased, administer another opioid dose, 50% to 100% higher than the initial dose.

- Similar to the parenteral guidelines, if the pain is decreased but still inadequately controlled, repeat the same dose, and if the pain is improved and adequately controlled, continue at current effective dose as needed over initial 24 hours. Refer as appropriate, described above.[6]

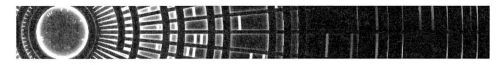

CASE 4.2

●●

Acute Pain Management in an Opioid-Tolerant Patient

CB is a 48-year-old woman admitted to hospice care with end-stage breast cancer. She has been receiving MS Contin 30 mg by mouth every 12 hours, with oral morphine solution 5 mg for moderate pain every 2 hours as needed, or 10 mg for severe pain every 2 hours as needed. The hospice nurse visits the patient Monday morning, only to learn that the patient has had a miserable weekend, with pain fluctuating between moderate and severe intensity. The nurse reviews the patient's pain diary and learns that the patient has continued her long-acting morphine and taken an average of 80-mg oral morphine for breakthrough pain per 24 hours on both Saturday and Sunday (e.g., total daily dose [TDD] for both Saturday and Sunday was 140-mg oral morphine each day). The nurse completes a history and physical and determines the patient's pain complaint is consistent with her previous complaint of pain, just increased in severity. The nurse has no reason to suspect a new pain syndrome (e.g., nerve compression or pain from a new metastatic site). The patient reports that when she takes the 10-mg morphine, she does feel a little bit better. The hospice nurse discusses the patient's situation with the hospice medical director and they agree to a plan. The nurse administers oral morphine solution 20 mg (this is 14% of the previous 24-hour morphine use, in the middle of the 10% to 20% recommendation); the patient rated her pain as a 9 at the time of morphine administration, and after 1 hour, the pain was reduced to an 8 (on a 0–10 scale; 0 = no pain, 10 = worst imaginable pain). The nurse repeated the 20-mg oral morphine dose, and 1 hour later the patient reported the pain was a 6 or 7. After discussing with the hospice medical director, the patient's opioid regimen was changed to MS Contin 60 mg by mouth every 12 hours to cover the majority of her recent increased use of morphine, with oral morphine solution 20 mg as needed every 2 hours. The hospice team will closely monitor the patient's response in the next couple of days and fine-tune the opioid regimen as appropriate.

Dose-Finding Around-the-Clock Opioid Therapy

Many patients transition from nonopioid therapy to opioid therapy by the addition of an "as needed" order for an IR (immediate release), meaning it's not *sustained-release* or *long-acting*; see Sidebar, "Definitions"). An example is "Percocet (5-mg oxycodone/ 325-mg acetaminophen per tablet), one tablet every 4 hours as needed for moderate-to-severe pain." If there is a concern about approaching or exceeding the maximum daily dose of the nonopioid component (e.g., acetaminophen), the prescriber could order "oxycodone 5 mg, one tablet every 4 hours as needed for moderate-to-severe pain." Alternately, morphine 5 mg, hydromorphone 2 mg, or oxymorphone 2.5 mg could be ordered. Doses need to be reduced and adjusted accordingly for vulnerable populations such as pediatrics, frail elderly, and those with hepatic or renal impairment.

If the patient is having continuous or persistent pain (meaning pain around-the-clock, not just occasional pain) necessitating around-the-clock opioid therapy, many expert guidelines recommend using an IR opioid regularly as a *dose-finding tool*.[2,3] The NCCN guidelines recommend starting with an IR opioid, as described above.[6] Guidance from the European Association for Palliative Care (EAPC) acknowledges the long-standing practice of using IR oral morphine every 4 hours based on the pharmacokinetics of oral morphine (e.g., time to peak approximately 1 hour, half-life of elimination approximately 2 to 3 hours, and duration of effect approximately 4 hours).[3] The guidelines state that IR formulations allow more flexible dosing than long-acting opioid formulations and are better suited for dose titration when pain is poorly controlled. Using a scheduled dose of IR morphine (or an alternate opioid if desired) every 4 hours, with the same dose available for additional pain relief as needed every 1 or 2 hours, the practitioner can determine the TDD of opioid necessary to control the pain. Because morphine has an elimination half-life of 2 to 3 hours, the patient would be at *steady-state* (which is where the rate in of opioid equals the rate out [of the body], resulting in a steady serum concentration of the opioid) within 24 hours. Therefore, it would be permissible to increase the opioid dose every 24 hours. Twenty-four hours after achieving good pain control, the patient could be transitioned to a long-acting oral or transdermal formulation for ease of administration.

Although many practitioners feel that it would be inappropriate to initiate therapy for persistent pain with a sustained-release opioid product in an opioid-naïve patient, research has shown that this strategy may be just as good or even better. Klepstad and colleagues randomized cancer patients who had continued pain despite treatment with codeine or propoxyphene to receive either four hourly doses of IR morphine, or a once-daily sustained-release formulation of morphine (both with rescue doses available).[7] The primary end-point of their study was time needed to achieve adequate pain relief (2.1 days for IR, 1.7 days for sustained-release); secondary end-points included other symptoms, health-related quality of life, and patient satisfaction. Patients in the IR morphine arm reported statistically significantly more tiredness after dosage titration, and no differences were shown in other secondary end-points. The authors pointed out that advantages of using sustained-release morphine from day one include increased patient convenience, less confusion about medication administration, and eliminated the need to convert from IR to sustained-release morphine subsequently. Of course, it is important to remember that vulnerable populations who would be started on a TDD of opioid *lower* than that which could be administered with commercially available sustained-release products cannot use this strategy. The EAPC guidelines state (as a weak recommendation) that either an IR or slow-release formulation of morphine (or alternate opioid) can be used for opioid initiation and titration (with an oral IR opioid available for breakthrough pain).[3] Let's look at a case illustrating these principles.

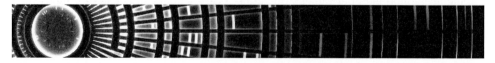

CASE 4.3
• •

Switching an IR Opioid to a Sustained-Release Opioid

VW is a 49-year-old man diagnosed with lung cancer. He developed pain that increased over several weeks to the point that he is using Tylenol #3 (acetaminophen and codeine) three to four tablets per day and has significant persistent pain despite this. His prescriber wants to switch him to around-the-clock morphine. What are two potential dosing strategies you could recommend for VW?

Strategy 1—Discontinue the Tylenol #3, and begin 5-mg oral morphine solution every 4 hours around the clock, and 5-mg oral morphine solution every 2 hours as needed for additional pain relief. Have VW keep a pain diary, documenting all doses of morphine taken. After 24 hours, calculate VW's TDD of morphine, and divide by 6. For example, if VW had taken his six scheduled doses and three additional doses of morphine, this is a TDD of 45-mg oral morphine. On day 2, VW's standing dose of morphine could be increased to 7.5 mg every 4 hours (his TDD of 45 mg divided into six equal doses), and either keep the "as needed" dose at 5 mg or increase it to 7.5 mg every 2 hours. Continue with this strategy until VW has achieved good pain control with minimal use of the "as needed" doses of morphine, and then switch to sustained-release morphine. For example, 5 days later, a review of VW's diary shows that an eventual increase to 10-mg oral morphine solution every 4 hours has controlled his pain with no need for additional morphine doses over the past 2 days. It would be appropriate to switch VW to a sustained-release morphine regimen based on this stable dose with one of the following:

- MS Contin 30 mg by mouth every 12 hours

- Kadian 60 mg by mouth once daily

- Kadian 30 mg by mouth every 12 hours

In all of these cases, you would also keep the IR morphine for breakthrough pain, which we will discuss in the next section.

Strategy 2—VW was taking three or four Tylenol #3 tablets per day and had persistent pain despite this. If he was taking four tablets per day that would be 120 mg of oral codeine per day, which is approximately equivalent to 15 mg of oral morphine per day (refer to Chapter 3 for an explanation of the mathematics involved). Minimally, VW needs a dosage increase—anywhere from 25% to 100%. We could start him on Kadian 20 mg by mouth per day (a 25% increase), or we could switch to MS Contin 15 mg by mouth every 12 hours, which would be appropriate (the lowest strength of MS Contin, which is a 100% increase in the TDD of oral morphine). Of course, you would also have an IR oral morphine product available for additional pain, such as 5-mg oral morphine solution every 2 hours as needed. Again, you would ask VW to maintain a pain diary. If on day 2 you find that VW has taken four or five doses of the oral morphine solution (20–25 mg of oral morphine) in the past 24 hours in addition to the MS Contin 15 mg twice daily (30-mg oral morphine; TDD 50–55 mg of oral morphine), it would be appropriate to increase his MS Contin to 30 mg by mouth every 12 hours. Similarly, you could have used Kadian as well.

BREAKTHROUGH PAIN

In the previous section, we discussed dosing opioids around the clock for **persistent pain**. Other terms used to describe this type of *always-present pain* include *baseline*, *basal*, *continuous*, *intractable*, and *constant*. On top of this, up to 90% of cancer and noncancer pain patients have a different or additional pain that comes and goes, referred to globally as **breakthrough pain**, presumably because it breaks through the persistent pain and around-the-clock analgesic the patient is taking (see Sidebar, "Characterizing Breakthrough Pain"). Breakthrough pain is also referred to as *episodic, incident,* or *transient* pain.[8] An early definition of breakthrough pain described the phenomenon as "a transitory increase in pain to greater than moderate intensity, which occurs on a baseline pain of moderate intensity or less."[9] Because clinicians and researchers through the years have defined *breakthrough pain* differently, it is difficult to compare epidemiologic studies concerning breakthrough pain.

Mercadante and Portenoy summarized 25 years of study concerning breakthrough pain and identify several elements that characterize breakthrough pain, and have gained some measure of consensus for definition, as follows:

- "Patient must be receiving a stable opioid regimen, and baseline pain must be controlled over some period.

- A precipitating event is not required to designate a breakthrough pain, but instead should be used to describe the subtype of breakthrough pain as spontaneous or incident type."[9]

An important point in this definition is that the background pain (the persistent or basal pain) is *controlled* over some period of time. If the persistent pain is not controlled, then, by definition, the presence of breakthrough pain cannot be determined (because you just have a red-hot mess of poorly controlled pain). Clearly the first order of business is to control the persistent pain, and that is what the focus of our exercises have been so far in this chapter, where the breakthrough dose of medication has been a "given." Now we will closely look at why ensuring breakthrough medication availability is essential in a good analgesic plan and how we magically determine the doses of the rescue opioid. On with the hunt!

As described above, breakthrough pain can be classified as **spontaneous pain** (idiopathic, occurring with no known stimulus; generally slower in onset and more

Table 4-1
Types of Breakthrough Pain

	Characteristics	Management Strategies
Spontaneous	Pain that requires no precipitating stimulus. Can occur without warning and be acutely severe. Spontaneous pain commonly has a neuropathic component.	IR opioid on an as-needed basis. Consider use of a co-analgesic (particularly if neuropathic).
Incident pain; volitional (or predictable)	Consistent temporal causal relationship with identifiable causes that are under the patient's control such as patient-precipitated movement, wound care, or personal care.	Nonopioid or IR opioid, on an as-needed basis prophylactically; rest; ice; patient education
Incident pain; nonvolitional (or unpredictable)	Consistent temporal causal relationship with identifiable causes that are not under the patient's control such as sneezing, bladder spasm, or coughing.	IR opioid on an as-needed basis
End-of-dose	Pain that recurs before the next scheduled dose of the around-the-clock analgesic. Likely due to a subtherapeutic dose of analgesic.	Increase in dose and/or frequency of around-the-clock analgesic

DEFINITIONS

We use terms such as *immediate release* and *sustained release* when we talk about opioid formulations, so it's important that we all have the same understanding about these terms.

- An **immediate-release (IR) opioid** is an unmodified formulation, such as an oral solution, a plain film-coated tablet, or a simple capsule. Examples include oral morphine solution (e.g., Roxanol), generic morphine or oxycodone tablets or capsules, or hydromorphone tablets. An IR tablet or capsule begins to dissolve after ingestion, or an oral solution delivers opioid readily available for absorption, and the opioid begins to work within 30 minutes or so. Morphine, hydromorphone, and oxycodone are examples of opioids that are widely used as IR formulations, and they are generally dosed every 4 hours or more frequently when used for breakthrough pain. Oxymorphone is also available as a 5-mg IR tablet; combination tablets and capsules such as hydrocodone/acetaminophen, oxycodone/acetaminophen, and others are also available as IR formulations.

- Within IR opioid tablets and capsules, we can further break these products down into *short-onset* and *rapid-onset*. For example, oral morphine, oxycodone, oxymorphone, and hydromorphone tablets or capsules are swallowed and start to act in about 30 minutes following dissolution and absorption. Fentanyl can be administered in the buccal cavity (known as transmucosal administration), and the onset of analgesia is 5 to 10 minutes. Therefore, transmucosal fentanyl (frequently referred to as *transmucosal immediate-release fentanyl*, TIRF) would be considered *rapid-onset* and oral morphine, oxycodone, hydromorphone, and oxymorphone would be considered *short-onset*.

- A **sustained-release opioid** is a tablet or capsule that is used to control persistent or around-the-clock pain. Sustained-release oral formulations have been pharmaceutically altered to allow dosing every 12 or 24 hours. Examples include long-acting morphine (e.g., MS Contin, Kadian, Arymo ER), oxycodone (OxyContin), and hydromorphone (Exalgo). The transdermal fentanyl patch (Duragesic and generic versions) is another sustained-release product designed to maintain blood levels of fentanyl within the therapeutic range for 72 hours. Transdermal buprenorphine (Butrans) is also a sustained-release product that is changed once a week.

Knowing if a tablet or capsule is IR or sustained release is an important consideration when treating persistent versus breakthrough pain. If a patient took an extra dose of MS Contin for breakthrough pain, not only would the painful episode be over long before an analgesic effect could be realized, but it would place the patient at risk of overdose once peak levels were reached after several hours.

Methadone is an unusual beast compared to most of the other mu-opioid agonists we have been discussing—it is rapid onset (onset of analgesia in 10–15 minutes), but it's long acting while not being a sustained-release formulation. I know you've got your head cocked to the side re-reading that last sentence, but it's true! The long-lasting properties of methadone are not due to pharmaceutical manipulation of the oral dosage formulation; methadone (and levorphanol) is *inherently* long acting, although the elimination half-life is highly variable. A further discussion on the use of methadone can be found in Chapter 6.

prolonged) or **incident pain** (secondary to a stimulus, which the patient may or may not be able to control).[9] Examples of incident pain (triggered by an identifiable event, and usually of short onset and short duration that can be predictable or unpredictable) include movement-induced bone pain and swallow-induced oropharyngeal pain from mucositis.[9] More controversial is whether **end-of-dose failure pain** (pain at the end of the dosing interval of the long-acting opioid) should be considered as breakthrough pain. A description of these terms and usual management options are shown in Table 4-1. Breakthrough pain can occur multiple times per day, lasting seconds to more than an hour, typically peaking within 10 to 30 minutes in patients with noncancer pain.[10,11] The patient is unable to predict the occurrence of approximately half of all

CHARACTERIZING BREAKTHROUGH PAIN

Imagine you have advanced cancer and a complicated pain picture. Your healthcare team has switched your analgesics several times, which now provides you with good pain control. You feel like you can't relax, however, because you know that two to four times a day a lightning bolt of pain will hit you, leaving you tearful and shaken. How can you enjoy the time you have left living with this threat hanging over your head?

Portenoy and Hagen studied a cohort of patients with cancer pain and showed that 64% of patients reported breakthrough pain, described as transient flares of severe pain.[8] The median number of breakthrough pain episodes was four per patient per day (range was 1–3,600). A little less than half of these episodes were paroxysmal (the "out of the blue" experience; spontaneous pain) and the rest were more gradual in onset. Duration of pain was a median of 30 minutes (range 1–240 minutes). Not quite one-third of the episodes were end-of-dose pain; 55% were precipitated by some event. Of these, most were volitional incident pain (e.g., patient-initiated activity), and the remainder were nonvolitional incident pain (e.g., flatulence or coughing). The pain was thought to be somatic or neuropathic in about one-third of the cases, and visceral or mixed in about 20% of the cases.

Looking at hospice patients specifically, Fine and Busch found that 86% of patients experienced breakthrough pain, averaging 2.9 episodes per day each.[12] Average pain intensity was 7 (compared to a baseline pain rating of 3.6 during the day and 2.6 at night) on a 0-to-10 scale (0 = no pain, 10 = worst imaginable pain), with an average of 30 minutes to pain relief. Zeppetella and colleagues found similar results in a hospice population, showing about half of episodes occurred suddenly, 59% were unpredictable, and 75%

of patients were dissatisfied with their pain control.[13] Interestingly, Gagnon and colleagues evaluated the impact of delirium on the circadian distribution of breakthrough analgesia in advanced cancer patients and found that patients without delirium used more breakthrough analgesics in the morning, while those with delirium used more in the evening and at night.[14]

The situation is just as grim with chronic pain patients. Seventy-four percent of opioid-treated chronic noncancer pain patients experience severe to excruciating breakthrough pain.[10] Half of the patients studied had low back pain, and the pathophysiology was characterized as somatic in a little more than one-third of episodes, neuropathic in about 18%, visceral in 4%, and mixed in 40% of events. The majority of these patients could identify a precipitating event for the pain, with 92% related to some activity. Looking at patients with chronic back pain specifically, Bennett and colleagues conducted a telephone survey of 117 patients with controlled baseline back pain.[15] Of these, 74% experienced breakthrough pain; the median number of episodes was two per day, median time to maximum intensity was 10 minutes, and median duration was 55 minutes. The vast majority of these patients used short-acting opioids to manage the breakthrough pain, but many found these agents to be unsatisfactory in controlling these painful episodes.

It's easy to imagine how pain patients can become fearful and withdrawn, always waiting for the other shoe to drop. It is imperative that healthcare practitioners carefully characterize the nature of the patient's breakthrough pain(s) and strategize preemptive and reactive plans to address the pain. Questions used to assess the presence and nature of breakthrough pains are shown in Table 4-2.[16]

episodes of breakthrough pain.[11] Uncontrolled breakthrough pain has a negative impact on quality of life and makes patients fearful and sedentary, leading to further deconditioning and disability.[11]

Therapeutic Options for Breakthrough Pain

First, it is important not to overlook nonpharmacologic options that may be useful in treating breakthrough pain. This includes strategies such as pacing activities (not overdoing activities to the point of invoking pain), ice or heat applications, wraps/braces/corsets, physical therapy interventions, massage therapy, transcutaneous electrical nerve stimulation (TENS), and nerve blocks. Pharmacologic therapy

Table 4-2

Assessing Breakthrough Pain

Do you ever have pain that is different from your baseline, persistent, "always there" pain? If so, can I ask you a few questions about that pain?

Precipitating Events	• Do you notice anything in particular that brings on this pain? Examples include movement, light touch, rolling over in bed, walking or standing, physical therapy, wound care, or other activities. • Does the pain occur without any identifiable provocation? • Does the pain consistently occur right before the next scheduled dose of your pain medication?
Palliating Events	• What have you tried to prevent or relieve the pain, such as resting, ice/heat application, repositioning, avoiding activities, and so forth?
Previous Treatment or Therapy	• What medications have you tried to prevent or treat this pain? How well did they work? • Did you have any side effects from the medication?
Quality	• What words would you use to describe this pain?
Region/Radiation	• Where on your body does this pain occur? • Does the pain move anywhere?
Severity	• Using a 0-to-10 scale (0 = no pain, 10 = worst imaginable pain), how would you rate the severity of this pain?
Temporal	• How often does this pain occur? Daily? Multiple times per day? Approximately how many episodes per day? Per week? • How long does it take the pain to reach its worst, and how long does the pain last altogether?
Associated Symptoms	• Does this pain keep you from doing any of your desired activities? • Has this pain had an effect on your mood, appetite, ability to sleep, and provide self-care? • Can you do all the things you want to do, or does this pain prevent those activities?

will likely still be necessary, but these nondrug measures may reduce the frequency or amount of opioid required.

As stated earlier, one of the most important principles of treating pain is to ensure that baseline persistent pain is controlled effectively with around-the-clock analgesics, usually with a sustained-release product. Nonopioid analgesics such as acetaminophen or a nonsteroidal anti-inflammatory agent may be used for breakthrough pain, but there are several disadvantages to this strategy. Most important, the patient will probably not achieve sufficient pain relief. Patients who require around-the-clock opioid therapy for persistent pain will likely need an opioid for breakthrough pain as well. Second, the nonopioid analgesics have a longer onset of action, a dose-related ceiling effect, and dose-related toxicities. Don't overlook the importance of co-analgesics (adjuvants), however. Spontaneous pain commonly has a neuropathic component, and a co-analgesic may significantly reduce episodes of spontaneous breakthrough pain.

The opioids used most often for breakthrough pain include morphine, oxycodone, hydromorphone, and fentanyl. Oxymorphone is also available in an IR formulation and may be used for breakthrough pain, and IR combination analgesics (e.g., hydrocodone/acetaminophen or oxycodone/acetaminophen) may also be used, although practitioners must be mindful of the dose limitations of the nonopioid component.

Selecting the Best Opioid for Breakthrough Pain

Several considerations go into making the decision of *which* opioid to use for breakthrough pain. Most practitioners tend to use the same opioid for treating persistent, around-the-clock pain as they do for breakthrough pain (e.g., MS Contin with IR morphine). This practice tends to make the calculation easier and keeps things "cleaner." Patients may, however, end up on two different opioids for a variety of reasons. For example, a patient may be using a transdermal fentanyl patch for persistent pain, but oral morphine or oxycodone solution for breakthrough pain. Alternately, a patient may be receiving MS Contin around the clock, but using fentanyl buccal tablets for breakthrough pain for quicker onset of action. A bit more controversial is the use of two different opioids based on the concept of genetic polymorphism of opioid receptors. We already know that there are a *bunch* of mu-opioid receptors (probably 25 or more), and different opioids (e.g., morphine versus oxycodone) may bind or activate receptors slightly differently, giving a different therapeutic effect. For the most part, if the patient can swallow oral tablets, capsules, or solutions, it is probably easier to use the same opioid for persistent pain and breakthrough pain, unless the pain is not optimally controlled, and usual and customary interventions do not rectify the situation.

Practitioners may be tempted to select an opioid for breakthrough pain based on the speed of onset, particularly for nonvolitional incident pain or idiopathic pain that peaks quickly. For example, the more hydrophilic opioids such as morphine, oxycodone, and hydromorphone are thought to have an onset of analgesia of about 30 minutes, while more lipophilic opioids such as methadone or fentanyl have a much more rapid onset (e.g., 10–15 minutes).[16] But let's not be so quick to throw morphine and its hydrophilic friends out the window. Mercadante and colleagues compared fentanyl pectin nasal spray (FPNS) to oral morphine (OM) in breakthrough cancer pain.[17] Fifteen minutes post-opioid administration, 71.9% of FPNS patients had a ≥33% reduction in pain, compared to 58.8% of OM patients. This difference was not statistically significant. At 30 minutes, those experiencing ≥33% reduction in pain was almost identical (93.9% versus 92.9% of patients, respectively). There was a bigger difference (which was statistically significant) when looking at a ≥50% reduction in pain at 15 minutes (52.4% of FPNS patients versus 14.1% OM patients). Results were similar at 30 minutes (86.6% and 82.3%). Further, the authors report a decrease in pain intensity from a baseline of 7.6 (on a 0–10 scale) to 4.4 with FPNS and 4.9 with OM at 15 minutes; and 2.8 with FPNS and 3.1 with OM at 30 minutes. A difference of 0.5 and 0.3 (at 15 and 30 minutes respectively) may be statistically significant, but it is unlikely to be clinically significant on a 0–10 pain severity rating scale. These results show us that FPNS is probably a bit quicker out of the gate, but it's important to note that OM reduced pain by ≥33% in almost 60% of patients—that's pretty darned quick onset as well. Bhatrager and associates evaluated the efficacy and safety of oral transmucosal fentanyl citrate (OTFC) and OM in breakthrough cancer pain, reporting the reduction of pain on a 0-to-10 scale at 5, 15, 30, and 60 minutes post-dose.[18] While the results were statistically significantly different, we have to consider the clinical importance of these differences. Improvement in breakthrough pain intensity on the 0-to-10 numeric rating scale comparing OTFC to OM was 1.44 versus 0.85 at 5 minutes; 2.97 versus 2.44 at 15 minutes; 4.56 versus 4.04 at 30 minutes; and 5.91 versus 5.15 at 30 minutes. Again, the OTFC did show quicker onset, but is the half-point reduction in pain (noted at 15 and 30 minutes) clinically apparent to patients? Continuing on this theme, Webster compared the fentanyl buccal tablet (FBT) to IR oxycodone (OxyIR) for breakthrough cancer pain and noncancer pain.[19] When evaluating "meaningful pain relief" at 15 minutes, there was no difference between the two treatments (17% of FBT patients versus 16% of OxyIR patients). There was a statistically significant difference at 30 minutes; 46% of FBT patients versus 38% OxyIR patients. Ashburn showed similar results comparing FBT to OxyIR, showing 41% of FBT patients experiencing ≥33% reduction in pain intensity at 30 minutes, as compared to 32% of OxyIR patients.[20] Those with a ≥50% reduction in pain at 30 minutes were 21% of FBT versus 16% OxyIR. Some have speculated that oxycodone may have a slight edge over morphine in treating breakthrough pain due to more selective and rapid uptake in the brain.[21,22]

Last, we must also consider the economic implications of selecting an opioid for breakthrough pain. For example, Fallon and colleagues compared FPNS to OM tablets for breakthrough cancer pain.[23] At 10 minutes post-dose, 33.9% of FPNS-treated patients experienced a 33% reduction in pain, as compared to 28.3% of OM-treated patients. At 15 minutes post-dose, this reduction was seen in 55.4% of FPNS patients versus 47.3% of OM patients. Davis subsequently published an *astonishing* letter in response to this trial.[24] First, he pointed out that the number needed to treat to benefit one patient with FPNS at 10 minutes is 18, and 12 at 15 minutes, versus OM. Second, using the cost of morphine and FPNS at the time of publication (2012; $0.30/dose OM; $60/dose FPNS—note, as of this writing in 2018, prices are approximately $1/dose OM and $138/dose FPNS), he speculated that the cost per year to benefit one patient using FPNS instead of OM for two episodes of breakthrough pain per day would be $777,600 if aiming for the 10-minute difference, or $518,000 for the 15-minute improvement. It boggles the mind to do this cost comparison using 2018 pricing (ok, the devil made me do it—it's between $1.2 and $1.8 million/year!). This benefit-burden analysis doesn't even include the increased risk of adverse effects associated with FPNS as opposed to OM. We'd better start rolling our quarters.

So, a lot goes into this decision. I would argue that the majority of patients will achieve good results or "close enough for government work" results with morphine, oxycodone, or hydromorphone. We should reserve the more rapid-acting transmucosal fentanyl products, which are considerably more expensive, for those cases where that small degree of faster onset is clinically necessary.

Determining the Dose of Rescue Opioid

There are many suggested guidelines for determining the dose of an opioid for breakthrough pain, assuming the patient is receiving an oral long-acting opioid (e.g., morphine, hydromorphone, or oxycodone) for the baseline pain. The consensus based on original research and guideline recommendations is to offer 10% to 20% of the TDD of the same opioid for rescue, using a short-acting formulation.[6,25–29] For example, if a patient were receiving MS Contin 30 mg by mouth every 12 hours, the TDD of *scheduled* morphine is 60 mg. Ten percent of 60 mg is 6 mg, and 20% is 12 mg. Both 6 and 12 are goofy numbers for a dose, so it would be likely we'd recommend either 5 mg or 10 mg. Therefore, a sample order would be MS Contin 30 mg by mouth every 12 hours, and morphine oral solution 10 mg by mouth every 2 hours as needed for breakthrough pain.

Often practitioners want to give patients a little latitude in selecting their own break-through opioid dose. For example, it's not uncommon that specific predictable types of incident pain, such as wound care, may require a higher dose of opioid than other episodes of breakthrough pain. To allow this degree of flexibility, the prescriber could write two prescriptions: morphine 5 mg by mouth every 2 hours as needed for moderate pain, and morphine 10 mg by mouth every 2 hours as needed for severe pain. Note that accrediting organizations (e.g., The Joint Commission) find "range" orders for dose or dosing interval (e.g., take 5–10 mg every 1–2 hours) difficult to consistently interpret. The Institute for Safe Medication Practices (ISMP) suggests giving range orders only if they are associated with objective measures (e.g., morphine 5 mg for moderate pain, or morphine 10 mg for severe pain, as needed every 2 hours). If the patient can take the breakthrough opioid every hour, the "every 2 hours" part of the order becomes mean-ingless. In addition, selecting between doses without clear direction (e.g., moderate pain versus severe pain) is beyond the scope of practice for a nurse, and certainly for a patient!

If the patient were receiving his or her around-the-clock opioid as an IR product dosed every 4 hours, additional opioid could be offered for breakthrough pain in between doses (e.g., every 1–2 hours). The dose should be 25% to 50% of the scheduled 4-hourly around-the-clock dose. For example, if the patient were receiving oxycodone 10 mg every 4 hours around the clock, an additional 2.5 or 5 mg of oxycodone could be made available for breakthrough pain, including volitional incident pain (e.g., physical therapy) administered preemptively.

The dose of the rescue opioid should be adjusted based on the patient's response. With volitional incident pain, the best way to assess the appropriateness of the rescue dose is to assess the pain rating *before and after* the incident. For example, if Mrs. Smith knows that jumping into the passenger side of a car to go to the Wendy's drive-through for a Frosty causes pain, she could premedicate with morphine about 45 to 60 minutes before leaving home. Hmmmm . . . a Frosty with morphine beads sprinkled on top! Add some Senna sprinkles and you're all set! If Mrs. Smith were able to go to Wendy's after taking 10 mg of oral morphine and her pain never exceeded a 3 (on a 0–10 scale; 0 = no pain, 10 = worst imaginable pain) and she was content with her pain control, that's an appropriate dose. On the other hand, if she says despite 10 mg of oral morphine, the pain increased to a very uncomfortable 6 or 7, it might be appropriate to increase the dose of opioid to perhaps 15 or even 20 mg. The goal is patient comfort, short of adverse effects. It is not uncommon for the dose of opioid used to prevent volitional incident pain to be disproportionately higher than what may be required for spontaneous pain (e.g., greater than the 10% to 20% of the TDD, or perhaps equivalent to the 4-hourly standing dose of opioid).

A word about the dosing interval for opioid rescue dosing: As briefly discussed previously, most short-acting opioids generally have a duration of 4 hours. Unfortunately, many practitioners will order a short-acting opioid such as morphine, hydromorphone, or oxycodone as every 4 to 6 hours. In the majority of patients, these three opioids do not provide pain relief for 6 hours, and the pain may recur and last until the next dose may be administered. Even giving a short-acting opioid every 4 hours may result in the pain recurring. It is probably best to allow administration of the rescue short-acting opioid every 1 to 2 hours (particularly in patients with advanced illness and/or unstable pain). In the case of volitional incident pain, the patient will be administering the short-acting opioid 45 to 60 minutes before the event that triggers the pain.

The best way to assess the appropriateness of the rescue dose of opioid for nonvolitional incident pain or spontaneous pain is to compare the pain rating before taking the rescue opioid dose, and 1 hour after administering the rescue dose. For example, let's suppose Mr. Johnson tells you his background persistent pain is usually an acceptable 2 or 3 (on a 0–10 scale; 0 = no pain, 10 = worst imaginable pain), and the spontaneous pain he experiences several times a day shoots it up to a 7 or 8. If he tells you his pain comes back down to a 3 or 4 one hour after taking 10 mg of short-acting oral morphine, and he is content with this, then your dose is appropriate. On the other hand, if he tells you the pain 1 hour after administration is still a 5 or 6, you would want to increase the dose of breakthrough analgesic by 50% to 100%.

Note the following rules of thumb:

- If the rescue dose relieves less than 50% of the pain, double the rescue dose.
- If greater than 50% of the pain is relieved (but still not at goal), increase the rescue dose by 50%.
- Close to 100% pain relief (or otherwise acceptable to the patient) indicates no change is necessary.

Remember: A 30% to 50% reduction in pain or greater is considered to be clinically important pain relief.

What about patients who require a more lipid-soluble opioid to treat breakthrough pain that comes on very quickly? As mentioned above, two possibilities are methadone and fentanyl. Methadone is an extremely useful opioid to have in our arsenal, and the onset of analgesia is 10 to 15 minutes. However, the duration of effect is 4 to 8 hours, which is probably longer than needed for breakthrough pain. However, methadone has been used successfully in this manner and will be discussed in detail in a subsequent chapter.

Fentanyl administered by the transmucosal route (TIRF; transmucosal immediate-release fentanyl) has an onset of analgesia of 5 to 10 minutes, and a short duration of action (1–2 hours). There are three primary transmucosal routes of administration—buccal, sublingual, and intranasal.[30]

At present, there are six TIRFs on the market:

1. Compressed lozenge oral transmucosal fentanyl citrate (OTFC) (Actiq)
2. Fentanyl effervescent buccal tablet (FBT) (Fentora)
3. Buccal soluble film (FBSF) (Onsolis)
4. Sublingual oral disintegrating transmucosal fentanyl citrate (ODT) (Abstral)
5. Intranasal fentanyl spray (INFS) (Lazanda)
6. Sublingual spray (SUBSYS)[23]

Unfortunately, the dose of a TIRF cannot be determined as a percentage of the around-the-clock opioid the patient is receiving, whether it's a fentanyl product or not. A *Cochrane Review* on the use of opioids for the management of breakthrough pain in cancer patients found no meaningful relationship between the successful dose of a TIRF and the around-the-clock oral or transdermal opioid medication.[31] The authors recommended determining the most appropriate dose of a TIRF by appropriate titration to determine the most successful dose. Table 4-4 shows recommendations for the dosing and titration of all six TIRFs, including approved switches from Actiq to several of the other TIRFs.[32-37]

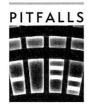

PITFALLS Fentora Precautions

In September 2007, the Food and Drug Administration (FDA) reported receiving reports of death and life-threatening side effects in patients who have taken Fentora. According to this Public Health Advisory, Fentora was prescribed for patients who were not appropriate candidates, received unapproved doses, and were inappropriately switched between OTFC (Actiq) and Fentora.

In response to these reports, the FDA issued the following Public Health Advisory:

- "Fentora should only be used for breakthrough pain in opioid-tolerant patients with cancer.
  - Fentora should not be used to treat any type of short-term pain including headaches or migraines, postoperative pain, or pain due to injury.
  - Fentora should not be used by patients who only take narcotic pain medications occasionally.
- The dosage strength of fentanyl in Fentora is NOT equal to the same dosage strength of fentanyl in other fentanyl-containing products.
  - Healthcare professionals must not directly substitute Fentora for other fentanyl medicines, including Actiq (e.g., on a mcg-per-mcg basis; see prescribing information).
  - Doctors must select the Fentora dose carefully for each patient.
- Patients who take Fentora and their caregivers must understand how to use it safely and follow the directions exactly. Directions for taking Fentora are provided in the Medication Guide for patients.
- Healthcare professionals who prescribe Fentora and patients who use Fentora and their caregivers should be aware of the signs of fentanyl overdose. Signs of fentanyl overdose include trouble breathing or shallow breathing; tiredness, extreme sleepiness or sedation; inability to think, talk, or walk normally; and feeling faint, dizzy, or confused. If these signs occur, patients or their caregivers should get medical attention right away."[38]

Elements of this warning are now reflected in the prescribing information for all six TIRF products.

Types of Breakthrough Pain

As discussed previously, there are several types of breakthrough pain. *Incident pain* that the patient can control and/or predict is best treated with a preemptive strike. The patient can use a more cost-effective short-acting opioid such as morphine, oxycodone, oxymorphone, or hydromorphone, taking a dose 45 to 60 minutes before the painful activity. The dose is usually 10% to 20% of the TDD of the around-the-clock opioid, but the dose should be increased or decreased as needed to keep the patient comfortable.

Nonvolitional incident pain and spontaneous breakthrough pain should be treated by administering the dose as soon as the breakthrough pain is experienced, or pain begins to worsen. If the pain is very rapid in onset, it may be appropriate to use a TIRF product. The TIRFs have demonstrated superiority over oral opioids in terms of onset of action, shorter duration of action, and cancer patient preference.[30] This is a considerably more expensive option, and formulary considerations may limit their utility. However, for patients with very quick-onset severe pain that significantly impacts their quality of life, use of a more expensive medication may be appropriate. One other strategy is to increase the around-the-clock opioid dose above that required to control baseline pain. Mercadante and colleagues demonstrated this with 25 patients with movement-related episodic pain due to bone metastases.[39] The dose of opioid was escalated beyond that required for pain control at rest, but short of adverse effects. This approach was successful, and only a small minority of patients required treatment of opioid-induced adverse effects or a decrease in opioid dose.

End of dose failure—the last type of breakthrough pain—may be treated with the use of rescue opioid doses, by giving the around-the-clock opioid more frequently, or by increasing the dose of the regularly scheduled (around-the-clock) opioid. Fewer doses per day are preferred; therefore, it would be worth a trial of an increased dose using the original dosing schedule.

A final word about titrating the around-the-clock opioid regimen based on the use of rescue medication. If a patient is *routinely* using his or her rescue medication, it is important to do a careful reassessment of the pain complaint. Perhaps a co-analgesic would be appropriate to add to the regimen. Alternatively, the patient could be experiencing disease progression and a higher dose of their scheduled opioid is required. When the patient is consistently using two, three, or four doses of rescue opioid per day, it would be appropriate to recalculate the TDD of opioid necessary to keep the patient comfortable (this calculation includes the standing dose and rescue doses used on average per day) and increase the regularly scheduled dose. It is likely that you will need to readjust the rescue dose as well (to keep the same ratio that already worked for the patient; for example, 20% of the TDD of scheduled opioid to be available for breakthrough pain). These principles will be illustrated in the next section of this chapter as we continue on this amazing mathematical journey!

Table 4-4

Dosing and Titration of Oral Transmucosal Fentanyl for Breakthrough Cancer Pain

Transmucosal IR Fentanyl Dosing Guidance[32-37]	

Black-box warnings, contraindications and warnings that apply to all transmucosal fentanyl products
 	
• Actiq
• Fentora
• Subsys
• Abstral
• Onsolis
• Lazanda
	• May only be prescribed for opioid-tolerant patients. Defined as patients taking around-the-clock opioid therapy of at least a week or longer:
	  • 60-mg oral morphine per day
	  • 25-mcg/hr transdermal fentanyl
	  • 30-mg oral oxycodone per day
	  • 8-mg oral hydromorphone per day
	  • 25-mg oral oxymorphone per day
	  • 60-mg oral hydrocodone per day
	  • Equianalgesic dose of another opioid taken daily
	• Contraindicated in management of acute or postoperative pain
	• Indicated *only* for the management of BTcP in patients with cancer, 18 years and older (Actiq in 16 years or older)
	• Do not substitute for any other fentanyl products.
	• Do not convert patients on a mcg per mcg basis from any other fentanyl products.
	• Keep out of the reach of children and dispose of unneeded medication properly.
	• Concomitant use with CYP3A4 inhibitors (or discontinuation of CYP3A4 inducers) can result in a fatal overdose of fentanyl.
	• Once titrated to an effective dose, patient should generally only use one TIRF unit of the appropriate strength per BTcP episode.
	• If the patient experiences greater than four BTcP episodes per day, the dose of the maintenance (around-the-clock) opioid used for persistent pain should be reevaluated.

Actiq	
Dosage Formulation and Strengths	• Solid oral transmucosal lozenge • 200 mcg, 400 mcg, 600 mcg, 800 mcg, 1,200 mcg, 1,600 mcg
Initial Dosing	• Initial dose is 200 mcg. • May repeat same dose 15 minutes after completion of Actiq unit (30 minutes after start). • Maximum of two Actiq for any episode of BTcP • Wait ≥4 hours before treating another episode of BTcP with Actiq.
Dose Titration	• Try the 200-mcg dose for several episodes of BTcP as described above. • If insufficient, increase dose to next highest strength with next episode of BTcP. • Maximum of two Actiq for any episode of BTcP • Wait ≥4 hours before treating another episode of BTP with Actiq
Maintenance Dose	• May repeat dose 15 minutes after completion of Actiq unit with same strength. • Must wait 4 hours before treating another episode of BTcP with Actiq.
Fentora	
Dosage Formulation and Strengths	• Buccal tablets • 100 mcg, 200 mcg, 400 mcg, 600 mcg, 800 mcg

Table 4-4
Dosing and Titration of Oral Transmucosal Fentanyl
for Breakthrough Cancer Pain (continued)

Transmucosal IR Fentanyl Dosing Guidance[32-37]

Initial Dosing	• Initial dose is 100 mcg; may repeat same dose in 30 minutes as needed with the only exception of patients already using Actiq (see below).
	• Maximum of two Fentora for any one episode of BTcP
	• Wait ≥4 hours before treating a subsequent episode of BTcP with Fentora.
	• If switching from Actiq to Fentora, use the following starting doses (these are not conversions per se):
	• Current Actiq dose 200 mcg → Fentora 100-mcg tablet
	• Current Actiq dose 400 mcg → Fentora 100-mcg tablet
	• Current Actiq dose 600 mcg → Fentora 200-mcg tablet
	• Current Actiq dose 800 mcg → Fentora 200-mcg tablet
	• Current Actiq dose 1,200 mcg → Fentora 2 × 200-mcg tablet
	• Current Actiq dose 1,600 mcg → Fentora 2 × 200-mcg tablet
Dose Titration	• Try the 100-mcg dose for several episodes of BTcP as described above.
	• If insufficient, increase dose to next highest strength with next episode of BTcP.
	• Patients whose initial dose is 100 mcg and who need to titrate to a higher dose can be instructed to use two 100-mcg tablets (one on each side of the mouth in the buccal cavity) with their next BTcP episode.
	• If two 100-mcg tablets are not an effective dose, in the next BTcP episode, the patient may be instructed to place two 100-mcg tablets on each side of the mouth in the buccal cavity (total of four 100-mcg tablets). Titrate using multiples of the 200-mcg Fentora tablets for doses above 400 mcg (600 mcg and 800 mcg) for subsequent BTcP episodes.
	• Maximum of two Fentora doses for any one episode of BTcP
	• Wait ≥4 hours before treating a subsequent episode of BTcP with Actiq.
Maintenance Dose	• May repeat dose 30 minutes after completion of Fentora with same strength for the same episode of BTcP.
	• Must wait 4 hours before treating another episode of BTcP with Fentora.
Subsys	
Dosage Formulation and Strengths	• Sublingual spray
	• 100 mcg, 200 mcg, 400 mcg, 600 mcg, 800 mcg
Initial Dosing	• Initial dose is one 100-mcg spray sublingually, with patients using Actiq being the only exception (see below).
	• If pain is not relieved after 30 minutes, patients may take only one additional dose of 100 mcg.
	• Maximum of two doses Subsys for any episode of BTcP
	• Wait ≥4 hours before treating another episode of BTcP with Subsys.
	• If switching from Actiq to Subsys, use the following starting doses (these are not conversions per se):
	• Current Actiq dose 200 mcg → 100-mcg Subsys spray
	• Current Actiq dose 400 mcg → 100-mcg Subsys spray
	• Current Actiq dose 600 mcg → 200-mcg Subsys spray
	• Current Actiq dose 800 mcg → 200-mcg Subsys spray
	• Current Actiq dose 1,200 mcg → 400-mcg Subsys spray
	• Current Actiq dose 1,600 mcg → 400-mcg Subsys spray

(continued)

Table 4-4

Dosing and Titration of Oral Transmucosal Fentanyl for Breakthrough Cancer Pain (continued)

Transmucosal IR Fentanyl Dosing Guidance[32-37]

Dose Titration	• From the 100-mcg initial dose, closely follow patients and change the dosage level until the patient reaches a dose that provides adequate analgesic using a single Subsys dose per BTcP episode with tolerable side effect.
	• Titration steps are as follows:
	   • 100 mcg (1 x 100-mcg unit)
	   • 200 mcg (1 x 200-mcg unit)
	   • 400 mcg (1 x 400-mcg unit)
	   • 600 mcg (1 x 600-mcg unit)
	   • 800 mcg (1 x 800-mcg unit)
	   • 1,200 mcg (2 x 600-mcg units)
	   • 1,600 mcg (2 x 800-mcg units)
	• Maximum of two doses of Subsys for any one BTcP episode
	• Wait ≥4 hours before treating a subsequent episode of BTcP with Subsys.

Maintenance Dose	• May repeat dose 30 minutes after completion of Subsys with same strength. • Must wait 4 hours before treating another episode of BTcP with Subsys.

Abstral

Dosage Formulation and Strengths	• Sublingual tablet • 100 mcg, 200 mcg, 300 mcg, 400 mcg, 600 mcg, 800 mcg

Initial Dosing	• Initial dose is one 100 mcg, with the only exception of patients already using Actiq (see below).
	• If pain is not relieved after 30 minutes, patients may take only one additional dose of 100 mcg.
	• Maximum of two doses Abstral for any episode of BTcP
	• Wait ≥2 hours before treating another episode of BTcP with Abstral.
	• If switching from Actiq to Abstral, use the following starting doses (these are not conversions per se):
	   • Current Actiq dose 200 mcg → Abstral 100-mcg tablet
	   • Current Actiq dose 400 mcg → Abstral 200-mcg tablet
	   • Current Actiq dose 600 mcg → Abstral 200-mcg tablet
	   • Current Actiq dose 800 mcg → Abstral 200-mcg tablet
	   • Current Actiq dose 1,200 mcg → Abstral 200-mcg tablet
	   • Current Actiq dose 1,600 mcg → Abstral 400-mcg tablet

Dose Titration	• If adequate analgesia was not obtained with the first 100-mcg dose, continue dose escalation in a stepwise manner over consecutive BTcP episodes until adequate analgesic with tolerable side effects is achieved. • Increase the dose by 100-mcg multiples up to 400 mcg as needed. • If adequate analgesia is not obtained with a 400-mcg dose, the next titration step is 600 mcg; the next titration step is 800 mcg. • During titration, patients can be instructed to use multiples of 100-mcg tablets and/or 200-mcg tablets for a single dose. Instruct patients not to use more than four tablets at one time.
Maintenance Dose	• May repeat dose 30 minutes after completion of Abstral with same strength for any one episode of BTcP. • Must wait 2 hours before treating a subsequent episode of BTcP with Abstral.

Table 4-4

Dosing and Titration of Oral Transmucosal Fentanyl for Breakthrough Cancer Pain (continued)

Transmucosal IR Fentanyl Dosing Guidance[32-37]

Onsolis	
Dosage Formulation and Strengths	• Buccal soluble film • 200 mcg, 400 mcg, 600 mcg, 800 mcg, 1,200 mcg
Initial Dosing	• Initial dose is one 200-mcg film. • Only use one film per BTcP episode. • Patients must wait at least 2 hours before treating another episode of BTcP with Onsolis.
Dose Titration	• Follow patients and change the dosage strength until the patient reaches a dose that provides adequate analgesia with tolerable side effects. • If adequate pain relief is not achieved after one 200-mcg Onsolis film, titrate using multiples of the 200-mcg Onsolis film (for doses of 400, 600, or 800 mcg). • Increase the dose by 200 mcg in each subsequent episode of BTcP until the patient reaches satisfactory dose. • Do not use more than four of the 200-mcg Onsolis films simultaneously. • When multiple 200-mcg Onsolis films are used, they should not be placed on top of each other and may be placed on both sides of the mouth. • If adequate pain relief is not achieved after 800-mcg Onsolis (e.g., four 200-mcg Onsolis films), and the patient has tolerated the 800-mcg dose, treat the next episode by using one 1,200-mcg Onsolis film. • Doses above 1,200 mcg should not be used. • Patients must wait at least 2 hours before treating a subsequent episode of BTcP with Onsolis.
Maintenance Dose	• Single doses should be separated by at least 2 hours. • Onsolis should only be used once per BTcP episode; Onsolis should not be redosed within an episode. • During any episode of BTcP, if adequate pain relief is not achieved after Onsolis, the patient may use a rescue medication (after 30 minutes) as directed by his or her healthcare provider.
Lazanda	
Dosage Formulation and Strengths	• Nasal spray • Each spray delivers 100 mcL of solution containing either 100-mcg or 400-mcg fentanyl base.
Initial Dosing	• Initial dose is one 100-mcg spray of Lazanda (one spray in one nostril). • During any episode of BTcP if there is inadequate pain relief after 30 minutes following Lazanda dosing or if a separate episode of BTcP occurs before the next dose of Lazanda is permitted (e.g., 2 hours), the patient may use a rescue medication directed by their healthcare providers. • Do not switch patients from any other fentanyl products to Lazanda. • Patient must wait at least 2 hours before treating a subsequent episode of BTcP with Lazanda.

Dose Titration	• Titration steps should be as follows:
	  • Lazanda dose 100 mcg (1 × 100-mcg spray; one spray in one nostril).
	  • Lazanda dose 200 mcg (2 × 100-mcg spray; one in each nostril).
	  • Lazanda dose 400 mcg (4 × 100-mcg spray; two in each nostril—alternate nostrils) or 1 × 400-mcg spray.
	  • Lazanda dose 800 mcg (2 × 400 mcg; one in each nostril).

(continued)

Table 4-4

Dosing and Titration of Oral Transmucosal Fentanyl for Breakthrough Cancer Pain (continued)

Transmucosal IR Fentanyl Dosing Guidance[32-37]

Maintenance Dose	• Once an appropriate dose has been established, instruct patients to use that dose for each subsequent BTcP pain episode.
	• Limit Lazanda use to four or fewer doses per day.
	• During any episode of BTcP, if there is inadequate pain relief after 30 minutes following Lazanda dosing or if a separate episode of BTcP occurs before the next dose of Lazanda is permitted (e.g., 2 hours), the patient may use a rescue medication directed by their healthcare providers.

BTcP = breakthrough cancer pain; TIRF = transmucosal immediate-release fentanyl.

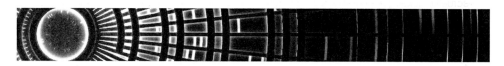

CASE 4.4
. . . .

Preempting Volitional Incident Pain

EY is an 82-year-old woman with end-stage dementia and multiple pressure ulcers. She has a long-standing history of severe osteoarthritis pain for which she receives Kadian 60 mg by mouth every 24 hours. Although EY is not able to provide a pain rating due to her dementia, the nurse observes that when she is doing a dressing change, EY moans, cries out, and becomes very tense, holding her body very stiffly. The nurse clearly suspects that the dressing change is causing EY additional pain.

Clearly, this is *volitional incident pain*. It's volitional in that the pain is caused by an activity that *could* be predicted and controlled; obviously, EY herself cannot prevent the dressing change, but it's not an incident beyond *everyone's* control (e.g., unpredictable provocation of pain caused by coughing or sneezing). With volitional incident pain, the best strategy is to administer a dose of rescue opioid 30 to 45 minutes before the precipitating event. Our rule of thumb is 10% to 20% of the TDD of the regularly scheduled (around-the-clock) opioid. In this case, the patient is receiving 60 mg of oral morphine per day. Ten to 20 percent would be 6- to 12-mg; the nurse recommends starting with 5 mg of morphine prior to dressing changes and allowing a repeat dose if ineffective, which the prescriber approves.

During the next dressing change, 5 mg of morphine was administered 45 minutes before-hand, and it had little-to-no effect on EY's behavior, so the procedure was stopped until the additional 5 mg was given, and allowed time to take effect. This was the ticket—EY did not exhibit the behaviors previously associated with the dressing change, and she took a short nap afterward, but was easily arousable. Subsequently, the nurse administered 10-mg oral morphine 45 minutes before wound care with good success.

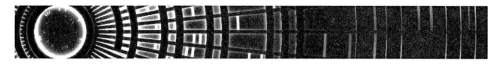

CASE 4.5

Dosing Transmucosal Fentanyl

MJ is a 42-year-old man with lung cancer, who is using a transdermal fentanyl (TDF) patch 75 mcg every 3 days to control his pain. The TDF mostly controls his pain, but several times a day he unexpectedly experiences an unprovoked "grabbing" sensation in his lower back that feels like a hot poker branding him, which is exquisitely painful. The pain lasts for about 15 minutes, leaving him completely drained for the next 30 minutes or so. He has morphine oral solution 20 mg every 2 hours available for breakthrough pain, which MJ says he takes, but it doesn't kick in quickly enough to address the pain. In fact, the morphine actually makes the post-episode exhaustion worse. MJ is extremely anxious about this situation, because he feels like he's on "pins and needles" all day waiting for this lightning bolt.

To better match the onset of analgesia with the temporal nature of the pain, you decide to switch MJ to an FBT (Fentora). Because there is no consistent correlation between the around-the-clock opioid dose and FBT, you prescribe the lowest dose, 100-mcg FBT, and advise MJ to insert one tablet between his cheek and upper molar the instant the pain occurs. If the pain has not resolved 30 minutes after inserting the tablet in the buccal cavity, MJ can take one additional 100-mcg tablet. After several days, MJ tells you that this approach has been more successful, but he is requiring two tablets every time he has the breakthrough pain. To make things simpler for MJ, you prescribe the 200-mcg FBT for future episodes of this spontaneous breakthrough pain.

Determining Rescue Dosing with Transdermal Fentanyl

FAST FACTS When a patient is receiving TDF, how does the prescriber come up with the dose of morphine oral solution for breakthrough pain? As you will learn in Chapter 5, most practitioners consider 2 mg per day of oral morphine to be approximately equivalent to 1 mcg per hour of TDF. Therefore, a TDF 75-mcg patch would be approximately equal to oral morphine 150-mg per day. Using our 10% to 20% rule for rescue opioid dosing, this would be 15 to 30 mg of oral morphine. The 20-mg oral morphine dose is right in the middle of the range; this dose would be adjusted (up or down) per patient response.

OPIOID DOSE ESCALATION STRATEGIES

Surprisingly, there is not much evidence-based research on opioid dose escalation. This primarily leaves us with the standard of practice as a guideline. An important part of the rule of thumb commonly used in practice is the recognition that the analgesic effect is a logarithmic function of the opioid dose; therefore, dosage increases are done as a percentage of the current TDD, not increasing by a specific milligram amount. Practitioners routinely use this strategy when increasing from one to two tablets of a combination product, for example, "Increase from one Percocet tablet every 4 hours to two Percocet tablets." This represents a 100% increase in the regularly scheduled opioid dose. When put in those terms, you're probably holding your head thinking, "Whoa!" But if you think about it, as Dr. David Weissman has said, practitioners don't increase a furosemide dose from 10 mg to 11 mg, but that's what practitioners like to do with opioids, especially parenteral infusions (increase from 4 mg/hr to 5 mg/hr).[40] Dr. Weissman further points out that patients generally do not notice a change in analgesia when dose increases are less than 25% above baseline. Going from 4 mg/hr to 5 mg/hr of parenteral morphine is only a 20% dosage increase. *So where does this leave us?* Let's consider oral opioids and parenteral opioids separately. Methadone, fentanyl, and continuous opioid infusions will be discussed in later chapters.

Oral Opioid Regimens

Many patients are receiving an oral long-acting opioid plus an IR opioid for breakthrough pain. Probably the most common strategy used to titrate the oral opioid regimen is to use the rescue opioid to titrate to a comfortable level, then calculate the TDD of opioid (long acting and short acting) and adjust the long-acting opioid dose to deliver all or the majority of this TDD. Of course, as you increase the dose of the long-acting opioid, you will need to increase the dose of the rescue opioid (still 10% to 20% of the TDD). This strategy is recommended by the NCCN guidelines, or if the patient cannot get comfortable using their current rescue opioid, to defer to their recommendation of giving 10% to 20% of the total opioid used in the previous 24 hours, and reassessing in 60 minutes.[6] Let's look at an example both ways.

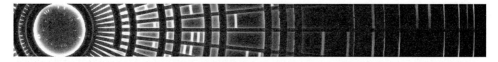

CASE 4.6
• •

Opioid Dose Escalation—Oral Opioids

A patient is taking OxyContin 20 mg by mouth every 12 hours, with OxyIR 5 mg by mouth every 2 hours as needed for additional pain. If the patient tells you that taking four doses of the OxyIR 5 mg, along with the OxyContin 20 mg by mouth every 12 hours, keeps him comfortable, you would calculate the TDD of oxycodone (60 mg in this case) and readjust his regimen to OxyContin 30 mg by mouth every 12 hours, and OxyIR 10 mg by mouth every 2 hours as needed for additional pain.

If, on the other hand, the patient tells you he is taking six doses of the 5-mg OxyIR rescue opioid in addition to the OxyContin, but his pain is still a 6 or 7 (on a 0–10 scale; 0 = no pain, 10 = worst imaginable pain), you could give 10% to 20% of the TDD now (which would be 9–18 mg of oxycodone) and reevaluate pain control in 60 minutes. We give the patient 10 mg, and in 1 hour his pain rating is still a 6. We then give the patient 15 mg, and in 1 hour his pain is down to a 4 or 5. Over the next 2 days, the patient reports requiring at least five doses of the 15-mg OxyIR, in addition to his OxyContin 20 mg by mouth every 12 hours. This is a TDD of 115 mg of oxycodone, so you adjust his OxyContin to 60 mg by mouth every 12 hours and leave the OxyIR at 15 mg by mouth every 2 hours as needed for additional pain.

A rule of thumb that is commonly followed in clinical practice for patients who continue to have pain despite their opioid regimen is as follows:[40]

- *For ongoing moderate-to-severe pain*, increase opioid TDD by 50% to 100%, regardless of starting dose.

- *For ongoing mild-moderate pain*, increase opioid TDD by 25% to 50%, regardless of starting dose.

- Short-acting, IR single-ingredient opioids (e.g., morphine, oxycodone, hydromorphone) can be safely dose-escalated every 2 hours.

- Long-acting, oral sustained-release opioids such as morphine, oxycodone, or hydromorphone, can be increased every 24 hours (does not include transdermal opioids and methadone, which are discussed in other chapters).

These guidelines assume the patient has normal renal and liver function; if this is *not* the case, dosage escalation recommendations should be reduced.

Wells and colleagues evaluated a variation of the above guidelines by designing a standard opioid titration order sheet for nurses to use to manage pain in ambulatory cancer patients.[41] The protocol was as follows:

- *For patients with controlled pain* (pain rated as 4 or less with four or fewer rescue doses per 24 hours, and meeting these criteria for 3 consecutive days), their long-acting opioid was adjusted by an amount equal to the daily rescue dose to decrease the frequency of short-acting opioid administration.

  - *Example:* MS Contin 30 mg by mouth every 12 hours plus morphine sulfate immediate release (MSIR) 10 mg every 2 hours as needed, using three doses per day for 3 days (pain controlled) → change to MS Contin 45 mg by mouth every 12 hours and continue MSIR 10 mg every 2 hours as needed.

- *Patients with moderate pain* (5–6) had their long-acting opioid increased to 125% of their average TDD (long-acting opioid plus short-acting opioid) over the past 3 days.

  - *Example:* OxyContin 40 mg by mouth every 12 hours plus OxyIR 15 mg every 2 hours, using three doses per day for 3 days (pain average 5–6) → change to OxyContin 80 mg by mouth every 12 hours plus OxyIR 20 mg by mouth every 2 hours as needed. The OxyContin 80 mg by mouth every 12 hours represents a 25% increase in the patient's total daily dose of oxycodone of 125 mg.

- ***Patients with severe pain*** (≥7) had their long-acting opioid increased to 150% of their average TDD (long-acting opioid plus short-acting opioid) over the past 3 days.

  - *Example:* Kadian 80 mg by mouth every 24 hours plus MSIR 10 mg every 2 hours, using two doses per day for 3 days (pain average ≥7) → change to Kadian 150 mg by mouth every 24 hours plus oral morphine 20 mg by mouth every 2 hours as needed. Kadian 150 mg by mouth per day represents a 50% increase in the patient's total daily dose of morphine of 100 mg by mouth.

Results from this study included 39 study nurse titration interventions in 17 patients over the 4-week trial. No adverse effects were observed in any of the dosage increases, and opioid toxicities, worst pain, usual pain, and pain-related distress declined from baseline to the end of the study.[41]

When adjusting the opioid dose, there are several additional issues the practitioner must consider. First, the Cleveland Clinic guidelines recommend *not* including rescue doses taken for volitional incident pain; volitional (predictable) incident pain is under the patient's control, so if the patient chooses not to participate in those pain-precipitating activities, then including the IR morphine taken in response to those activities may result in an overdose.[1] Second, we have all seen patients who seem to be *emotionally attached* to their short-acting opioid. You get the feeling you could increase their MS Contin to a million milligrams every 12 hours, and they would still feel the need to take their short-acting morphine. If this is the case or if the patient doesn't clearly understand the purpose and intended outcome of increasing the MS Contin, you may be better off leaving the regimen as is.

Even though this book is about the opioid math, one last thing must be addressed—WHY isn't the patient's pain improving, and is increasing the opioid really the best strategy? Not all pain is opioid-responsive; some types of pain don't respond to opioid therapy at all, and some respond partially. Most importantly, when the patient takes their rescue opioid, does the pain improve? Is the patient's functional status improving on this opioid regimen? If the patient's functional status is not improving, you could be barking up the wrong tree altogether and more opioid won't fix that. This is why the Centers for Disease Control and Prevention (CDC) proposed total daily oral morphine equivalent limits—for the practitioner to pause for a moment and say "Am I going down the right road here? Is this helping the patient meet his or her goals? Is the patient *doing* better on this opioid regimen, such that increasing would move us closer to the goal?" Granted, the CDC guidelines were written for chronic noncancer pain, but the principle applies to all pain situations.[42]

Parenteral Opioid Regimens

We can use the same strategies discussed above for patients receiving regular doses of an opioid by the IV or sub-Q route of administration. For example, around-the-clock and rescue doses (not counting those for volitional incident pain) given over the past 24 hours can be totaled, and the new every 4-hourly, or continuous infusion hourly dose determined accordingly. For moderate pain, this new 24-hour dose could be increased by 25%; for severe pain, the new 24-hour dose could be increased by 50%. For very acute severe pain, we can follow the dosing guidelines presented at the beginning of this chapter (Acute Severe Pain in the Opioid-Naïve Patient) and adjust the dose as appropriate. Again, please refer to Chapter 7 for a complete review of parenteral opioid administration and titration.

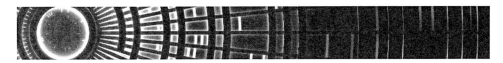

CASE 4.7

Opioid Dosage Escalation—Let's Practice One More!

HB is a 54-year-old woman who works as an administrative assistant to the Dean at the local community college. HB has significant osteoarthritis pain and was referred to you for evaluation of her analgesic regimen. She was receiving Percocet (7.5-mg oxycodone/325-mg acetaminophen), one tablet every 4 hours as needed (taking five tablets per day), gabapentin 300 mg by mouth three times daily, and Celebrex 200 mg by mouth daily. She told you that her pain rating ranged between 4 and 6 (on a 0–10 scale; 0 = no pain, 10 = worst imaginable pain) during the day while she was at work and when she took a walk in the evening with her dog. You decided to start her on OxyContin 20 mg by mouth every 12 hours, and keep the Percocet for breakthrough pain. After 2 weeks, she returns to your office and tells you that when she takes an additional three tablets of Percocet during the day she has an average pain rating of 2 or 3, which she finds acceptable. She asks you if there is a way she can stop taking the Percocet, however, because she doesn't like taking analgesics while at work.

She is taking oxycodone 40 mg per day from the long-acting OxyContin and an additional 22.5 mg from the Percocet, for a TDD of 62.5 mg. It would be reasonable to increase the OxyContin to 30 mg by mouth every 12 hours and keep the Percocet for breakthrough pain, although it is less likely she will need to take it during the workday.

DECREASING OPIOID DOSES

Just as practitioners need to understand how to titrate safely and efficiently opioid regimens *up*, they also need to understand how to taper safely and efficiently opioid regimens *down*. Why might a practitioner feel the need to reduce the opioid regimen? ***Bottom line—when the burden is greater than the benefit. Several examples include the following:***

- Taper opioids after surgery as acute postoperative pain improves.
- Patients in remission from cancer and opioids are no longer necessary or warranted.
- Introduce an opioid-sparing co-analgesic or use of a nonpharmacologic intervention (which could slowly provide benefit over time, such as exercise or physical therapy, or have a more immediately pain-relieving effect such as radiation or a nerve block).
- Patient may be experiencing adverse effects from the opioid regimen.
- Patient is not meeting his or her pain management goals with the opioid regimen.

- Patient has been receiving opioid therapy for a long period of time, and the practitioner would like to attempt opioid reduction.

- There are unexpected or confirmed results on urine drug testing.

- Patient using opioid to cope with anxiety or depression.

- There is confirmed criminal activity or diversion of opioid therapy.

Contemporary issues such as opioid abuse, misuse, diversion, and death compel this author to point out that "tapering opioids in pain patients is a very different process than detoxifying opioid addicts, and often takes a lot longer (several months versus several weeks) depending on the dose they begin with and the extent of their pain" per Dr. Forest Tennant.[43] In this editorial, Dr. Tennant cites a survey conducted through social media that reported over two-thirds of almost 2,000 patients say their opioid dose was decreased or stopped since the CDC released its opioid prescribing guidelines.[43,44] It is critically important that opioid reduction is done for a valid reason and be conducted in a safe fashion. The CDC guidelines did *not* imply or recommend automatically stopping opioids for all patients, but rather the decision should be based on the patient's pain relief and functional abilities.[42]

What guidance do we have for decreasing opioid dosage regimens? The Cleveland Clinic offers the following guidelines:[1]

- For patients with good pain control, but experiencing dose-related excessive side effects on an oral opioid regimen, it would be appropriate to reduce the around-the-clock opioid dose by 30%, but keep the rescue dose unchanged.

- For patients with continued pain but experiencing an opioid-induced adverse effect, consider adding a co-analgesic and reducing the around-the-clock opioid by 30% to 50%. Of course, switching to an entirely new opioid is also a consideration.

- If the patient undergoes a definitive pain-relieving procedure, it would be appropriate to reduce the regularly scheduled opioid dose by 50% immediately, and continue dose reductions every third day until the opioid is entirely discontinued. The rescue dose should remain available during this downward titration period for unexpected breakthrough pain.

Kral, Jackson, and Uritsky provide excellent guidance on opioid tapering for patients taking consistent opioid therapy (at least 60-mg morphine equivalent per day for at least 7 consecutive days) in a nonaddiction setting.[45]

A summary of their recommendations are as follows:

- ***Acute care setting***—Patients who were opioid naïve prior to surgery are generally discharged with a limited quantity of short-acting opioids, and generally self-taper as their pain resolves over the next few days to a week. The second group includes patients who had extensive surgery, or those who were opioid tolerant prior to surgery, and may require a tapering schedule postoperatively.

- ***Outpatient setting***—The authors describe two different likely patient populations. One group includes those who take low-dose short-acting opioids sparingly or sporadically (<8 tablets/day); this group will likely not require a formal tapering schedule. Patients who are receiving an oral long-acting opioid plus short-acting opioids for breakthrough pain on a daily basis will likely require a more structured tapering regimen to avoid withdrawal symptoms.

- *Complicated history*—The authors point out that the more complicated the patient's history is with opioid therapy, the more important it is to provide psychosocial support during the taper. Providing support and clear explanations of the process has been shown to be very beneficial when reducing or withdrawing opioid therapy.[46,47]

- *Consensus opinion*—Kral and colleagues reviewed all guidance published for recommendations on opioid tapering and concluded that there isn't one magical answer. The prime directive is to avoid symptoms of opioid withdrawal; but a slower, more individualized approach may be necessary for patients with significant comorbid conditions (e.g., cardiorespiratory disease, anxiety, psychological dependence on opioids).

- *Dosage formulations for tapering*—It is recommended that long-acting oral opioids be used to taper, by administering on a set schedule (e.g., every 8 or 12 hours). Do not use "as needed" short-acting opioids.

- *Dosing recommendations*—Recommendations for the actual taper are disparate ranging from reduce dose by 10% per week, up to 50% per week. For example, the American Pain Society/American Academy of Pain Medicine recommends a slow taper as 10% reduction weekly, or a more rapid taper which is a 25% and 50% reduction every few days (greater reduction at higher doses, slower taper with oral morphine equivalent of 60–80-mg daily).[48]

- *Emergency situations (bad weather or other circumstances)*—suggest the patient reduce his or her opioid dose by 25% every day or every other day. This may not entirely prevent withdrawal symptoms, but may reduce them. Opioid withdrawal won't kill someone (although it may feel that way!).

How can we tell if the taper is too rapid? Certainly, the first clue would be pain escalation. If the patient finds he or she is using the rescue medication consistently (if that is even permitted), it may be prudent to go back up on the dose of the regularly scheduled opioid a bit, and resume decreasing the opioid dose with a slower/lower taper. The second indication is the development of signs or symptoms of the opioid withdrawal syndrome, including any combination of the following: restlessness/irritability/agitation/dysphoric mood, abdominal pain/cramping, pupillary dilatation, lacrimation, rhinorrhea, piloerection (goosebumps), yawning, sneezing, anorexia, nausea, vomiting, and diarrhea.[49] There are several instruments used in clinical practice to diagnose physical dependence and assess opioid withdrawal, including the Objective Opioid Withdrawal Scale (OOWS), the Subjective Opioid Withdrawal Scale (SOWS), the Clinical Opiate Withdrawal Scale (COWS), the modified Finnegan scale, and the neonatal abstinence syndrome scoring card. These instruments can be viewed at https://www.ncbi.nlm.nih.gov/books/NBK143183/.[50] The COWS scale, for example, assigns a numerical rating to resting pulse rate, sweating, restlessness, pupil size, bone or joint aches, runny nose or tearing, gastrointestinal upset, tremor, yawning, anxiety, or irritability, and gooseflesh skin. When tapering opioids, it is probably not necessary to rate the patient using one of these scales, but instead to be mindful of the presenting symptoms of opioid withdrawal.

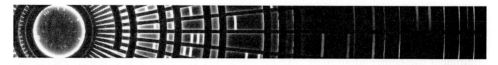

CASE 4.7

Opioid Dosage Reduction

EK is a 72-year-woman with chronic back pain, who has failed several nonopioid analgesics, and was recently started on morphine 5 mg by mouth every 4 hours. She was eventually titrated to MS Contin 30 mg by mouth every 8 hours, but she complained that this made her too sleepy and nauseated. She was switched to OxyContin 30 mg by mouth every 12 hours with OxyIR 10 mg by mouth every 2 hours as needed for breakthrough pain, but the sedation and nausea have persisted. Several antiemetics and methylphenidate have been tried with minimal success. You have decided to reduce her opioid regimen to see if this helps alleviate her complaints.

Using the guideline described above, it is worth reducing the regularly scheduled opioid by 30%. When you reduced the OxyContin to 20 mg by mouth every 12 hours (keeping the OxyIR 10 mg by mouth every 2 hours as needed), her nausea was reduced to an acceptable level and the sedation completely cleared, returning to her normal level of alertness. EK is content with this regimen, and she knows she can use the OxyIR if she has a flare in the pain.

This has certainly been an action-packed chapter! You've been putting out fires all over the place! We've discussed how to manage acute severe pain in an opioid-naïve patient, how to perform dose-finding for a regularly scheduled opioid regimen, how to design an opioid regimen for breakthrough pain, and how to increase and decrease opioid regimens. You might want to take a nap before you go on to the next chapter!

PRACTICE PROBLEMS

P4.1: Acute Severe Pain in an Opioid-Naïve Patient

JK is a 62-year-old woman with adenocarcinoma of the descending colon, who presented to the ED several days before her scheduled colon resection surgery complaining of sudden-onset, severe supra-clavicular swelling and pain. JK takes only an occasional acetaminophen and is not receiving opioids. She rates this pain as the worst imaginable pain possible (she says it's "at least" 10 out of 10), and states it started abruptly at this intensity. The pain started about an hour and a half ago, and her physician directed her to the ED. JK tells you she has a history of itching when given morphine, but she has taken hydromorphone successfully in the past. How would you go about controlling JK's pain? What would you monitor?

P4.2: Switching from an IR to Sustained-Release Oral Opioid

WM is an 82-year-old woman living in a long-term care facility, with advanced osteo-arthritis pain that has made it difficult for her to ambulate. Nonopioid medications do not provide any degree of significant relief; however, she has responded to 2.5-mg oral oxycodone in the past. WM despises taking medication, and says "if I can't take it just once a day, I'm not going to take it." When WM was given 5 mg of oxycodone, it made her very somnolent, leaving her fairly distrustful of opioids in general. However, WM complains constantly about her persistent pain. WM also has mild hepatic impairment. What do you recommend?

P4.3: Calculating Oral Opioid Rescue Doses

LP is a 64-year-old man with end-stage lung cancer. He is receiving MS Contin 200 mg by mouth every 12 hours and naproxen 500 mg by mouth every 12 hours, as well as Percocet (5-mg oxycodone/325-mg acetaminophen), one to two tablets every 4 hours as needed for breakthrough pain. LP tells you that when he experiences unanticipated, unprovoked breakthrough pain, he takes two Percocet tablets, but they are not particularly effective (bringing pain rating down from an 8 to about a 6). LP is growing weaker and is now experiencing shortness of breath occasionally as well. Your formulary has IR oxycodone, morphine, and hydromorphone available. What do you recommend?

P4.4: Switching from OTFC Lozenges to FBTs

FM is a 24-year-old man with a glioblastoma, receiving methadone 20 mg by mouth every 8 hours around the clock for persistent pain. He had been using an OTFC lozenge (Actiq), 600 mcg as needed for spontaneous breakthrough pain. He was originally able to use the lozenge correctly, continuously moving it through his cheeks coating the mucosal tissues to optimize absorption giving him good pain relief. Now, however, he has grown too weak to do so, and his pain relief from each lozenge is not as great. You've heard about FBTs (Fentora), which do not require this kind of physical manipulation. The prescriber is agreeable and asks what the starting dose should be, because she heard that there is no consistent correlation between the around-the-clock opioid and the starting dose of Fentora. What do you recommend?

P4.5: Parenteral Opioid Dosage Escalation

QN is 47-year-old woman with end-stage breast cancer admitted to your inpatient hospice unit for pain control. She was taking three or four Lortab tablets (5-mg hydrocodone bitartrate/325-mg acetaminophen) per day and was complaining of moderate-to-severe pain. On admission, she was switched to parenteral hydromorphone and is now receiving 4 mg every 4 hours with 2 mg every 2 hours for breakthrough pain. QN has been getting approximately five extra doses of the 2-mg hydromorphone, and her pain persists between a 7 and an 8 (on a 0–10 scale; 0 = no pain, 10 = worst imaginable pain). She has been examined and her complaint carefully assessed, and you do not feel any additional co-analgesics would provide additional relief. How should you adjust her parenteral hydromorphone? Assuming this does the trick, what dose of oral hydromorphone should you send her home on assuming she is NOT using the breakthrough hydromorphone (I know, tricky, asking you to do drug math from previous chapters!)?

P4.6: Opioid Dosage Reduction

RR is a 49-year-old man diagnosed with pancreatic cancer. He has failed chemotherapy and has been referred to hospice. He is complaining of severe pain, which he describes as a sharp pain between shoulder blades that radiates straight through his back, as well as pain in both the right and left upper quadrant. His opioid regimen was increased over a week to MS Contin 90 mg by mouth every 12 hours with minimal relief. The physician has decided to send RR for a celiac plexus block. Over the 12 to 24 hours after receiving the block, RR cries "It's a miracle—the pain is gone! I have my life back. Now I don't need this morphine!" You interrupt RR as he's doing the happy dance to inform him that he cannot stop the morphine cold, because it would most likely cause symptoms of opioid withdrawal. How should you taper RR off this morphine regimen?

Could I Get That to Go, Please? Bottom Line It for Me . . .

▶ Severe, acute pain in an opioid-naïve patient must be treated promptly and aggressively. As an example, Cleveland Clinic guidelines recommend morphine 1 mg IV every minute for up to 10 minutes, followed by a 5-minute respite; repeat cycle two more times as necessary. Importantly, the therapeutic endpoint is a 2 to 4 drop in pain, *not* complete pain relief (because you're dose-stacking).

▶ The NCCN guidelines for treating pain in adult cancer patients provide guidance on managing acute pain in the opioid-tolerant patient. Administer 10% to 20% of the average 24-hour total of opioid used, and reassess pain in 15 minutes (if IV) or 60 minutes (if oral). Repeat as appropriate, and adjust opioid regimen accordingly per patient response.

▶ Patients often start opioid therapy with an "as needed" short-acting opioid. If the patient is using this opioid regularly, determine the 24-hour average dose and convert to the long-acting oral formulation of the same opioid to provide equivalent pain relief.

▶ Breakthrough pain is described as a superimposed pain in a patient receiving a stable opioid regimen and baseline pain that is generally controlled. A precipitating event is not required to designate breakthrough pain, but helps to distinguish the breakthrough pain as spontaneous (which could be predictable or unpredictable) or incident type.

▶ If the patient is receiving an oral long-acting opioid, the same opioid may be made available as the unmodified, short-acting formulation, dosed as 10% to 20% of the total daily scheduled opioid dose (e.g., for morphine, oxycodone, hydrocodone, hydromorphone).

▶ TIRF products may be used for breakthrough cancer pain and may match the temporal characteristics of the breakthrough pain better than an oral opioid, and is preferred by patients. These formulations tend to be more expensive and less likely to be covered by insurance. There is no equianalgesic conversion available for the TIRF products.

▶ When escalating opioid dosage regimens, one strategy is to use the short-acting opioid (the "prn" dose), titrating to good pain control. Add the 24-hour opioid total dose and offer as the scheduled, long-acting opioid. Provide an adequate dose of the short-acting opioid for breakthrough pain.

▶ For ongoing moderate-to-severe pain, increase total daily opioid dose by 50% to 100%; for ongoing mild-to-moderate pain, increase total daily opioid dose by 25% to 50%.

▶ Short-acting, IR single-ingredient opioids (e.g., morphine, oxycodone, hydromorphone) can be dose escalated every 2 hours.

▶ Long-acting, oral sustained-release opioids (e.g., morphine, oxycodone, hydromorphone) can generally be increased every 24 hours.

▶ Several opioid tapering recommendations are available, reducing TDD from 10% to 50% per week. Patients should receive psychosocial support and be closely monitored for pain recurrence and symptoms of opioid withdrawal.

REFERENCES

1. Walsh D, Rivera NL, Davis MP, et al. Strategies for pain management: Cleveland Clinic Foundation guidelines for opioid dosing for cancer pain. *Support Cancer Ther.* 2004;1(3):157-164.

2. Mercadante S. Opioid titration in cancer pain: a critical review. *Eur J Pain.* 2007;11:823-830.

3. Caraceni A, Hanks G, Kaasa S, et al. Use of opioid analgesics in the treatment of cancer pain: Evidence-based recommendations from the EAPC. *Lancet Oncology.* 2012;13:e58-e68.

4. Davis MP, Weissman DE, Arnold RM. Opioid dose titration for severe cancer pain: a systematic evidence-based review. *J Palliat Med.* 2004;7(3):462-468.

5. Davis MP, Lasheen W, Gamier P. Practical guide to opioids and their complications in managing cancer pain: what oncologists need to know. *Oncology.* 2007;21(10):1229–1238.

6. National Comprehensive Cancer Network. NCCN Clinical Practice Guidelines in Oncology. Adult Cancer Pain, v.2.2017. https://www.nccn.org/professionals/physician_gls/pdf/pain.pdf. Accessed February 21, 2018.

7. Klepstad P, Kaasa S, Jystad A, et al. Immediate- or sustained-release morphine for dose finding during start of morphine to cancer patients: a randomized, double-blind trial. *Pain.* 2003;101:193-198.

8. Portenoy RK, Hagen NA. Breakthrough pain: definition, prevalence and characteristics. *Pain.* 1990;41:273-281.

9. Mercadante S, Portenoy RK. Breakthrough cancer pain: twenty-five years of study. *Pain.* 2016;157(12): 2657-2663.

10. Portenoy RK, Bennett DS, Rauck R, et al. Prevalence and characteristics of breakthrough pain in opioid-treated patients with chronic noncancer pain. *J Pain.* 2006;7:583-591.

11. Portenoy RK, Payne D, Jacobsen P. Breakthrough pain: characteristics and impact in patients with cancer pain. *Pain.* 1999;81:81:129-134.

12. Fine P, Busch MA. Characterization of breakthrough pain by hospice patients and their caregivers. *J Pain Symptom Manage.* 1998;16:179-183.

13. Zeppetella G, O'Doherty CA, Collins S. Prevalence and characteristics of breakthrough pain in cancer patients admitted to a hospice. *J Pain Symptom Manage.* 2000;20:87-92.

14. Gagnon B, Lawlor P, Mancini IS, et al. The impact of delirium on the circadian distribution of break-through analgesia in advanced cancer patients. *J Pain Symptom Manage.* 2001;22:826-833.

15. Bennett DS, Simon S, Brennan M, et al. Prevalence and characteristics of breakthrough pain in patients receiving opioids for chronic back pain in pain specialty clinics. *J Opioid Manage.* 2007;3(2):101-106.

16. Vellucci R, Mediati RD, Gasperoni S, et al. Assessment and treatment of breakthrough cancer pain: from theory to clinical practice. *J Pain Research* 2017;10:2147-2155.

17. Mercadante S, Aielli F, Adile C, et al. Fentanyl pectin nasal spray versus OM in doses proportional to the basal opioid regimen for the management of breakthrough cancer pain: a comparative study. *J Pain Symptom Manage.* 2016;52:27-34.

18. Bhatnager S, Devi S, Vinod NK, et al. Safety and efficacy of oral transmucosal fentanyl citrate compared to morphine sulphate immediate release tablet in management of breakthrough cancer pain. *Indian J Pall Care.* 2014;20(3):182-187.

19. Webster LR, Slevin KA, Narayana A, et al. Fentanyl buccal tablet compared with immediate-release oxycodone for the management of breakthrough pain in opioid-tolerant patients with chronic cancer and noncancer pain: a randomized, double-blind, crossover study followed by a 12-week open-label phase to evaluate patient outcomes. *Pain Med.* 2013;14:1332-1345.

20. Ashburn MA, Slevin KA, Messina J, et al. The efficacy and safety of fentanyl buccal tablet compared with immediate-release oxycodone for the management of breakthrough pain in opioid-tolerant patients with chronic pain. *Anesth Analg.* 2011;112(3):693-702.

21. Bostrom E, Simonsson USH, Hammarlund-Udenaes M. In vivo blood-brain barrier transport of oxycodone in the rat: indications for active influx and implications for pharmacokinetics/pharmacodynamics. *Drug Metab Dispos.* 2006;34:1624-1631.

22. Bostrom E, Hammarlund-Udenaes J, Simonsson USH. Blood-brain barrier transport helps to explain discrepancies in in vivo potency between oxycodone and morphine. *Anesthesiology* 2008;108:495-505.

23. Fallon M, Reale C, Davies A, et al. Efficacy and safety of fentanyl pectin nasal spray compared with immediate-release morphine sulfate tablets in the treatment of breakthrough cancer pain: a multicenter, randomized, controlled, double-blind, double-dummy multiple-crossover study. *J Support Oncol.* 2011;9:224-231.

24. Davis MP. Are there cost benefits to fentanyl for breakthrough pain? *J Pain Symptom Manage.* 2012;44(#):e1-e2.

25. Davies AN, Dickman A, Reid C, et al. The management of cancer-related breakthrough pain: Recommendations of a task group of the Science Committee of the Association for Palliative Medicine of Great Britain and Ireland. *Eur J Pain.* 2009;13:331-338.

26. Green E, Zwaal C, Beals C, et al. Cancer-related pain management: A report of evidence-based recommendations to guide practice. *Clin J Pain.* 2010;26;449-462.

27. Mercadante S, Intravaia G, Villari P, et al. Intravenous morphine for breakthrough (episodic-) pain in an acute palliative care unit: a confirmatory study. *J Pain Symptom Manage.* 2008;35:307-313.

28. Mercadante S, Villari P, Ferrera P, et al. Transmucosal fentanyl vs. intravenous morphine in doses proportional to basal opioid regimen for episodic-breakthrough pain. *Br J Cancer.* 2007;96:1828-1833.

29. Mercadante S, Villari P, Ferrera P, et al. The use of opioids for breakthrough pain in acute palliative care unit by using doses proportional to opioid basal regimen. *Clin J Pain.* 2010;26:306-309.

30. Brant JM, Rodgers BB, Gallagher E, et al. Breakthrough cancer pain. *Clin J Oncol Nurs.* 2017;21(3 Suppl):71-80.

31. Zeppetella G, Ribeiro MDC. Opioids for the management of breakthrough (episodic) pain in cancer patients. Cochrane Database Syst Rev. 2006; I1, Art. No.: CD004311. DOI: 10.1002/14651858.CD004311.pub2.

32. Actiq Prescribing Information. http://www.actiq.com/pdf/ActiqDigitalPlandMedGuide.pdf. Accessed February 21, 2018.

33. Fentora Prescribing Information. http://www.fentora.com/pdfs/pdf100_prescribing_info.pdf. Accessed February 21, 2018.

34. Abstral Prescribing Information. https://www.accessdata.fda.gov/drugsatfda_docs/label/2014/022510s013lbl.pdf. Accessed February 21, 2018.

35. Subsys Prescribing Information. https://www.subsys.com/assets/subsys/client_files/files/PrescribingInfo.pdf. Accessed February 21, 2018.

36. Onsolis Prescribing Information. https://www.accessdata.fda.gov/drugsatfda_docs/label/2009/022266s000lbl.pdf. Accessed February 21, 2018.

37. Lazanda Prescribing Information. http://www.lazanda.com/sites/all /themes/lazanda/pdfs/Lazanda_Prescribing_Information.pdf. Accessed February 21, 2018.

38. Healio HemOnc Today. FDA warns doctors about dentanyl buccal. https://www.healio.com/hematology-oncology/practice-management/news/print/hemonc-today/%7B8665a1c1-b1aa-4013-a9a3-f9320ac6ec39%7D/fda-warns-doctors-about-fentanyl-buccal. Accessed February 22, 2018.

39. Mercadante S, Villari P, Ferrera P, et al. Optimization of opioid therapy for preventing incident pain associated with bone metastases. *J Pain Symptom Manage.* 2004;28:505-510.

40. Weissman DE. Fast facts and concepts #20 opioid dose escalation. Palliative Care Network of Wisconsin Website. https://www.mypcnow.org/blank-it0kw. Updated May 2015. Accessed February 22, 2018.

41. Wells N, Murphy B, Douglas S, et al. Establishing the safety and efficacy of an opioid titration protocol. *J Opioid Manage.* 2005;1(1):41-48.

42. Dowell D, Haegerich TM, Chou R. CDC guideline for prescribing opioids for chronic pain—United States, 2016. *MMWR Recomm Rep.* 2016;65(No. RR-1):1-49.

43. Tennant F. A plea for proper opioid tapering. *Practical Pain Management.* 2017;17(6). https://www.practicalpainmanagement.com/treatments/pharmacological/opioids/plea-proper-opioid-tapering. February 22, 2018.

44. Anson P. Survey: opioids reduced or stopped for most patients. Pain News Network website. https://www.painnewsnetwork.org/stories/2016/8/4/survey-opioids-stopped-or-reduced-for-most-patients. August 4, 2016. Accessed February 22, 2018.

45. Kral LA, Jackson K, Uritsky TJ. A practical guide to opioid tapering. *Mental Health Clin.* 2015;5(3):102-108.

46. Matthias MS, Johnson NNL, Shields CG, et al. I'm not gonna pull the rug out from under you: Patient-provider communication about opioid tapering. *J Pain.* 2017;18(11):1365-1373.

47. Sullivan MD, Turner JA, DiLodovico C, et al. Prescription opioid taper support for outpatients with chronic pain: A randomized controlled trial. *J Pain.* 2017;18(3):308-318.

48. Chou R, Fanciullo GJ, Fine PG, et al. Clinical guidelines for the use of chronic opioid therapy in chronic noncancer pain. *J Pain.* 2009;10(2):113-130.

49. Prommer E. Opioid withdrawal: creating more problems. *J Pain Symptom Manage.* 2007;33(2):114-115.

50. NCBI Bookshelf. Guidelines for the Psychosocially Assisted Pharmacological Treatment of Opioid Dependence. Geneva, Switzerland: World Health Organization; 2009. https://www.ncbi.nlm.nih.gov/books/NBK143185/. Accessed February 22, 2018.

SOLUTIONS TO PRACTICE PROBLEMS

P4.1: Establish IV access and administer hydromorphone 0.2 mg every minute for 10 minutes. The prescriber should be bedside monitoring the patient's sensorium (level of alertness/sedation), respiratory rate, and pain rating. After 10 injections, the prescriber should wait 5 minutes and continue to assess patient. If pain is still not controlled after the 5-minute respite, continue administering hydromorphone 0.2 mg every minute for up to 10 additional minutes while monitoring the therapeutic and potential response. This cycle can be repeated one more time (for a total of 30 doses of 0.2-mg hydromorphone); if pain still is not relieved, the patient should be further evaluated as to the cause of the pain. In this case, after controlling JK's pain subsequent imaging and cytology of the lesion showed it to be a metastasis to the right clavicle that resulted in this pathological fracture.

P4.2: Clearly WM would benefit from around-the-clock opioid therapy given her complaint of persistent pain. She is sensitive to the effects of opioids (e.g., 5-mg oral oxycodone made her very somnolent), and she doesn't want to take medication frequently. WM has almost tied your hands—but you're smarter than the average bear, and you recommend Kadian 10 mg by mouth once daily. This is the lowest strength sustained-release oral morphine product available (equivalent to 1.7-mg oral morphine every 4 hours). You could also recommend she continue the 2.5-mg oral oxycodone if needed (although it's unlikely she'll take it). Given WM's history of mild hepatic impairment, it would be prudent to wait at least 1 week before considering a dosage increase. Because WM probably won't take the "as needed" oral oxycodone, it would be best to assess her complaint of pain and her functional status after 1 week on the Kadian 10 mg once daily, and if she is tolerating it well but there is room for improvement, recommend increasing to Kadian 20 mg by mouth once daily (the equivalent of 3.3 mg every 4 hours). Don't forget the bowels, or WM will *really* get cranky!

P4.3: Let's consider why two Percocet tablets aren't giving LP sufficient relief. He is taking 400 mg per day of oral morphine. Ten to 20% of this would be 40 to 80 mg of oral morphine as breakthrough. This is approximately equivalent to 32 to 64 mg of oral oxycodone. Two Percocet (5-mg oxycodone/325-mg acetaminophen) tablets only provide 10-mg oral oxycodone. Sherlock Holmes rides again—it's not enough opioid! Your formulary options for IR oral opioids include morphine, oxycodone, and hydromorphone. We have no reason to suspect that LP wouldn't respond to morphine (because it's working for the persistent pain), plus morphine has a very strong track record in treating dyspnea, which LP is starting to experience. An appropriate dose of rescue morphine would be 40 to 80 mg of oral morphine available as 15- and 30-mg tablets, or a variety of oral solutions. You decide to use the oral concentrated solution, 20 mg/mL, and recommend a starting dose of 40 mg (2 mL) for breakthrough pain or dyspnea. If LP becomes too weak to swallow the oral concentrated solution, it can be instilled in the buccal cavity (perhaps 1 mL in each side of the buccal cavity).

P4.4: The prescriber is correct that there is no consistent correlation between the dose of the regularly scheduled opioid and the appropriate dose for the FBT; however, we do have dosing guidelines to switch from OTFC to FBT (see Table 4-4). FM was using a 600-mg OTFC lozenge, and the recommended dose to convert to FBT is 200 mcg. The prescriber orders six 200-mcg FBTs with instructions to insert one tablet in between the cheek and gum when the patient experiences breakthrough pain. If the pain has not resolved 30 minutes later, FM may administer a second 200-mcg FBT. If this is not sufficient, FM must wait 4 hours before using FBT again, at which time he can use two 200-mcg FBTs (one on each side of the mouth in the buccal cavity). If 400 mcg of FBT is the appropriate dose, the prescriber should order the 400-mcg FBT for FM.

P4.5: The first thing to do is calculate QN's TDD of IV hydromorphone. She is getting 4-mg every 4 hours, plus five doses per day of the 2-mg dose, for a TDD of 34 mg. She is rating her pain as severe (7 or 8); therefore, it would be appropriate to increase her TDD by 50%, which would be 51 mg. If we continue giving the hydromorphone every 4 hours, this is 8.5 mg. We would recommend 8-mg hydromorphone IV every 4 hours with 4 mg every 2 hours as needed for breakthrough pain.

If the 8 mg every 4 hours controls QN's pain, this is a TDD of 48 mg. Consulting our Equianalgesic Opioid Dosing table (Table 1-1) we see that 2-mg parenteral hydromorphone is approximately equivalent to 5-mg oral hydromorphone. Therefore, her TDD of oral hydromorphone would be 120 mg, or 20 mg every 4 hours (with 10 mg every 2 hours as needed for breakthrough pain).

P4.6: Using the guideline presented in this chapter, we can reduce RR's morphine dose by up to 50% every third day. On day 1, we can reduce it to MS Contin 45 mg by mouth every 12 hours. On day 4, we can reduce it to MS Contin 30 mg by mouth every 12 hours. On day 7, we can reduce it to MS Contin 15 mg by mouth every 12 hours, then discontinue the MS Contin on day 10. Meanwhile, we will continue his oral morphine solution 20 mg by mouth every 2 hours as needed for breakthrough pain, or even lower the dose as the days pass. As the week progresses, you would monitor RR for recurrent pain (and encourage use of the rescue dose) and for signs or symptoms of opioid withdrawal. Don't forget to reduce or discontinue any bowel regimen RR is receiving when you discontinue the opioid (if appropriate).

CHAPTER 5

Transdermal and Parenteral Fentanyl Dosage Calculations and Conversions

INTRODUCTION

Fentanyl is a synthetic phenylpiperidine derivative with pharmacologic properties similar to morphine, hydromorphone, oxycodone, and other opioids. Fentanyl has potent mu-opioid receptor activity and some activity at the δ- and κ-opioid receptors as well. Important differences about fentanyl include its high degree of potency (about 75–100 times more potent than morphine on an mg-to-mg basis), and high lipid solubility (far greater than morphine). Fentanyl has a large volume of distribution (approximately 6 L/kg) and is rapidly distributed from the plasma into highly vascularized compartments and eventually redistributed to muscle and fat tissue.[1] The lipophilic nature of fentanyl also facilitates rapid diffusion across the blood-brain barrier, resulting in a quick onset of action once the drug is absorbed from the administration site.[1] The transfer half-life from the systemic circulation to the central nervous system (CNS) is 4.7 to 6.6 minutes.[2]

OBJECTIVES

After reading this chapter and completing all practice problems, the participant will be able to:

1. Describe the pharmacokinetics of fentanyl, and variables that can influence transdermal and parenteral dosing.

2. Recommend an appropriate dose of transdermal fentanyl when switching from other opioids, including rescue opioid dosing. The participant will be able to describe the appropriate timing of this conversion.

3. Recommend a strategy for switching from transdermal fentanyl to another opioid regimen, including dosing and appropriate timing.

4. Describe how to transition between parenteral fentanyl and transdermal fentanyl.

Practitioners commonly think of parenteral fentanyl as fast onset and short acting and morphine as slower onset and longer acting, but actually fentanyl and morphine have similar elimination half-lives (2–4 hours for morphine and 3–7 hours for fentanyl).[3] Fentanyl, as described above, is a *fast-in, fast-out* drug, crossing the blood-brain barrier quickly in a bidirectional fashion. Morphine, however, is described as a *slow-in, slow-out* drug when crossing the blood-brain barrier.[3]

As described in the Equianalgesic Opioid Dosing table in Chapter 1, when fentanyl is administered as a single intravenous (IV) bolus, it has a redistribution-limited short duration of action. However, with prolonged exposure to fentanyl (multiple boluses or continuous infusion), elimination is clearance limited.[4] With repeated doses or continuous infusion, the duration of effect of fentanyl is longer than that seen with a single IV bolus due to accumulation in the muscle and fat tissue compartments.[1] Fentanyl is extensively metabolized by the cytochrome P450 isoenzyme system, primarily by the CYP3A4 enzyme.[4] Predictably, fentanyl is subject to altered serum concentrations when co-administered with a CYP3A4 enzyme inducer or inhibitor.

Because fentanyl is a small and highly lipophilic molecule with low ionization and has the ability to pass through cellular barriers reaching the capillary bed, it is well suited for absorption across biological membranes (e.g., transdermal and transmucosal), demonstrating bioavailability ranging from 50% to 90%.[1,3]

Because of these properties, fentanyl is available in several dosage formulations and may be administered by the following routes for a variety of pain-related indications:

- *Parenteral*—Fentanyl may be given by IV injection, IV infusion, subcutaneous (sub-Q) infusion, or intramuscular (IM) injection (although we already agreed that an IM analgesic is an oxymoron, and this practice is discouraged). It is used parenterally pre-operatively, intra-operatively, and postoperatively, and is occasionally used for the management of severe acute and chronic pain in other clinical situations. Preservative-free fentanyl has been injected or infused epidurally or intrathecally by specialist practitioners.

- *Transdermal*—Transdermal fentanyl patches (TDF; also referred to as *fentanyl transdermal system*) have been available for many years; this formulation relies on passive diffusion [drug moving from an area of higher concentration (the transdermal patch) to an area of lower concentration (the skin)]. This formulation is indicated for the management of pain in opioid-tolerant patients, severe enough to require daily, around-the-clock, long-term opioid treatment.

- *Buccal* and *transmucosal*—As discussed in Chapter 4, these are immediate-release dosage forms approved to treat breakthrough pain in cancer patients.

- *Fentanyl iontophoretic transdermal system*—This system had been developed for the short-term management of acute postoperative pain in adults and was briefly on the market. The drug was delivered on patient demand, with an electrical charge driving the drug into the skin. The manufacturer voluntarily withdrew this product from the market in June 2017.[5]

Lötsch and colleagues provide an excellent diagram (Figure 5-1) and explanation of the differences in the sites of fentanyl absorption relative to the various routes of nonparenteral fentanyl administration. They state, "The actions of fentanyl are related to its concentrations at opioid receptors expressed within its main effect site, the CNS. Except for intranasal administration, whereby fentanyl is also directly delivered to the CNS, the extent and time course of its effects are a function of the time course of its plasma concentrations, $C_p(t)$."[2] They conclude by pointing out that the plasma concentration of fentanyl is influenced by the rate of fentanyl influx and the rate of fentanyl disposition (metabolism and excretion).

This chapter will focus on conversion calculations involving switching to and from TDF, and conversion calculations involving parenteral fentanyl.

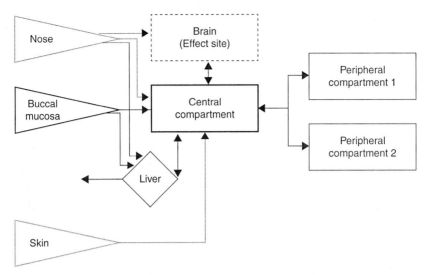

Figure 5-1. Schematic presentation of differences in the sites of fentanyl absorption in relation to different routes of nonintravenous fentanyl administration.

Source: Reprinted with permission of Springer Nature from Lötsch J, Walter C, Parnham MJ, et al. Pharmacokinetics of nonintravenous formulations of fentanyl. *Clinical Pharmacokinetics*. 2013;52:28.

TRANSDERMAL FENTANYL

Transdermal fentanyl patches were designed to provide long-lasting opioid therapy (3 days) for patients with stable chronic pain. Because fentanyl has a low molecular weight and high solubility in both fat and water, the drug is a good candidate for transdermal administration.

There are five commonly used patch strengths currently available:

- 12 mcg/hr (actually it delivers 12.5 mcg/hr, but is referred to as 12 mcg/hr to avoid a medication error by mistaking the intended dose to be 125 mcg/hr)
- 25 mcg/hr
- 50 mcg/hr
- 75 mcg/hr
- 100 mcg/hr

A generic pharmaceutical manufacturer also makes three "intermediate dosage strengths" of transdermal fentanyl: 37.5 mcg/hr, 62.5 mcg/hr, and 87.5 mcg/hr. The dose is determined by the surface area of the patch; therefore, the patches are larger as the dose increases.[6]

Pharmacokinetics

Transdermal fentanyl is formulated as both a gel-containing reservoir and a drug-in-adhesive matrix patch (see *Sidebar: Transdermal Fentanyl Patch Formulations*). Manufacturer's guidelines state that the TDF patch should be applied to an intact, non-irritated and nonirradiated flat skin surface such as the chest, back, flank, or upper arm. For young children or patients with cognitive impairment, consider applying TDF to the upper back to minimize risk of inappropriate patch removal. If necessary, hair should be clipped (not shaved) at the site of application. Fentanyl is absorbed through the skin, producing a drug depot in the upper skin layers, and then diffusing into the systemic circulation (see Figure 5-2). On average, minimally effective blood concentrations of fentanyl are seen in about 12 hours, and the time to maximum concentration is approximately 36 hours.[2,6] Approximately 3 to 6 days may be needed to ultimately reach steady-state serum concentrations with TDF.

It is important to recognize that transdermal drug delivery is fraught with variability from patient to patient. Even when considering any given patient, there are variables that can affect fentanyl absorption. For example, an elevated body temperature [e.g., 40°C (104°F)] increases fentanyl absorption by about one-third.[10,11] So, when you hear that a patient has been tucked into bed "snug as a bug in a rug," you might want to think about increased body temperature. This also applies to use of electric blankets, heating pads, tanning beds, sunbathing, hot baths, hot tubs, saunas, and heated water beds.[12] In one recent case from my practice, a patient on TDF for residual hip pain after a nasty construction accident (who insisted he had to apply his

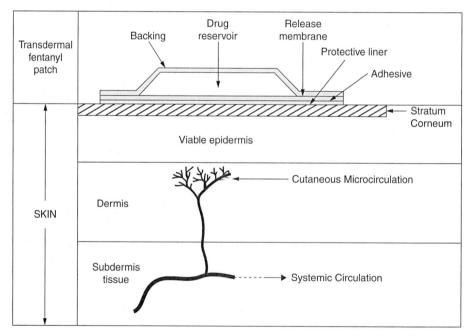

Figure 5-2. Fentanyl entering the systemic circulation. When TDF is initially applied, there is a lag time to benefit by a minimum of 12 hours as the drug makes its way out of the patch by passive diffusion, through the stratum corneum and epidermis to the dermis layer where it enters the cutaneous microcirculation, then to the subdermal tissue, and eventually into the systemic circulation. The time to maximum concentration is about 36 hours. Conversely, when the TDF patch is removed, it still takes hours for the serum fentanyl concentration to fall as there is already a significant amount of fentanyl on its way to the systemic circulation (e.g., in the epidermis, dermis, and subdermal tissue moving to the systemic circulation). It takes about 24 hours to see a 50% reduction in serum fentanyl levels after removing the source of fentanyl—the transdermal patch.[2,6,11]

Source: Adapted with permission from Varvel JR, Shafer SL, Hwang SS, et al. Absorption characteristics of transdermally administered fentanyl. *Anesthesiology.* 1989;70:928-934.

TRANSDERMAL FENTANYL PATCH FORMULATIONS

The first TDF product on the market was the branded product, Duragesic. This formulation is a gel-containing reservoir and shown in the diagram:

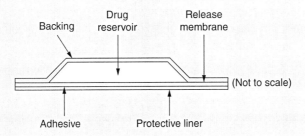

This formulation results in significant interindividual variability with 60% to 86% of the fentanyl absorbed in most patients. Conversely, 28% to 84.4% of the original fentanyl content remains in the patch after 3 days use. Subsequent to this initial formulation of TDF, newer formulations use a drug-in adhesive matrix layer (see below). These two formulations have been shown to be bioequivalent.[7-9]

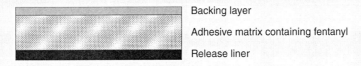

patch directly over the site of the pain, and refused to believe me when I said the drug didn't actually get sucked right into his hip) accidentally discovered the "bonus dose" effect of applying a heating pad directly over the patch. Obviously, this practice should be strictly discouraged, and I advised the patient accordingly after I recovered from my faint. There have been several fatalities reported due to nonadherence to this warning.

Another variable that is frequently talked about is the use of TDF in cachectic, low body weight patients. Many practitioners report that cachectic patients do not respond as well as expected to TDF and may report little or no improvement in pain when increasing the patch strength. Heiskanen and colleagues demonstrated lower plasma fentanyl concentrations at 48 and 72 hours in cachectic patients (mean body mass index [BMI] 16 kg/m^2) as compared to normal weight patients (mean BMI 23 kg/m^2).[13] Nomura and colleagues evaluated 19 patients being converted from continuous IV infusion to TDF, reporting on pharmacokinetics and pharmacodynamics observed in the switch.[14] As a secondary outcome, they sought to identify an association between serum albumin and the absorption of fentanyl from the transdermal patch. This secondary outcome showed the dose-adjusted serum fentanyl concentrations at 9, 12, 15, 18, and 24 hours were significantly lower in patients with low albumin (median 2.9 g/dL), as compared to patients with a normal albumin (medial 3.7 g/dL).[14] Davis provides comment on Nomura and colleagues' findings by explaining that fentanyl is 70% bound to protein, primarily albumin. Albumin is low in cachectic patients and reduced in cancer and inflammatory disorders due to "transcapillary leak into subcutaneous and muscle interstitial spaces."[15] Davis explains that transcapillary leak of albumin can increase up to 300% in patients with cancer cachexia, dramatically increasing the sequestration of albumin in the extravascular interstitial spaces. This interstitial albumin may bind to fentanyl and reduce plasma absorption of fentanyl.[15] Most importantly, if a cachectic patient has not responded to recent dosage increases in TDF, it may be wise to use the *last* effective patch strength on which to base conversion calculations and be liberal with rescue-opioid dosing (more on this later).

Another important pharmaco-kinetic parameter to consider when doing opioid conversion calculations involving TDF is how slowly the fentanyl serum concentration falls after patch removal. After removal, serum fentanyl levels decrease gradually, falling about 50% in the subsequent 20 to 27 hours.[11] Obviously it takes longer for the fentanyl serum concentration to fall after patch removal as compared to ending an IV infusion of fentanyl, because fentanyl continues to be absorbed from the depot in the upper layers of the skin, continuing to diffuse into the systemic circulation even after the patch is removed. Knowledge of this pharmacokinetic parameter is of particular importance when converting a patient *from* TDF to another opioid. For example, it would be prudent to wait 24 hours or longer before starting the full replacement dose of a different long-acting opioid after removing the TDF patch. Rather, the practitioner would encourage use of the rescue opioid during that time period if needed.

> **SIDEBAR BOX**: Clinicians have long recognized that cachectic cancer patients often do not receive the full-expected therapeutic benefit from TDF. In these situations, we often hear practitioners say, "I just need to find a little fat pad to place the transdermal fentanyl on so it will work." Finding a suitable "fat pad" for absorption likely isn't the only issue—failure to absorb the drug may not even be the primary issue. The issue is that cachectic patients are malnourished and hypoalbuminemic due to "transcapillary leak into subcutaneous and muscle interstitial spaces." The fentanyl goes with the albumin and is sequestered in extravascular interstitial spaces and thus unavailable for systemic circulation. It is preferable to avoid TDF in cachectic, hypoalbuminic patients.[9-11]

Other Important Considerations

We have seen that there are many misconceptions about the appropriate use of TDF among healthcare providers, occasionally resulting in avoidable morbidity and mortality. One recent survey questioned physician knowledge of TDF initial dosing strategies, use of rescue opioids with the patch, converting to and from TDF, and how to manage escalating pain in a patient receiving TDF.[16] Physicians who routinely prescribed TDF were more knowledgeable about the appropriate use of TDF compared to less-frequent prescribers, yet overall knowledge and confidence in using TDF was poor. Another study evaluated healthcare providers' ability to calculate an equivalent dose of various opioids, including TDF.[17] The results showed great disparity among providers, and lack of consistency in identifying the correct opioid conversions, including TDF. The bad news is that failure to understand completely these dosing principles may result in patient harm, including death. The good news is that they will probably want to buy this book!

In recent years, the Food and Drug Administration (FDA) released health advisories with safety warnings about TDF due to increased serious side effects and deaths from fentanyl overdose.

These precautions have resulted in labeling changes for TDF as follows:[11,18]

- The fentanyl patch is indicated for the management of pain in opioid-tolerant patients, severe enough to require daily, around-the-clock, long-term opioid treatment and for which alternative treatment options are inadequate.

- Patients considered opioid tolerant are those who are taking, for 1 week or longer, at least:
  - 60-mg morphine per day
  - 25-mcg TDF per hour
  - 30-mg oral oxycodone per day
  - 8-mg oral hydromorphone per day
  - 25-mg oral oxymorphone per day
  - 60-mg oral hydrocodone per day
  - An equianalgesic dose of another opioid
- Additional warnings address the risk of addiction, abuse, and misuse of fentanyl; life-threatening respiratory depression; accident exposure; neonatal opioid withdrawal syndrome; cytochrome CYP3A4 drug interactions; increased risk of toxicity with external heat; and increased risk with concurrent benzodiazepine administration.

Additional big "take-home" messages from these warnings are as follows: TDF is inappropriate for acute pain management or uncontrolled/unstable chronic pain and for intermittent or mild pain management, and should not be used in opioid-naïve patients. The prescribing information also recommends *all* other around-the clock opioids should be discontinued prior to beginning TDF. Our discussion of "starting doses" of TDF will focus on conversion calculations from other opioid regimens.

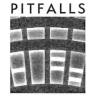

PITFALLS   TDF—Too Much of a Good Thing?

The Duragesic prescribing information warns about death and serious medical problems that have occurred when people were accidentally exposed to TDF.[11] Examples of accidental exposure include transfer of a TDF patch from an adult's body to a child while hugging, accidentally sitting on a patch, and possible accidental exposure of a caregiver's skin to fentanyl while applying or removing a patient's patch. One reported case of caregiver toxicity involved the mother of a 40-year-old patient receiving 600 mcg/hr of TDF every 36 hours.[19] Due to skin irritation, the caregiver sprayed the patient's skin with the corticosteroid fluticasone propionate prior to patch application and applied beclomethasone cream, another corticosteroid, to the application site when the patch was removed. The author hypothesized that the caregiver's opioid intoxication was exacerbated by the use of corticosteroids (which may have enhanced TDF absorption), the caregiver's application technique, and the high dosage involved.

It is also important to counsel patients, families, and caregivers on the appropriate disposal of used and unused TDF patches. The manufacturer of Duragesic TDF and the FDA recommend that unused patches should be folded in half so the adhesive side adheres to itself, and immediately flushed down the toilet after removal from the skin. Unused patches should be disposed of similarly. Simply folding the patch in half and discarding in the trash does not preclude a child or pet retrieving and playing with the patch, potentially leading to fatality. Practitioners should be aware of and adhere to any local or state guidelines regarding disposal of discontinued medications such as TDF, especially if they differ from the recommendations described here.

Converting to TDF—Equivalent Dosing

When converting to TDF, it is important that the patient's pain be under relatively stable control prior to the conversion. It is too difficult to chase increasing pain with a drug delivery system (e.g., transdermal patch) that can take up to 6 days to achieve steady-state serum levels. Initial dose finding with TDF takes longer to achieve pain relief and carries a greater risk of adverse effects as compared to using a short-acting oral opioid.

Given a patient with stable pain control, what is the process we use to convert to TDF? As you will see below, there are many approaches. We will start by examining what is reported in the Duragesic manufacturer's insert and then review selected literature that supports the conversion ratio most practitioners use today. *Hang in there with me and you'll be a pro in no time at all!*

Let's look at the conversion process suggested in the Duragesic package insert.[11]

- After ensuring the patient meets the definition of *opioid tolerant* as described above, determine the patient's 24-hour opioid requirement (don't forget to add in rescue medication consistently used for nonvolitional incident and spontaneous pain).

- If the patient was not already receiving oral morphine, convert the 24-hour opioid to oral morphine equivalents using a conversion chart and process as explained in previous chapters and shown in the Equianalgesic Opioid Dosing table (Table 1-1). (**Note**: Do *not* reduce the morphine equivalent amount to account for lack of complete cross-tolerance.)

- Consult a conversion table that provides an equianalgesic recommendation from oral morphine to TDF. The conversion chart provided by the manufacturer of Duragesic is shown in Table 5-1.[11]

Table 5-1
Conversion from Oral Morphine to Duragesic[11]

Recommended Initial Duragesic Dose Based on Daily Oral Morphine Dose	
Oral 24-Hour Morphine (mg/day)	Duragesic Dose (mcg/hr)
60–134	25
135–224	50
225–314	75
315–404	100
405–494	125
495–584	150
585–674	175
675–764	200
765–854	225
855–944	250
945–1,034	275
1,035–1,124	300

mcg = micrograms; mg = milligrams.

- Initiate treatment with the recommended dose and titrate dosage upward no more frequently than 3 days after administering the initial dose and every 6 days thereafter until analgesic efficacy is reached.

Sounds so straightforward, doesn't it? Well, you wouldn't be reading this chapter if it was *that* easy!

In the package insert for Duragesic, the manufacturer-provided conversion guideline has been criticized for including morphine ranges that are too broad and based on opioid conversions that have also been criticized.[20] For example, the equianalgesic potency conversions used in the package insert to arrive at the recommendations in Table 5-1 are 6:1 oral morphine:parenteral morphine instead of the more accepted 3:1 ratio associated with chronic morphine administration. Other cited inaccuracies include an oral morphine to oral hydromorphone ratio of 8:1 and an assumption that oral methadone is three times the potency of oral morphine and equipotent when given parenterally.[20] The consequences of underestimating the correct TDF strength are more than just merely an inconvenience necessitating increased use of the rescue medication. There have been at least four published case reports of patients experiencing a withdrawal syndrome when converting from oral opioids to TDF.[21] You would not be *wrong* to use this conversion guideline to switch to TDF, just recognize that it is extremely likely the TDF dose will be too low to meet patient needs. On the other hand, if a patient is taking a cytochromic P450 3A4-inhibiting medication (e.g., ketoconazole, erythromycin, nefazodone, diltiazem, grapefruit juice), use of this conversion chart may result in a TDF starting dose that will require less titration to achieve pain relief because the interacting drug will reduce fentanyl metabolism, resulting in an increased fentanyl serum level. Last, the manufacturer's guidelines are very clear that Table 5-1, which is admittedly conservative, should *not* be used to convert *from* TDF *to* oral morphine.[11] *If the table is purposefully conservative going to TDF, it would be too aggressive converting from TDF.*

We know that fentanyl is 75 to 100 times more potent than morphine.[22] **Keep your eye on the ball as we think this through:**

- 100-mg oral morphine per day ≈ 1-mg (1,000 mcg) fentanyl per day (transdermal or IV).
- Therefore, 60-mg oral morphine per day ≈ 0.6-mg (600 mcg) fentanyl per day.
- 0.6-mg (600 mcg) fentanyl per day (24 hr) = 25 mcg per hour (25 mcg/hr) fentanyl (transdermal or IV)—we just divided the total daily dose (TDD) by 24 to determine the hourly dose of fentanyl.

Therefore, **60-mg oral morphine per day** is about equivalent to **25 mcg per hour of TDF.**

Donner and colleagues evaluated this ratio in 98 cancer patients who were on sustained-release oral morphine and whose pain was stable, using the morphine:TDF equivalencies shown in Table 5-2.[22]

Patients were converted to TDF patches, which were changed every 72 hours and titrated to pain relief. Oral morphine solution was used for breakthrough pain. Their results showed that pain control was equivalent between sustained-release morphine and TDF, but that patients on TDF used more oral morphine solution for breakthrough pain. Slightly more than 40% of patients achieved sufficient pain relief with the initial TDF dose. The remainder required a dosage increase. The authors concluded that using

Table 5-2

Donner Recommended Conversion from Oral Morphine to Duragesic

Recommended Initial Fentanyl Doses Based on Daily Oral Morphine Dosage[22]	
24-Hour Oral Morphine Dose (mg/day)	Transdermal Fentanyl Dose (mcg/hr)
30–90	25
91–150	50
151–210	75
211–270	100
Every additional 60 mg/day	An additional 25 mcg/hr

mcg = micrograms; mg = milligrams.

the 100:1 (oral morphine:TDF) ratio is safe and effective, but that the actual ratio is probably closer to 70:1.

Are you still with me?—Here comes the best part! Building on the model that 60-mg oral morphine is approximately equivalent to 25 mcg/hr of TDF, and having research that shows even this is a bit conservative (although nowhere near as conservative as the manufacturer's recommendations), *it was a small leap to the conversion that most practitioners (including this author) use today, which is:*

- Use a 2:1 ratio → every 2 mg oral morphine per *day* ≈ 1 mcg per *hour* TDF.
- Another way to word this is the number of mcg per *hour* of TDF should be about half the number of milligrams of oral morphine per *day*.
- For example, 50 mg/day of oral morphine ≈ 25 mcg/hr TDF.

Breitbart and colleagues popularized this recommendation, offering the following process to convert to TDF:[23]

- Determine the TDD of oral morphine required to control the patient's pain (or the equivalent based on their current opioid regimen; refer to Table 1-1).
- Use a conversion of 2:1 (mg oral morphine per day to mcg/hr of TDF) to calculate the mcg/hr dose of fentanyl.
- Once an approximate mcg/hr dose for fentanyl is calculated, round up or down based on the most commonly available patch strengths (12 mcg/hr, 25 mcg/hr, 50 mcg/hr, 75 mcg/hr, or 100 mcg/hr), the patient's pain level, and overall clinical status. *If the patient's pain is well controlled, round down to the next patch strength. If the current opioid regimen is not adequately controlling the pain, consider rounding up to the next patch strength.*

The Palliative Care Network of Wisconsin (PC NOW) Fast Fact on Converting To/From Transdermal Fentanyl[24] cites both the manufacturer guidelines and Breitbart and colleagues. They further recommend that the 2:1 (mg oral morphine per day to mcg/hr of TDF) may be excessive in opioid-naïve patients and/or the elderly. (*Note:* We're not supposed to be starting TDF in opioid-naïve patients! Thought you had me, didn't you?!). When in doubt, they recommend rounding down to the closest patch strength and being liberal with rescue medication.

What more recent evidence do we have evaluating conversions to TDF? Reddy and colleagues retrospectively evaluated the opioid rotation ratio (ORR) conversion to TDF from other strong opioids.[25] They evaluated the conversion of 129 cancer patients from other opioids to TDF; the median opioid rotation ratio from net oral morphine equivalent daily dose (*net* meaning breakthrough doses were deducted from the TDD) to TDF (in mg/day) was 0.01 (range –0.02 to 0.04). The authors concluded that an opioid rotation ratio of 0.01 suggests that an oral morphine equivalent daily dose of 100 mg is equivalent to 1-mg TDF daily, or approximately 40 mcg/hr. This further suggests that the ratio between the oral morphine equivalent daily dose and TDF (in mcg per hour) is 2.5:1. The authors also pointed out that the large variability (from –0.02 to 0.04) of the ratio begs caution and close monitoring when rotating to TDF.

Can We Be Steadies?

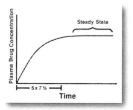

*Let's stop and consider evidence from crossover, **steady-state** trials of opioid conversions. These data are more robust than data based on single-dose crossover trials using an experimental pain model or based on bioavailability.*

*Reddy and colleagues evaluated the conversion ratio from strong opioids to TDF, and from TDF to strong opioids.[25,30] **Their results were as follows:***

▶ The median ORR from TDF mg/day to oral morphine equivalent daily dose (MEDD) is 100, and from TDF mcg/hr to MEDD is 2.4.

▶ The median ORR from MEDD to TDF in mg/day was 0.01.

BOTTOM LINE RECOMMENDATION: From TDF to oral MEDD is 2.4.

▶ TDF 100 mcg/hr ≈ 240-mg oral MEDD.

BOTTOM LINE RECOMMENDATION: From oral MEDD to TDF is 0.01.

▶ An oral MEDD of 100 mg is equivalent to 1-mg TDF daily, or approximately 40-mcg/hr TDF.

Have you thrown up your hands yet? *For a patient receiving a TDD of 100-mg oral morphine equivalent, we have the following possible conversions:*

• Duragesic package labeling would indicate TDF 25 mcg/hr.[11]

• Breitbart method would indicate TDF 50 mcg/hr.[23]

• Reddy method would indicate TDF 40 mcg/hr.[25]

Why don't I throw you right over the edge and tell you the patient is cachectic, has escalating pain, and is receiving a strong CYP3A4 inhibitor! This is another example of how we are calculating an *approximate* starting dose, and we must consider the entire patient scenario before selecting our final dose of TDF (or perhaps we will decide TDF is not even appropriate).

Before we jump into doing some calculations, I know you're scratching your head wondering why the manufacturer of Duragesic bothered to make a 12-mcg/hr patch, if the patient has to be taking at least 60-mg oral morphine a day for a week. Whether you go with the 2:1 or 2.5:1 (oral morphine daily dose in mg: TDF in mcg/hr), a 12-mcg/hr patch would be equivalent to 25- or 30-mg oral morphine per day (less than the FDA's mandate for a minimum of 60-mg oral morphine per day prior to switching to TDF). That's a head-banger alright! One possibility was to have flexibility in using two different strength patches to more finely titrate a dose (e.g., 37 mcg/hr = a 25-mcg/hr patch plus a 12-mcg/hr patch). The Scottish Palliative Care Guidelines state that you can use a 12-mcg/hr TDF in a patient receiving a 24-hour oral morphine dose between 30 and 60 mg, which seems reasonable mathematically.[26] Interestingly, PC NOW Fast Facts state that you can use the 12-mcg/hr TDF in an opioid-naïve patient, but practitioners must recognize that this is like starting an opioid-naïve patient on 25- or 30-mg oral morphine per day. For elderly or debilitated patients, this may be excessive. Friesen and colleagues evaluated all patients who were newly prescribed TDF in Manitoba between April 1, 2001, and March 31, 2013.[27] They calculated all prior opioid use to oral morphine equivalents, determining the average daily dose in the 7 to 30 days prior to initiating TDF. Results showed that fentanyl initiation was considered unsafe in 74.1% of cases due to inadequate prior opioid exposure. This was particularly common in women and patients over 65 years of age. The authors pointed out that older adults (who were the most egregious cases) are at the greatest risk of toxicity from this practice.

Although we have not described how these folks calculated an appropriate rescue opioid dose, we will do so during our case exercises. You didn't think I'd leave you hanging, did you? Well I can't speak for you, but I'm exhausted after thinking all that through! *Let's look at a case!*

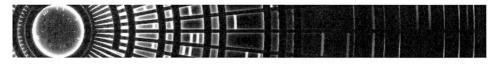

CASE 5.1

Switching from Oral Long-Acting Morphine to TDF

JR is a 62-year-old woman with esophageal cancer. Her pain has been well controlled on MS Contin 60 mg by mouth every 12 hours, with morphine oral solution 20 mg every 2 hours as needed for breakthrough pain. She has been using about three doses per day of the morphine oral solution, and this regimen has kept her comfortable. Unfortunately, she is having increased difficulty swallowing the MS Contin tablets. How would we convert her to TDF? Let's take a closer look—step by step, inch by inch.

STEP 1—*Assess the patient's pain:* We have assessed JR's pain, and it's well controlled. We are only switching her to TDF because of swallowing difficulties.

STEP 2—*Determine the patient's TDD of her current opioid:* JR is taking MS Contin 60 mg by mouth every 12 hours (120-mg oral morphine) plus three doses of morphine oral solution 20 mg (an additional 60 mg) for a grand total of 180-mg oral morphine per day.

STEP 3—*Decide which opioid to switch to and consult a conversion chart:* We already know we're switching to TDF. Using our guidelines of 2:1 oral morphine mg/day:TDF mcg/hr, we calculate a dose for TDF of 90 mcg/hr. Using the Reddy method of 2.5:1 (oral morphine mg/day:TDF mcg/hr), we calculate 72 mcg/hr.

STEP 4—*Individualize the dosage and ensure adequate access to breakthrough pain medication:* JR's preferred TDF starting dose is between 72 and 90 mcg/hr. Because her pain is well controlled, it seems reasonable to go with the 75 mcg/hr strength. We'll discuss the issue of breakthrough pain in a moment.

STEP 5—*Patient follow-up and reassessment:* We will discuss the timing of switching to and from TDF below, but we must always remember to monitor our patient carefully during and after the transition.

However, we're not done with JR! This case raises several additional issues. First, how do we time the transition from MS Contin to TDF? Also, what do we do for breakthrough pain?

Because it takes 12 to 16 hours to achieve therapeutic fentanyl serum levels, we must provide the patient with opioid coverage during the conversion period. In cases such as JR, she should take one last dose of MS Contin (60 mg) at the same time the TDF is applied. This last dose of sustained-release morphine (which lasts 8–12 hours) will be tapering off as the TDF is kicking in. JR should also continue to have the same dose of short-acting morphine (20 mg) available for breakthrough pain, as this dose has been effective for her.

If JR is too weak to swallow one last sustained-release morphine tablet prior to application of the TDF, she should receive at least two to three doses of short-acting morphine after the TDF is applied. In other words, instead of taking one last MS Contin 60-mg tablet, if she can't swallow it, she would be given oral morphine 20 mg at time zero (time of patch application), 4 hours after patch application, and 8 hours after patch application. These three 20-mg doses equal the 60-mg dose she would have received from that one last MS Contin tablet. And, of course, continue the oral morphine solution 20 mg every 2 hours as needed for additional pain.

This same principle should be followed for any patient who was receiving only short-acting opioids around the clock prior to TDF conversion. Let's look at a patient taking oral morphine 10 mg every 4 hours around the clock, with oral morphine 5 mg every 2 hours for additional pain, being switched to TDF 25 mcg/hr. When the 25-mcg/hr TDF patch is applied, the patient should continue to receive the regularly scheduled oral morphine 10 mg every 4 hours for at least two or three more doses. Keep the as needed oral morphine 5 mg every 2 hours order in place for additional pain relief.

This brings us to the question of *which* opioid to use for breakthrough pain when patients are using TDF for persistent pain. We discussed this at length in the previous chapter—our options are buccal or transmucosal fentanyl, short-acting/immediate-onset morphine, oxycodone, hydromorphone, or oxymorphone. There is no compelling reason why we *must* use the same opioid for the persistent pain and the breakthrough pain, and the transmucosal fentanyl products are fairly expensive compared to the more traditional opioids. However, if you decide the use of a rapid-acting fentanyl product is appropriate, follow the dosing guidelines as discussed in Chapter 4. Remember, there is *no* reliable correlation between the TDF patch strength and the appropriate starting dose of rapid-acting fentanyl. You must begin with the lowest dose/strength rapid-acting fentanyl dose and titrate per recommended guidelines.

If the patient had been using a short-acting opioid for breakthrough pain successfully prior to conversion to TDF, he or she can continue taking the same opioid at the same dose once he or she converts to TDF. This is permissible because the patient's pain is stable, and we are not increasing or decreasing the TDD of oral morphine (or equivalent dose of another opioid) other than to accommodate patch strength availability. However, if the patient did not have a short-acting opioid available, we can still calculate a ballpark starting dose for breakthrough pain. For example, if a patient had been receiving Kadian 100 mg by mouth per day prior to conversion to TDF, a reasonable dose of short-acting morphine would have been 10 to 15 mg (using our 10% to 15% of the TDD rule to determine the dose for break-through pain). If the patient was switched to TDF 50 mcg/hr, it would be appropriate to also recommend oral morphine 15 mg by mouth every 2 hours as needed for breakthrough pain. Of course, you would follow the same guidelines as discussed in Chapter 4 to determine if the dose is appropriate.

Let's look at another case, shall we?

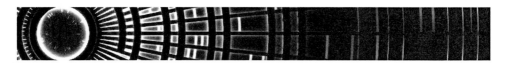

CASE 5.2

Switching from Multiple Opioids to TDF

KG is a 52-year-old woman with a history of pancreatic cancer, admitted to your hospital with a complaint of significant nausea with oral ingestion of food or medications and occa-sional vomiting. Her pain is fairly well controlled on her current analgesic regimen, which is as follows:

- TDF 25 mcg/hr
- OxyContin 20 mg by mouth every 12 hours
- Hydromorphone 4 mg by mouth every 2 hours as needed for breakthrough pain, using on average six doses per day

You would like to roll all of this into TDF due to the nausea, and the use of two long-acting opioids (OxyContin and TDF) is making all the little hairs on the back of your neck stand up. What's the first step? As I'm sure you recall, the first step is to do a careful assessment of the pain and determine if an opioid is the best treatment of KG's pain. Perhaps she needs a co-analgesic added. Let's assume we've done the assessment and feel that switching entirely to TDF is the best plan. Step 2 is to perform an accurate accounting of how she has been taking her opioids. With a complaint of nausea and occasional vomiting, it is impor-tant to determine how much of her opioid regimen she has received over the past 24 to 48 hours (e.g., to be alert for possible opioid withdrawal). Let's assume she has experienced only very occasional vomiting, and it hasn't significantly affected her total daily opioid use.

Step 3 is to convert her OxyContin and hydromorphone to an equivalent dose of oral morphine. Her TDD of oxycodone is 40 mg—how much oral morphine is this approximately equivalent to? Using method A (e.g., simple ratio), we know that the oral oxycodone:oral morphine ratio is 20:25 (see Table 1-1: Equianalgesic Opioid Dosing table). Using this, we calculate that 40-mg oral oxycodone is equivalent to 50-mg oral morphine. You can also use method B:

Actual Drug Doses: **Equianalgesic Data from Chart:**

$$\frac{\text{"X" mg TDD new opioid}}{\text{mg TDD current opioid}} = \frac{\text{equianalgesic factor of new opioid}}{\text{equianalgesic factor of current opioid}}$$

Let's fill in the numbers:

$$\frac{\text{"X" mg TDD oral morphine}}{\text{40 mg oral oxycodone}} = \frac{\text{25 mg oral morphine}}{\text{20 mg oral oxycodone}}$$

We cross-multiply:

$(25) \times (40) = (X) \times (20)$

$1,000 = 20X$

$X = 50$

This method also shows that 40-mg oral oxycodone per day is approximately equivalent to 50-mg oral morphine per day.

Now we need to do the same exercise with the oral hydromorphone the patient has been using for breakthrough pain. She is taking on average six doses of 4-mg hydromorphone, which gives us a TDD of 24-mg oral hydromorphone. *How much oral morphine is this approximately equivalent to?*

$$\frac{\text{"X" mg TDD oral morphine}}{\text{24-mg oral hydromorphone}} = \frac{\text{25 mg oral morphine}}{\text{5-mg oral hydromorphone}}$$

Cross multiply and solve for X:

$(25)(24) = (x)(5)$

$X = 120 \text{ mg}$

We see that 24-mg oral hydromorphone per day is approximately equivalent to 120-mg oral morphine per day.

If we add the oral morphine equivalent we got from the oxycodone calculation (50 mg) to the oral morphine equivalent from the hydromorphone calculation (120 mg), we have determined the patient is receiving an equivalent dose of 170 mg of oral morphine per day, in addition to the TDF 25 mcg/hr.

P E A R L S   ## A Critically Important Point to Note at this Juncture Is as Follows

When switching from one opioid to another, we discussed how we usually reduce the dose of the new opioid by 25 to 50% to allow for incomplete cross-tolerance.

We do not do this when doing the calculation for the purposes of converting to TDF. *The incomplete cross-tolerance factor has already been taken into account when making the jump from oral morphine (or oral morphine equivalent) to TDF. You will see this same concept discussed in Chapter 6 on methadone dosing. The converse holds true as well; when we convert* **from** *TDF* **to** *oral morphine, the "lack of cross tolerance" factor has already been considered.*

OK, back at the ranch—in addition to the TDF 25 mcg/hr, the patient is receiving approximately the equivalent of 170-mg oral morphine per day. Half of this is 85—which would represent 85-mcg/hr TDF. Using the Reddy method, it would be TDF 68 mcg/hr. A reasonable compromise is TDF 75 mcg/hr (this is Step 4—individualization for the patient). Also, don't forget the goal of this exercise was to combine all the opioids the patient was receiving into one opioid—TDF. She's already on TDF 25 mcg/hr. If we add 75 mcg/hr based on the calculations we've just done, we could discontinue the OxyContin and hydromorphone, and increase the TDF from 25 mcg/hr to 100 mcg/hr.

The next burning question is, "How do we time all this?" If she is able to swallow, the patient should receive her last OxyContin 20-mg tablet at the same time the TDF patch is changed from 25 mcg/hr to 100 mcg/hr (or a 75-mcg/hr patch added). If she is too nauseated to take anything by mouth, discontinue both the OxyContin and hydromorphone, and switch to TDF 100 mcg/hr. You will then need to rely on a nonoral route of administration to provide a rescue opioid. Your options are parenteral or rectal. How do we calculate the dose for both routes assuming we want to use morphine? *This is hurting your head to use skills you learned in previous chapters, isn't it? I know you can do it—keep the faith!*

OK, let's recap. We have calculated that TDF 100 mcg/hr will probably maintain the level of comfort she had initially on her three-opioid regimen (OxyContin, TDF, and hydromorphone for breakthrough pain). TDF 100 mcg/hr is approximately equivalent to 200 mg/day of oral morphine. Ten to 15% of this is 20 to 30 mg; therefore, we could offer morphine rectal suppositories 20 mg every 2 hours as needed for breakthrough pain, titrating to 30-mg rectal morphine as needed. Alternately, if you want to provide a sub-Q injection of morphine as needed, we need to convert the 200-mg TDD oral morphine to parenteral morphine. As you recall, 10-mg parenteral morphine is equivalent to 25-mg oral morphine; therefore, her TDD of parenteral morphine would be about 80 mg. Ten to 15% of 80 mg is 8 to 12 mg; therefore, an appropriate dose of sub-Q morphine would be 10 mg every 2 hours as needed for breakthrough pain.

One last note about the timing of this conversion. Let's say the patient had her current 25-mcg/hr TDF patch placed 24 hours ago. You have two options when converting to TDF 100 mcg/hr. You could add a 75-mcg/hr TDF patch now, and at the end of 48 additional hours you could remove *both* the 25- and 75-mcg/hr patches (which is technically a day earlier than when we would have to change the 75-mcg/hr patch) and replace with a 100-mcg/hr TDF patch. Or, you could remove the 25-mcg/hr TDF patch when you admitted the patient and switch immediately to a 100-mcg/hr TDF. As stated earlier, it will take a minimum of 12 hours to see a clinically meaningful increase in fentanyl serum concentrations with the new patch addition, and at least 36 hours (if not 3–6 days) to achieve maximum steady-state concentrations.[1] The last step is to carefully monitor the patient during and after this transition to ensure an optimal therapeutic outcome.

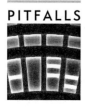

PITFALLS

"Set and Forget" Method Akin to "You Snooze, Your Patient May Lose"

Many providers feel that once a TDF patch is "set" in place on the patient, you can walk away and "forget" about the patient for 3 days. Wrong-O! You MUST continue to use good clinical judgment and monitor your patient regularly. If the patient is becoming overmedicated on fentanyl, you will need to take special precautions to reverse the opioid intoxication for hours and hours after patch removal. Similarly, TDF is not a cure-all; patients still need to be monitored for responsiveness and use rescue medications appropriately.

Titrating Transdermal Fentanyl

Once we have switched a patient to TDF, how do we titrate the dose up?—Let's consider both the dose and the timing. Let's start with how quickly we can increase the patch strength.

According to the guidelines in the prescribing information for Duragesic,

> Do not increase the Duragesic dose for the first time until at least 3 days after the initial application. Titrate the dose based on the daily dose of supplemental opioid analgesics required by the patient on the second or third day of the initial application. It may take up to 6 days for fentanyl levels to reach equilibrium on a new dose. Therefore, evaluate patients for further titration after no less than two 3-day applications (e.g., every six days) before any further increase in dosage is made.[11]

It makes sense that we cannot gauge the efficacy of the TDF dose within the first 24 hours after initial patch application (or dosage increase) because the serum fentanyl continues to rise during this period. One reference states TDF absorption is 47% complete at 24 hours, 88% complete at 48 hours, and 94% complete at 72 hours.[28] Therefore, we should look at average use of the rescue medication on days 2 and 3 and let that guide our titration decision making. If the patient requires more than three doses of his or her rescue medication for spontaneous pain in a 24-hour period to achieve good pain control, the patch strength should be increased. Titrating with TDF is challenging and often cumbersome due to the long onset and duration of action (I always use the analogy that it's like steering the *Titanic*, and we see how well THAT worked out!). The best rule of thumb is to change the dose when the pain is stable (note I didn't say the pain was *controlled*, but *stable*), but not more quickly than described above.

How much should we increase the patch strength? There are two ways you can do this: First, calculate how much of the rescue opioid the patient was using per day on average, and calculate the conversion to TDF. For example, consider a patient who was switched from an oral opioid regimen to 50 mcg/hr TDF with 15-mg oral morphine every 2 hours for breakthrough pain. Assume the patient took four doses of oral morphine on both days 2 and 3, for a TDD of 60-mg oral morphine. Half of this is 30 mcg/hr; therefore, it would be appropriate to increase the TDF to 75 mcg/hr. You can also use a rule of thumb to increase the TDF by 25 mcg/hr when at lower doses, but increase by 50 mcg/hr if the patient is using a greater amount of rescue medication, the pain is severe, and a 50 mcg/hr increase is within reason. For example, you would *not* increase from 25 mcg/hr to 75 mcg/hr—this would be a 200% increase. We discussed in a previous chapter that we increase by 25% to 50% for moderate pain, or 50% to 100% for severe pain. Therefore, in the face of more severe pain, you can comfortably increase by up to 100% while not exceeding the absolute increase by 50 mcg/hr. For example, a patient on 50 mcg/hr TDF who is using around-the-clock rescue medication and continues complaint of pain (assuming an opioid remains the appropriate analgesic) may be increased to 100 mcg/hr on day 4. It may also be reasonable to increase the dose of the rescue medication and observe the patient's response over the next 6 days before considering an additional dosage increase of TDF.

Transdermal fentanyl patches are approved for use for 3 continuous days (72 hours). Clinical practice and research have shown that about 20% of patients may require a shorter application interval of 48 hours.[29] If possible, an increase in the TDF dose is preferred (to be able to maintain the every 72-hour dosing interval), but if the patient consistently has more breakthrough pain during the last 24 hours of each cycle (e.g., using more than four doses of rescue opioid), changing to every 48-hour dosing would be appropriate. *Dosage intervals less than 48 hours in duration are inappropriate and should not be used in any patient, regardless of the circumstances. Also, if the patient is using more than one patch simultaneously, they should all be changed at the same time or day, not rotated like tires, which really increases the risk for error.*

Converting from TDF—Equivalent Dosing

Occasionally, we have a clinical situation where it would be in the patient's best interests to switch *from* TDF to a different opioid or route of administration. Alternately, it may be a formulary consideration driving this decision. In any case, what guidelines do we use to switch off TDF?

The manufacturer's guidelines offer the following recommendations for discontinuation of Duragesic:[11] "To convert patients to another opioid, remove Duragesic and titrate the dose of the new analgesic based upon the patient's report of pain until adequate analgesia has been attained. Upon system removal, 17 hours or more are required for a 50% decrease in serum fentanyl concentrations."

Can we use our 2-mg oral morphine per day:1 mcg/hr TDF guideline in reverse? If I was a bettin' woman, I'd say yes, but do we have any data to back this up? Why yes, our friend Reddy evaluated this very thing! Specifically, Reddy and colleagues sought to determine the ORR when switching off TDF to other strong opioids, as measured by the MEDD.[30] Their results showed the median ORR from TDF mg/day to oral MEDD is 100, and from TDF mcg/hr to oral MEDD is 2.4 (e.g., TDF 100 mcg/hr ≈ oral MEDD of 240 mg). This is a bit more aggressive than the 1 mcg/hr TDF:2-mg oral morphine/day guideline. *Let's look at the following case.*

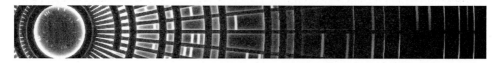

CASE 5.3
• •
Switching Off TDF: Timing Considerations

BL is a 52-year-old man admitted to your hospice program with a diagnosis of lung cancer; he is receiving 50-mcg/hr TDF with oral morphine 15 mg by mouth every 2 hours as needed for breakthrough pain. He is able to swallow tablets and capsules, and TDF is not on your formulary. BL is agreeable to switching to sustained-release morphine tablets. Using the data from Reddy, 50-mcg/hr TDF would be approximately 120-mg oral morphine per day.

Using the 1 mcg/hr TDF:2-mg oral morphine per day rule, you calculate an approximate total daily dose of oral morphine of 100 mg. Let's go with the more conservative estimate of 100-mg oral morphine per day.

But, how do we make this switch? How do we time taking off the patch and beginning the morphine therapy? An important part of answering this question is knowing the rate at which the fentanyl is eliminated from the body after patch removal, as follows:

- Seventeen hours after patch removal, 50% of fentanyl is eliminated from the body.

- Thirty-four hours after patch removal, 75% of fentanyl is eliminated from the body.

- Fifty-one hours after patch removal, 87.5% of fentanyl is eliminated from the body.

- Sixty-eight hours after patch removal, 93.5% of fentanyl is eliminated from the body.

Remember, even though fentanyl is a quick-onset, short-acting opioid, when administering by transdermal patch, it takes many hours for the drug to completely be absorbed from the site of application (the skin), enter the systemic circulation (see Figure 5.2), be metabolized and eliminated from the body.

One guideline published in the literature to prevent pain recurrence when switching from TDF to a different opioid/route of administration is as follows:[31,32]

- Calculate your new opioid regimen. (**Note:** If you're working with a home-based patient, *make sure the new opioid is in the home* before removing the patch; don't gamble on the time of delivery because if you're wrong the patient may end up in a pain crisis!)

- Remove the TDF patch.

- For the first 12 hours after patch removal, use *only* the previously prescribed rescue opioid for pain that occurs.

- Twelve hours after patch removal, begin with 50% of the calculated scheduled opioid regimen, and continue to offer the rescue opioid as needed.

- Twenty-four hours after patch removal, increase to 100% of the calculated scheduled opioid regimen, and continue to offer the rescue opioid as needed.

In the case of BL, even though we have a good idea that TDF 50 mcg/mL is equivalent to 100 mg/day of oral morphine, you decide to move first to using the oral morphine solution he has in the home on an around-the-clock basis before ultimately switching him to oral sustained-release morphine tablets. *So, let's take a look at how we do this.*

After removing the patch, you instruct the patient to wait 12 hours before taking *scheduled* doses of oral morphine; however, he is welcome to use the morphine 15 mg every 2 hours as needed for *breakthrough* pain. Based on our rule of thumb that TDF 50 mcg/hr is equivalent to 100-mg oral morphine per day, we determine the 4-hourly dose of oral morphine to be 15 mg. Twelve hours after the patch is removed, we instruct BL to take 50% of the calculated dose of morphine, which would be oral morphine 7.5 mg every 4 hours (with rescue opioid still available). After 24 hours, BL is instructed to increase to oral morphine 15 mg every 4 hours around the clock. After 2 days of this regimen, he is switched to sustained-release oral morphine 45 mg every 12 hours, keeping the oral morphine 15 mg every 2 hours as needed for breakthrough pain.

TDF in Older Adults and Cachectic Patients

As previously discussed, many variables affect the absorption of fentanyl from a transdermal system and age is no exception. By determining the amount of fentanyl left in the transdermal patch after 72 hours, Solassol and colleagues determined that patients >75 years of age absorbed 50% of fentanyl while patients <65 years of age absorbed 66% (difference was statistically significant).[33]

As briefly discussed earlier in this chapter, some practitioners who care for patients with advanced illnesses have noticed that cachectic patients occasionally seem to get less relief from TDF than expected, for which some evidence has become available.[13-15] Although there are no hard and fast guidelines on how to deal with this, we also know it makes no sense to actually try to teach a pig to whistle, so it would be imprudent to ignore this perceived lack of response. *Let's look at a case that illustrates this point.*

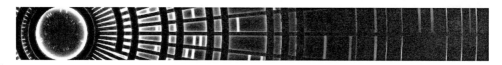

CASE 5.4
•••

TDF and Cachectic Patients

SW is a 92-year-old woman (5'5", 82 lb) admitted to hospice with a diagnosis of protein-calorie malnutrition. She has a long-standing history of osteoarthritis, affecting her knees, hips, and spine. She has painful diabetic neuropathy and a range of general aches and pains. Her pain did not adequately respond to nonopioid analgesics; therefore, she was started on morphine 5 mg by mouth every 4 hours, over time increasing to 15 mg by mouth every 4 hours. Her pain was fairly well controlled on this regimen, but the morphine made her nauseated. Her physician switched her to 50-mcg/hr TDF with good response for about 10 days. When she complained of increased pain, her physician increased the TDF to 75 mcg/hr, and then to 100 mcg/hr 6 days later. Neither dosage increase had any appreciable effect on her pain. You decide to switch her to sub-Q injections of morphine around the clock. This brings us to our burning question: Which strength patch do you base your calculations on? The 50-mcg/hr patch, the 75-mcg/hr patch, or the 100-mcg/hr patch?

Because SW did not show a response to either the 75-mcg/hr or 100-mcg/hr TDF, it would be prudent to base your calculations on the 50-mcg/hr patch. Therefore, a 50-mcg/hr TDF patch is about equal to 100-mg oral morphine, which is about equal to 40-mg parenteral morphine per day. If we decide to give the sub-Q injection every 4 hours, this calculates to a 6.67-mg dose, so reduce to 5 mg. In addition, you could even get an order for morphine 2.5 or 5 mg sub-Q every 2 hours as needed for breakthrough pain on top of the regularly scheduled doses of sub-Q morphine. Using the guidelines discussed above, for the first 12 hours after removing the patch, you would rely solely on the as needed order; during the next 12 hours, you could begin with morphine 2.5 mg sub-Q every 4 hours (plus the 5-mg every 2 hours as needed dose). After 24 hours, you would move to your full dose of morphine 5 mg sub-Q every 4 hours. After 24 to 48 hours of therapy, you will determine if this regimen is sufficient.

Importantly, this is not an evidence-based recommendation, it's based more on a violent objection to being thrown in jail for overdosing a LOL (little old lady) on opioids. As we have discussed from the beginning of this book, **"Safety first"** is our mantra. The second mantra is **"Make sure the patient has adequate rescue opioid available."**

PARENTERAL FENTANYL

As described in the beginning of the chapter, there are several routes for fentanyl administration. Use of parenteral fentanyl includes IV injection, IV infusion, IM injection (no, no, bad dog!), and sub-Q injection or infusion. In the hands of skilled practitioners, fentanyl has also been administered epidurally and intrathecally. The remainder of this chapter will be devoted to conversion calculations regarding parenteral fentanyl.

IV Fentanyl

In Chapter 7, we will discuss advanced opioid therapy including continuous infusions and neuraxial opioid therapy. However, because we're talking about fentanyl, let's look at a conversion from oral morphine to a continuous IV (or sub-Q) fentanyl infusion. As we discussed earlier in the chapter, fentanyl is approximately 70 to 100 times more potent than morphine on a mg-to-mg basis, but there is some debate over the exact morphine-fentanyl equivalency (of course, life would be too simple if that were not the case!). *Let's take a look at a case.*

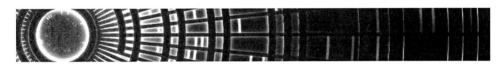

C A S E   5 . 5
• •
Switching from an Oral Opioid to IV Fentanyl

MB is a 48-year-old man with a history of a work-related injury resulting in chronic low back pain. His pain is currently treated with sustained-release morphine 120 mg by mouth every 12 hours with morphine sulfate immediate release (MSIR) 30 mg every 4 hours as needed for breakthrough pain (which he takes on average twice a day) with good pain control. He has been admitted to the hospital for back surgery, and the surgeon has asked you to convert his oral morphine regimen to a continuous IV fentanyl infusion prior to surgery. *No pressure there!*

Let's take a look at how we do this:

- Our first step is to assess the patient's pain; he has told you his current oral morphine regimen controls his pain.

- For our second step, we need to calculate his TDD of oral morphine. He is getting a total of 300-mg oral morphine per day ($120 \times 2 + 30 \times 2 = 240 + 60 = 300$).

- Our third step is the conversion calculation.

- Step 4 is individualizing the dose for the patient.

Three hundred milligrams a day of oral morphine is equivalent to 120 mg per day of parenteral morphine (recall that 25-mg oral morphine ≈ 10 mg parenteral morphine). If we were going to put him on a continuous IV morphine infusion, we would divide by 24 to get the hourly infusion rate, which would be about 5 mg/hr. Using the equivalency shown in the Equianalgesic Opioid Dosing table in Chapter 1 (10-mg parenteral morphine ≈ 0.15-mg parenteral fentanyl), we determine that 5-mg parenteral morphine ≈ 0.075-mg parenteral fentanyl. We can convert 0.075-mg fentanyl to mcg, which comes out to 75-mcg IV fentanyl/hr. However, as explained in the footnote in Table 1-1, many practitioners consider 4 mg/hr of IV morphine to be equivalent to 100 mcg/hr of IV fentanyl (a 1:40 equivalency).

Using this rule of thumb, MB's *300 mg of oral morphine per day* is approximately equivalent to *120 mg of parenteral morphine per day*, which is equal to *5 mg/hr of parenteral morphine*, which would be equivalent to *125 mcg/hr of IV fentanyl*.

So the answer to the question, "What hourly dose of parenteral fentanyl is equivalent to 300 mg a day of oral morphine?" is somewhere between 75 mcg/hr and 125 mcg/hr (of IV fentanyl). I vote we split the difference and go with 100 mcg/hr; but if you want to be conservative, you could start lower and allow for a generous bolus dose. For example, you could start the patient at 75 mcg/hr of IV fentanyl with a 35-mcg bolus every 15 minutes.

- Step 5 is closely monitoring your patient; within a few hours, you will be able to determine how many doses of breakthrough fentanyl the patient requires, and you can adjust your infusion rate accordingly. Because we are stopping a sustained-release oral opioid, we will allow MB to use the fentanyl bolus option for the first 6 hours, and then begin the continuous IV infusion of fentanyl.

Converting from Transdermal to IV Fentanyl

As stated earlier, the dose of TDF and IV fentanyl is the same. When you really think about it, transdermal drug delivery technically *is* parenteral drug delivery (it's not enteral unless you're doing weird things with the patch!). While you're wrapping your head around that, just recognize that 25 mcg/hr of TDF is equivalent to 25 mcg/hr of IV fentanyl, and 100 mcg/hr of TDF is equivalent to 100 mcg/hr of IV fentanyl, and so forth.

So, if the dosing equivalency is so straightforward, why are we taking time to discuss how to switch patients from TDF to IV fentanyl? Funny you should mention "time"—*it's all in the timing!* As stated earlier, once you remove a TDF patch, it takes about 17 hours to see a 50% decrease in the fentanyl serum concentration. Clearly, we don't want to wait 17 hours to start our IV fentanyl, so what is an appropriate way to work out this timing?

Most practitioners would use the following technique:
- Remove the TDF patch.
- For the next 6 hours, use as needed IV fentanyl for pain management.
- Six hours after TDF patch removal, begin an infusion of IV fentanyl at 50% the anticipated dose (in other words, 50% of the TDF patch strength). The as needed dose of IV fentanyl is still available.

- Twelve hours after TDF patch removal, increase the IV fentanyl infusion to 100% of the anticipated dose (which should be equivalent to the TDF patch strength). The as needed dose of IV fentanyl continues to remain available.

On occasion, patients receiving TDF experience rapidly escalating pain that cannot be managed with a transdermal system. In these cases, the practitioner may choose to switch the patient to IV fentanyl. Kornick and colleagues described their protocol for this conversion in patients with acute cancer-related pain.[34] Their protocol was as follows: All transdermal patches were removed from the patient, and a continuous infusion of IV fentanyl was begun at an equivalent hourly rate (1:1, transdermal:IV) at the time of patch removal. A patient-demand bolus of 50% to 100% of the hourly infusion rate was available every 15 to 20 minutes. In the published case series, 10 patients were switched from transdermal to IV fentanyl, the results of nine were reported. Eight of the nine patients reported pain in excess of 8 (on a 0–10 scale; 0 = no pain, 10 = worst imaginable pain) on presentation; seven of the nine had a significant decrease in pain intensity at 24 hours. One of the nine patients reported sedation 24 hours after starting IV fentanyl, which resolved by the next day. As discussed by the authors, during the initial hours after the switch from transdermal to IV fentanyl, the patient was actually receiving approximately twice as much fentanyl as the prescribed IV dose due to the continued absorption of fentanyl from the skin depot despite TDF patch removal. In the cases they described, this was useful because all the patients were in pain crisis. This would *not* be appropriate for a patient who was *not* in acute pain crisis.

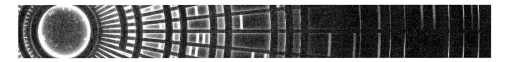

CASE 5.6
Switching from TDF to Parenteral Fentanyl

AL is a 62-year-old man with a history of prostate cancer, admitted to the hospital for a course of radiation. To have increased flexibility in treating his pain while hospitalized, the palliative care team has been asked to switch him from his current 50 mcg/hr TDF to a continuous IV infusion of fentanyl. AL's pain is currently well controlled on TDF along with a nonsteroidal anti-inflammatory agent. *How should we convert AL to a continuous IV fentanyl infusion?*

Based on the discussion above, AL is not in pain at this time, so clearly this is not a crisis situation. It would be appropriate to remove the TDF patch, establish IV access, and have a 25-mcg fentanyl bolus available every 20 minutes for the first 6 hours. At 6 hours, the continuous IV infusion of fentanyl should begin at 25 mcg/hr, and the bolus option is still available. Twelve hours after TDF patch removal, the IV infusion of fentanyl should be increased to 50 mcg/hr, and the bolus option remains in place. Should AL's pain increase or decrease over the next few days, the continuous infusion can be adjusted accordingly.

Converting from IV to Transdermal Fentanyl

When a patient's pain has been stabilized on a continuous infusion of fentanyl, it is common practice to want to switch the patient to a more convenient dosage formulation, such as TDF. Our friends Kornick and associates have kindly provided guidance in this area as well![35] They report on a series of adult patients with cancer-related pain who had been treated with continuous infusion fentanyl (with a patient-demand bolus at 50% to 100% of the hourly infusion rate, available every 15–20 minutes). All patients reported stable and acceptable pain control in the 12 hours prior to conversion to TDF. The protocol they used was to round the effective hourly infusion rate to the closest TDF patch strength, and apply the patch(es). Six hours after TDF patch application, the continuous fentanyl infusion rate was decreased by 50%, and was discontinued 6 hours thereafter. The demand bolus option remained in place at the same dose and lockout interval for at least 24 hours after TDF patch application. Fifteen patients were evaluated in this case series; only one patient reported unsatisfactory pain control at 6 and 12 hours, but acceptable pain control at 18 and 24 hours. Overall, all 15 patients had acceptable pain control using this two-step taper without significant increases in sedation or demand fentanyl bolus use; however, 20% of patients experienced an adverse effect.

Nomura and colleagues compared the 6- versus 12-hour conversion from IV fentanyl to TDF in chronic cancer pain.[36] In the 12-hour arm, the continuous IV infusion (CII) of fentanyl was decreased by 50% 6 hours after applying the TDF, and then stopped after another 6 hours (such as Kornick did, above). In the 6-hour arm, the CII dose rate was decreased by 50% 3 hours after applying the TDF patch and stopped after another 3 hours. A 1:1 conversion rate was used for the CII and TDF dose (e.g., 50 mcg/hr = 50 mcg/hr). Their results showed that the 6-hour method was superior to the 12-hour method. In the 12-hour arm, about 25% of patients experienced an adverse effect (somnolence, confusion, nausea, vomiting, diarrhea, fatigue; similar to Kornick), primarily occurring at hours 6 to 18. Patients in the 6-hour arm maintained pain control and had few adverse effects.

Rounding things out, Samala and colleagues also evaluated a 6-hour overlap method of IV fentanyl and TDF.[37] Using a 1:1 conversion, they overlapped a continuous, nontapered dose of IV fentanyl for 6 hours after TDF placement, then discontinued the IV fentanyl. They found this approach to be safe and effective, with pain control stable at the 6- and 24-hour marks, and a slight bump in pain intensity at 12 and 18 hours (which did not necessitate rescue analgesia and therefore considered not clinically important). Only one of 17 patients possibly had an adverse effect (tachycardia, dyspnea, nausea), and the authors concluded their method was as safe as those described by Kornick and Nomura. ***Don't forget to provide an immediate-release opioid for breakthrough pain***.

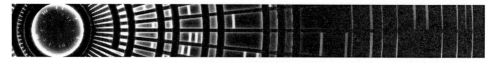

CASE 5.7
∙∙
Switching from Parenteral Fentanyl to TDF

AL, our 62-year-old man with prostate cancer from Case 5.6, has completed his course of radiation and is ready for discharge home. He is being maintained on a fentanyl continuous infusion at 70 mcg/hr; he has only used his bolus dose (35 mcg) once in the past 24 hours. He would like to resume TDF therapy. How do we handle this transition?

Well, I do love a menu of options. Per the research from Kornick and colleagues, we could round the hourly fentanyl amount to the closest TDF patch strength (75 mcg/hr in this case) and do a two-step taper over 12 hours. Alternatively, we could use the 6-hour transition, either by reducing the infusion to 50% at 3 hours as suggested by Nomura or simply continuing the infusion for 6 hours and stopping the infusion at 6 hours as Samala suggested. Regardless of which method we choose, we will, of course, be vigilant in monitoring AL for pain control and adverse effects, particularly oversedation.

In this chapter, we have explored conversions in the land of fentanyl—to and from transdermal fentanyl and to and from parenteral fentanyl. All that to-ing and fro-ing has left me a bit dizzy—hopefully you'll find our "to go" points helpful. In this summary table, you will find all the "pearls" we discussed when converting to and from TDF, and how to adjust the TDF dose. *What's not to love about a good cheat sheet?*

Could I Get That to Go, Please? Bottom Line It for Me . . .

Converting from an oral long-acting opioid (an 8- or 12-hour tablet or capsule) to TDF

▸ If patient is not taking oral morphine, convert to oral morphine.

▸ Using the 2-mg oral morphine/day ≈ 1 mcg/hr TDF rule, calculate the TDF patch strength. Alternatively, use the Reddy method, where 100-mg oral morphine per day ≈ TDF 40 mcg/hr.

▸ Advise patient to take one last dose of the oral 8- or 12-hour long-acting opioid at the same time the first TDF patch is applied.

▸ Increase TDF if necessary in 3 days, and every 6 days thereafter as needed.

Converting from an around-the-clock, oral, short-acting opioid to TDF

▸ If patient is not taking oral morphine, convert to oral morphine.

▸ Using the 2-mg oral morphine/day ≈ 1 mcg/hr TDF rule, calculate the TDF patch strength. Alternatively, use the Reddy method, where 100-mg oral morphine per day ≈ TDF 40 mcg/hr.

▸ Advise patient to take two or three scheduled doses of their oral short-acting opioid after TDF patch application: one dose at the time of application, another dose 4 hours later, and if needed, a third dose 4 hours later. Rescue opioid should be available throughout.

▸ Increase TDF if necessary in 3 days, and every 6 days thereafter as needed.

Titrating TDF upward

▸ After initiation of TDF therapy, evaluate use of rescue opioid on days 2 and 3. If patient is using more than three doses of rescue opioid, calculate TDD of rescue opioid, and increase TDF patch strength in an equivalent amount.

▶ Increase by 25 to 50 mcg/hr, but not to exceed a 100% increase. Also, no dosage increase should exceed 50 mcg/hr.

  ▶ Increase from 25 mcg/hr to 50 mcg/hr.

  ▶ For patients on 50 mcg/hr or higher, increase by no more than 50 mcg/hr.

Converting from TDF to an oral opioid

▶ Based on TDF patch strength, calculate oral morphine equivalent (or other opioid equivalent). If converting to oral morphine, use the 1 mcg/hr TDF ≈ 2-mg oral morphine/day rule. Alternatively, use the Reddy method, where TDF 100 mcg/hr ≈ 240-mg oral MEDD.

▶ Once the new opioid product is in the patient's home, remove the TDF patch.

▶ For the first 12 hours after patch removal, use only the previously prescribed rescue opioid.

▶ Twelve hours after patch removal, begin with 50% of the calculated scheduled opioid regimen; rescue opioid continues to be available.

▶ Twenty-four hours after patch removal, increase to 100% of the calculated scheduled opioid regimen; rescue opioid continues to be available.

Converting from TDF to IV fentanyl

▶ Remove the TDF patch.

▶ Establish IV access and allow an as needed bolus dose of fentanyl.

▶ Six hours after TDF patch removal, begin 50% of IV fentanyl infusion (which should be 50% of the TDF patch strength); bolus option remains in place.

▶ Twelve hours after TDF patch removal, increase IV fentanyl infusion to 100% of prescribed amount (which should be equal to the TDF patch strength); bolus option remains in place.

Conversion from IV fentanyl to TDF

▶ Apply TDF patch in the same strength as IV fentanyl infusion.

▶ Option A: Three hours after application of TDF, reduce IV fentanyl infusion by 50%; bolus option remains in place. Discontinue IV infusion at 6 hours.

▶ Option B: Continue IV fentanyl infusion for 6 hours after applying TDF; discontinue infusion after 6 hours.

▶ Don't forget about a rescue analgesic!

PRACTICE PROBLEMS

P5.1: Switching from Oral Morphine to TDF

TS is a 72-year-old man with severe osteoarthritis pain. His prescriber has him on a regimen of morphine oral solution, 20 mg every 4 hours around the clock. When TS remembers to take all six doses of morphine per day, his pain is very well controlled. Unfortunately, when he forgets to take doses, he ends up in pain crisis. His prescriber asks your help in converting TS from oral morphine to TDF. What do you recommend, and specifically how should the switch be timed?

P5.2: Switching from Oral Long-Acting Oxycodone to TDF

HH is a 62-year-old woman with chronic low back pain, currently taking OxyContin 40 mg by mouth every 12 hours with OxyIR 10 mg every 2 hours (takes about four times per day). This reduces HH's pain to about a 4 (on a 0–10 scale; 0 = no pain, 10 = worst imaginable pain). Unfortunately, HH complains that she cannot afford the OxyContin tablets, and she would like to switch to generic TDF. What do you recommend?

P5.3: Switching from TDF to Oral Morphine

DW is a 48-year-old man who just moved to the area for a new job. He has a 10-year history of chronic low back pain for which he receives 100-mcg/hr TDF. Unfortunately, his new prescription plan does not cover TDF, and he has been referred to you for conversion to oral morphine. What do you recommend?

P5.4: Switching from TDF to IV Fentanyl

TJ is a 58-year-old man with end-stage lung cancer, who has been admitted to your inpatient hospice unit in a pain crisis. He is currently receiving 75-mcg/hr TDF with MSIR 15 mg by mouth every 2 hours for breakthrough pain. He rates his pain as a 9 (on a 0–10 scale; 0 = no pain, 10 = worst imaginable pain), where it has been for the past 24 hours. He has taken several doses of the MSIR but tells you "that stuff doesn't work, so I quit taking it." You would like to switch him to a continuous IV infusion of fentanyl. What is your dosing strategy?

P5.5: Switching from IV Fentanyl to TDF

TJ, the 58-year-old man with end-stage lung cancer described in Case P5.4, was admitted and switched to a continuous fentanyl infusion. Several days later, his pain is very well controlled on 120 mcg/hr of fentanyl with a 40-mcg bolus every 15 minutes as needed for breakthrough pain. He has used four doses of the rescue fentanyl over the past 24 hours. He would now like to be transitioned back to TDF so he can return home. What do you recommend, and how do you make a smooth transition?

REFERENCES

1. Schug SA, Ting S. Fentanyl formulations in the management of pain: An update. *Drugs.* 2017;77:747-763.
2. Lötsch J, Walter C, Parnham M, et al. Pharmacokinetics of non-intravenous formulations of fentanyl. *Clin Pharmacokinet.* 2013;52:23-36.
3. Taylor DR. The pharmacology of fentanyl and its impact on the management of pain. *Medscape Neurology:* Pharmacologic Management of Pain Expert Column. 2005. https://www.medscape.org/viewarticle/518441_1. Accessed February 24, 2018.
4. Mather LE. Clinical pharmacokinetics of fentanyl and its newer derivatives. *Clin Pharmacokinet.* 1983;8:422-446.
5. The Medicines Company. Re: Voluntary discontinuation and withdrawal from market of IONSYS® (fentanyl iontophoretic transdermal system), CII. http://www.ionsys.com/pdfs/IONSYS_Discontinuation_Letter.pdf. Accessed February 24, 2018.
6. Muijsers RBR, Wagstaff AJ. Transdermal fentanyl: an updated review of its pharmacological properties and therapeutic efficacy in chronic cancer pain control. *Drugs.* 2001;61(15):2289-2307.

7. Lane ME. The transdermal delivery of fentanyl. *Eur J Pharm Biopharm.* 2013;84:449-455.

8. Marquardt KA, Tharratt RS, Musallam NA. Fentanyl remaining in a transdermal system following three days of continuous use. *Ann Pharmacother.* 1995;29:969-971.

9. Freynhagen R, von Giesen HJ, Busche P, et al. Switching from reservoir to matrix systems for the trans-dermal delivery of fentanyl: a prospective, multicenter pilot study in outpatients with chronic pain. *J Pain Symptom Manage.* 2005;30:289-297.

10. Carter KA. Heat-associated increase in transdermal fentanyl absorption. *Am J Health-Syst Pharm.* 2003;60:191-192.

11. Duragesic (Fentanyl Transdermal System) Prescribing Information. http://www.janssenlabels.com/package-insert/product-monograph/prescribing-information/DURAGESIC-pi.pdf. Accessed February 24, 2018.

12. McLean M, Fudin J. Optimizing pain control with fentanyl patches. *Medscape Pharmacists.* 2008. www.medscape.com/viewarticle/576398. Accessed February 24, 2018.

13. Heiskanen T, Mätzke S, Haakana S, et al. Transdermal fentanyl in cachectic cancer patients. *Pain.* 2009;144:218-222.

14. Nomura M, Inoue K, Matsushita S, et al. Serum concentration of fentanyl during conversion from intravenous to transdermal administration to patients with chronic cancer pain. *Clin J Pain.* 2013;29(6):487-491.

15. Davis M. *F1000Prime* Recommendation of [Nomura M et al., *Clin J Pain.* 2013;29(6):487-491]. *F1000Prime Rep,* 03 Jun 2013. doi: 10.3410/f.718013602.793477405.F1000Prime.com/718013602#eval793477405.

16. Welsh J, Reid A, Graham J, et al. Physicians' knowledge of transdermal fentanyl. *Palliat Med.* 2005;19:9-16.

17. Rennick A, Atkinson T, Cimino NM, et al. Variability in opioid equivalence calculations. *Pain Med.* 2016;17:892-898.

18. FDA. Extended-release (ER) and long-acting (LA) opioid analgesics risk evaluation and mitigation strategy (REMS). 2015 June. https://www.fda.gov/downloads/Drugs/DrugSafety/PostmarketDrugSafetyInformationforPatientsandProviders/UCM311290.pdf. Accessed February 24, 2018.

19. Gardner-Nix J. Caregiver toxicity from transdermal fentanyl. *J Pain Symptom Manage.* 2001;21:447-448.

20. Anderson R, Saiers JH, Abram S, et al. Accuracy in equianalgesic dosing: conversion dilemmas. *J Pain Symptom Manage.* 2001;21:397-406.

21. Skaer TL. Practice guidelines for transdermal opioids in malignant pain. *Drugs.* 2004;64:2629-2638.

22. Donner B, Zenz M, Tryba M, et al. Direct conversion from oral morphine to transdermal fentanyl: a multicenter study in patients with cancer pain. *Pain.* 1996;64:527-534.

23. Breitbart W, Chandler S, Eagel B, et al. An alternative algorithm for dosing transdermal fentanyl for cancer-related pain. *Oncology.* 2000;14:695-705.

24. Weissman DE, Rosielle D. *Converting to Transdermal Fentanyl,* 2nd ed. Fast Fact and Concept #2: November 2014, Palliative Care Network of Wisconsin (PC Now). https://www.mypcnow.org/blank-rdun4. Accessed February 4, 2018.

25. Reddy A, Tayjasanat S, Haider A, et al. The opioid rotation ratio of strong opioids to transdermal fentanyl in cancer patients. *Cancer.* 2016;122:149-156.

26. Fentanyl Patches. Scottish Palliative Care Guidelines, Healthcare Improvement Scotland, January 31, 2018. http://www.palliativecareguidelines.scot.nhs.uk/guidelines/medicine-information-sheets/fentanyl-patches.aspx. Accessed February 4, 2018.

27. Friesen KJ, Woelk C, Bugden S. Safety of fentanyl initiation according to past opioid exposure among patients newly prescribed fentanyl patches. *CMAJ.* 2016;188(9):648-653.

28. Portenoy RK, Southam MA, Gupta SK, et al. Transdermal fentanyl for cancer pain. Repeated doses phar-macokinetics. *Anesthesiology.* 1993;78:36-43. Abstract.

29. Donner B, Zenz M, Strumpf M, et al. Long-term treatment of cancer pain with transdermal fentanyl. *J Pain Symptom Manage.* 1998;15:168-175.

30. Reddy A, Yennurajalingam S, Reddy S, et al. The opioid rotation ratio from transdermal fentanyl to "strong" opioids in patients with cancer pain. *J Pain Symptom Manage.* 2016;51(6):1040-1045.

31. Abrahm JL. *A Physician's Guide to Pain and Symptom Management in Cancer Patients.* 2nd ed. Baltimore, MD: The Johns Hopkins University Press; 2005:249.

32. ABHB Prescribing Guideline: Use of Transdermal Fentanyl Patches. May 2013. http://www.wales. nhs.uk/sites3/Documents/814/ABHBprescribingGuidance-FENTANYLpatchesMay2011Update.pdf. Accessed February 4, 2018.

33. Solassol I, Caumette L, Bressole F, et al. Inter- and intra-individual variability in transdermal fentanyl absorption in cancer pain patients. *Oncol Rep.* 2005;14:1029-1036.

34. Kornick CA, Santiago-Palma J, Schulman G, et al. A safe and effective method for converting patients from transdermal to intravenous fentanyl for the treatment of acute cancer-related pain. *Cancer.* 2003;97:3121-3124.

35. Kornick CA, Santiago-Palma, Khojainova N, et al. A safe and effective method for converting cancer patients from intravenous to transdermal fentanyl. *Cancer.* 2001;92:3056-3061.

36. Nomura M, Kamata M, Kojima H, et al. Six- versus 12-h conversion method from intravenous to trans-dermal fentanyl in chronic cancer pain: a randomized study. *Support Care Cancer.* 2011;19:691-695.

37. Samala RV, Bloise R, Davis MP. Efficacy and safety of a six-hour continuous overlap method for convert-ing intravenous to transdermal fentanyl in cancer pain. *J Pain Symptom Manage.* 2014;48(1):132-136.

SOLUTIONS TO PRACTICE PROBLEMS

P5.1: Importantly, TS's pain is well controlled when he takes all the morphine prescribed for him, which is 120 mg per day (morphine 20 mg by mouth every 4 hours around the clock). Using our 2-mg oral morphine/day:1-mcg/hr TDF guideline, this works out to be 60-mcg/hr TDF. Using the Reddy method, it calculates to TDF 48 mcg/hr. Our decision at this point is to either round up to 75-mcg/hr TDF or down to 50-mcg/hr TDF. Given TS's age and the fact that his pain was very well controlled (when he took the morphine), it would be appropriate to round down to 50-mcg/hr TDF. ***Specific timing would be as follows:***

8 a.m.: Apply 50-mcg/hr TDF patch.

8 a.m.: Take oral morphine 20 mg.

12:00 p.m.: Take oral morphine 20 mg.

4:00 p.m.: Make a conscious decision about taking a dose of morphine 20 mg.

Offer oral morphine 20 mg every 2 hours as needed from 8 a.m. onward.

P5.2: First, we calculate HH's TDD of oral oxycodone. OxyContin 40 mg by mouth every 12 hours = 80, plus OxyIR 10 mg × 4 doses per day = 40 mg, for a TDD of 120-mg oral oxycodone. Using one of our ratio equations, we determine that 120-mg oral oxycodone is approximately equivalent to 150-mg oral morphine. Using our 2-mg oral morphine/day:1-mcg/hr TDF rule of thumb, this works out to be 75-mcg/hr TDF. Using the Reddy method, it calculates to TDF 60 mcg/hr. Therefore, we must either round down to 50-mcg/hr TDF or go with the 75-mcg/hr TDF. Because HH's pain control could be improved, it would be appropriate to go with the 75-mcg/hr TDF. For breakthrough pain, we can continue to use the OxyIR, giving 10% to 15% of the TDD (120-mg oxyco-done)—15 mg every 2 hours as needed for breakthrough pain would be appropriate. HH should take one last OxyContin tablet when she applies the 75-mcg/hr TDF patch, and use her rescue opioid as needed.

P5.3: DW is using a 100-mcg/hr TDF patch, which is approximately equivalent to 200 mg per day of oral morphine. Using the Reddy method, TDF 100 mcg/hr ≈ 240-mg oral morphine per day. If we gave the oral morphine using the short-acting formulation, this would be 33 to 40 mg every 4 hours, and a rescue dose of 20 mg every 2 hours as needed. *We recommend the following conversion plan for DW:*

- Remove 100-mcg/hr TDF patch at 8 a.m.
- For the next 12 hours, use short-acting morphine 20 mg every 2 hours as needed for pain.
- For the next 12 hours (hours 13–24), patient should take oral morphine 20 mg every 4 hours, and an extra 20 mg as needed every 2 hours.
- Starting at 24 hours, take oral morphine 30 mg every 4 hours around the clock, and an extra 20 mg as needed every 2 hours. If we find that this is too low, we can increase the 4-hourly morphine dose to 35 or 40 mg.

After 3 days on oral morphine 30 mg every 4 hours around the clock, he had good pain control (rated as a 3 or 4 [on a 0–10 scale; 0 = no pain, 10 = worst imaginable pain]) and did not need any rescue doses. He was switched to MS Contin 100 mg every 12 hours, with oral morphine 20 mg every 2 hours as needed.

P5.4: As was described in the Kornick study, because TJ is in pain crisis, it would be appropriate to remove the 75-mcg/hr TDF patch, and immediately begin a continuous IV infusion of fentanyl at 75 mcg/hr. The patient should also have a demand bolus available at 50% to 100% of the continuous infusion hourly rate; therefore, it would be appropriate to offer 40 mcg every 20 minutes as needed. Of course, the palliative care practitioners will have to closely monitor TJ for sedation, as well as pain control and other adverse effects. TJ will also have to be carefully assessed to determine why he is having a pain crisis (e.g., pathological fracture).

P5.5: TJ's pain is well controlled on 120 mcg/hr of IV fentanyl; therefore, we will apply one 100-mcg TDF and one 25-mcg/hr TDF patch at 8 a.m. We will continue the infusion at 120 mcg/hr and keep the bolus option in place. At 11 a.m. (3 hours after patch application), we reduce the continuous infusion to 60 mcg/hr but keep the same bolus option in place. At 2 p.m. (6 hours after patch application), we discontinue the continuous infusion, but keep the same bolus option in place, or you could switch to an oral opioid for breakthrough pain. Alternately, you could apply the 100- and 25-mcg/hr patches at 8 a.m., continue the continuous infusion at 120 mcg/hr (and keep bolus in place), and discontinue the infusion at 2 p.m., and use an oral opioid for breakthrough pain.

CHAPTER 6

Methadone: A Complex and Challenging Analgesic, But It's Worth It!

INTRODUCTION

Ah methadone, magical, mystical, mischievous methadone! Dosing of no other opioid fuels controversy and heated debate as does methadone, yet one has to admire methadone's sheer cheekiness. Many are drawn to the cost-effectiveness of oral methadone, but methadone is clearly not for the uninitiated or uneducated practitioner. From an intellectual point of view, we could probably teach students in pharmacy school for 4 years just using methadone as the example drug. We have drama (the pharmacodynamics of methadone), we have intrigue (why DO we have so many conversion charts), excitement (wow—look at all those drug interactions), and we have danger (QT interval prolongation?). Despite, or in spite of, the good, the bad, and the ugly sides of methadone, its use is growing, particularly in serious illness. Despite the lack of well-designed clinical trials, evaluation of the available literature on using methadone for chronic noncancer pain shows that the majority of patients achieve effective pain control.[1] In this chapter, we will review the pharmacodynamics and pharmacokinetics of methadone, dosing of methadone in opioid-naïve patients, conversion calculations to and from methadone, and a look at the use of intravenous (IV) methadone. That should keep us out of trouble!

OBJECTIVES

After reading this chapter and completing all practice problems, the participant will be able to:

1. Describe the pharmacodynamics and pharmacokinetics of methadone.

2. Explain the mechanism of pharmacodynamic and pharmacokinetic drug interactions with methadone, list medications that commonly induce or inhibit methadone metabolism, and describe strategies for dealing with these interactions.

3. Describe appropriate and inappropriate candidates for methadone therapy.

4. List variables that increase the risk for methadone-induced QTc prolongation.

5. Determine a starting dose of methadone for an opioid-naïve patient, as well as a recommendation for rescue medication.

6. Calculate an appropriate dose of methadone for a patient converting to and from another opioid regimen.

7. Given an actual or simulated patient receiving methadone, describe a monitoring plan designed to detect methadone toxicity.

8. Describe the conversion process to and from oral to parenteral methadone and recommended dosing parameters for methadone delivered via patient-controlled analgesia.

9. Describe dosing strategies when using methadone as an adjunctive analgesic.

PHARMACODYNAMICS OF METHADONE

Methadone is a synthetic opioid agonist developed over 60 years ago, best known (sometimes to our disadvantage in pain management) for its use in treating opioid use disorder. Thanks to the long duration of action, efficacy, and low cost, methadone is enjoying increased popularity in the treatment of persistent pain.

Methadone is a mu-opioid receptor agonist (like morphine, oxycodone, and hydromorphone), and it also binds to the kappa- and delta-opioid receptors. Additional mechanisms of action include inhibiting the reuptake of serotonin and norepinephrine (which is how antidepressants act to treat pain). Additionally, methadone works as an antagonist at the N-methyl-D-aspartate (NMDA) receptor, thought to prevent central sensitization and reduce opioid tolerance, and possibly increase its effectiveness in treating neuropathic pain as compared to other opioids. Methadone is a racemic mixture of R- and S-methadone. R-methadone has a 10-fold affinity at the mu receptor, is up to 50 times more potent than S-methadone, and is responsible for most of its action.[2] S-methadone is responsible for serotonin and norepinephrine reuptake inhibition, and NMDA antagonism.[3]

PHARMACOKINETICS OF METHADONE

Absorption

Methadone may be given by a variety of routes of administration and dosage formulations. Routes of administration include oral, rectal, IV, intramuscular (IM? no, no, bad dog!), subcutaneous (sub-Q although it is quite irritating; see discussion later in chapter), epidural, and intrathecal (spinal administration is *not* Food and Drug Administration [FDA] approved).

Methadone is a basic and lipophilic drug that is detected in the blood 15 to 45 minutes after oral administration with peak plasma concentrations achieved in 2.5 to 4 hours.[4] Oral bioavailability is approximately 70% to 80% (range 36% to 100%), and absorption of oral methadone tablets and solution is equivalent.[5] Studies in healthy normal subjects who received methadone rectally, orally, and intravenously showed an absolute bioavailability of 76% (rectal) and 86% (oral), respectively.[6]

Distribution

Being highly lipophilic (fat-soluble), methadone is widely and quickly distributed throughout the body to the brain, gut, kidney, liver, muscle, and lung. Methadone is retained in these tissues and slowly released back into the plasma during redistribution and elimination. Due to these properties, methadone has a very long elimination half-life (time it takes for half the drug to be eliminated from the body). Methadone binds to alpha 1-acid glycoprotein, as well as albumin and globulin to a lesser degree. The portion of drug that is *free* or *unbound* is that which results in the pharmacologic actions of the drug; this portion varies fourfold among patients.[5] The range in protein binding could partially explain the extreme variability in patient responsiveness to methadone. For example, methadone 5 mg twice a day prescribed for me may result in a different response than methadone 5 mg twice a day prescribed for you (therapeutic or toxic).

Metabolism

Methadone is extensively metabolized, primarily by N-demethylation, to pharmaco-logically inactive metabolites, which are eliminated in the urine and feces.[4] Metabo-lism takes place primarily in the liver, with some also occurring in the gut. There is significant variation in how methadone is metabolized among individuals. The cyto-chrome P450 (CYP450) enzymes responsible for the metabolism of methadone in the liver include CYP3A4, 2B6, 2C8, 2C9, 2C19, and 2D6.[5] When evaluating methadone turn-over and EDDP (2-ethyl-1,5-dimethyl-3,3-diphenylpyrroline) formation, 2B6 shows the most activity (2B6 > 3A4 > 2C19 > other enzymes). However, after abundance scaling (accounting for relative amount of enzyme present), the 3A4 accounts for greater than two-thirds of methadone metabolism.[6–11] Medications that alter the activity of some of these enzyme systems significantly influence the metabolism of methadone, resulting in either increased or decreased methadone metabolism in many cases. Drugs metabo-lized by the 2B6 or 2D6 enzyme systems are also subject to genetic variability. Interest-ingly, patients who are extensive metabolizers through CYP2C19 may have an increased risk of QTc prolongation, which may be associated with EDDP accumulation (so maybe it's not as "inactive" as originally thought!).[12] Finally, methadone even induces its own metabolism in the liver (OK, that's pretty wild!). We will discuss drug interactions with methadone more extensively later in the chapter.

Elimination

As discussed above, the inactive metabolites of methadone are eliminated in the urine and feces. Because the metabolites are inactive, methadone is a useful opioid in patients with renal impairment. However, a cautious approach to dosing (start with a lower dose, allow longer time to achieve steady-state) is recommended with severe renal impairment. Approximately 1% of methadone is removed with peritoneal or hemodialysis.[3] Again, the clinical implications of the presence of extensive CYP2C19 activity is unclear, possibly culminating in increased risk for EDDP-associated QTc prolongation.

Methadone has a very long elimination half-life, ranging from 5 to 130 hours, with a mean of about 20 to 35 hours.[4] The long half-life of methadone can result in toxicity due to accumulation in the body. Given this long and variable half-life, it can take 4 to 10 days to achieve a steady-state concentration of methadone in the serum. *Steady-state* is where *the rate of drug in = the rate of drug out* and the serum concentration is fairly steady. If the dose of methadone is increased or decreased, or a new medica-tion is started that increases or decreases methadone metabolism, it will take *another 4 to 10 days* to achieve the new steady-state. Some of the variables that influence (and alter) the metabolism and elimination of methadone have been discussed above. Addi-tional variables worth mentioning are patient gender (e.g., women metabolize metha-done faster than men) and urine pH.[13]

Drug Interactions with Methadone

A *drug interaction* describes a clinical scenario where one drug alters the phar-macologic effect of another drug given at the same time (e.g., in the same drug regimen).[14] Drug interactions can alter the pharmacokinetics or pharmacodynamics of a drug.

When we talk about a *pharmacodynamic drug interaction*, we are referring to one medication increasing or decreasing the therapeutic effectiveness or adverse effects of another drug. Giving methadone with other opioids would be a pharmacodynamic drug interaction—we will see increased analgesia (which is usually a good thing), but it could be *too* much of a good thing due to the additive toxicities such as respiratory depression and sedation. We may see increased central nervous system (CNS) depression when alcohol, neuroleptics, or other psychoactive medications (e.g., benzodiazepines, antidepressants) are used with opioids, including methadone. Another example of a pharmacodynamic drug interaction is administering methadone along with another medication that may prolong the QTc, such as an antiarrhythmic or antipsychotic agent, and selected antibiotics and antidepressants.[14]

Pharmacokinetic drug interactions affect or alter the absorption, distribution, metabolism, or elimination of the target drug. For example, there are some medications that compete with methadone for protein-binding sites. If methadone has a lower affinity for the protein-binding site than does the competing drug, methadone will be less likely to bind to the protein (because protein binding is competitive), resulting in a higher percentage of methadone that is *unbound* or *free*. This will result in a greater pharmacologic effect, both therapeutic and possibly toxic. The tricyclic antidepressants and neuroleptic medications can compete with methadone for binding on alpha 1-acid glycoprotein.[14] This represents a pharmacokinetic drug interaction affecting the distribution (and ultimately pharmacodynamics) of methadone.

As described previously, methadone is extensively metabolized in the intestines and liver by the CYP enzyme system. The primary enzymes responsible for the metabolism of methadone are CYP2B6 and CYP3A4 with less involvement of the other enzymes mentioned above. Even without the influence of interacting medications, the level of activity of the 3A4 enzyme varies significantly among individuals—with up to a 30-fold difference in the liver 3A4 enzymes and an 11-fold difference in the intestinal 3A4 enzymes.[4,15] Pharmacogenetics also complicate methadone pharmacokinetics; various phenotypes of the CYP2B6 and 2D6 can result in methadone metabolism ranging from poor to ultrarapid. CYP2B6 has up to 16 allelic variants reports, across a spectrum of ethnic distributions.[10,16–19]

Next, we must consider the influence of medications that can *induce* (increase) the activity of enzymes, and those that *inhibit* (reduce) the activity of enzymes, thus affecting the serum level of the object drug metabolized (methadone in this case), known as the *substrate*. Enzyme induction usually takes 1 to 2 weeks, while enzyme inhibition occurs much more quickly.[14] This means you may see an increase in methadone serum levels and adverse effects within a day or two of the patient starting a new medication that reduces methadone metabolism (an inhibitor). Conversely, it may take 1 to 2 weeks to see a decrease in methadone serum levels and an increase in pain after introducing a medication that induces methadone metabolism. Table 6-1 will help you understand the effect of giving methadone along with another medication known to be an enzyme *inhibitor* or enzyme *inducer*.

How can practitioners determine which other medications interact with methadone? Practitioners are strongly encouraged to use a drug interaction program

Table 6-1
Effect of Enzyme Inhibitors and Inducers on Methadone Metabolism

What's the Situation?	What Happens in This Situation?	What Does This Mean for My Patient?	What Should You Do About It?
Taking methadone with medications known to be enzyme *inhibitors*	The enzyme-inhibiting medication will slow the metabolism of methadone, resulting in an *increased* methadone serum level.	The patient may become toxic from a methadone overdose.	When converting to methadone and patient is already taking a medication known to inhibit methadone metabolism, reduce your calculated methadone dose by 25% or more. Encourage use of the rescue opioid as needed.
Taking methadone with medications known to be enzyme *inducers*	The enzyme-inducing medication will *increase* the metabolism of methadone, resulting in a *decreased* methadone serum level.	The dose of methadone may be insufficient, and the patient can experience increased pain.	Because this effect cannot be easily quantified, go with your calculated methadone dose but strongly encourage use of rescue opioid. Methadone dosage increase may be appropriate after patient achieves steady-state.

to screen for potential interactions with any patient in whom methadone is going to be used. One example is at the Indiana University School of Medicine website (http://medicine.iupui.edu/clinpharm/ddis/).[20] There are many other sources that may be helpful, such as smartphone apps, reference books on drug interactions, and primary literature. *To be safe*, it would be prudent to empirically reduce the calculated methadone dose by 25% or more for patients whose drug regimen contains a medication known to inhibit methadone metabolism. However, clinicians are encouraged to review the drug interaction literature to make their own determination regarding proactive dose reduction specific to a given CYP enzyme inhibition interaction.

One good place to start: Ask about the **three As**—amiodarone, anti-infectives, or antidepressants (Figure 6-1). The three As represent a significant portion of drug interactions with methadone. Refer to Table 6-2 for selected drug interactions with methadone.[4,14] This is by no means an exhaustive list of drugs that interact with methadone.

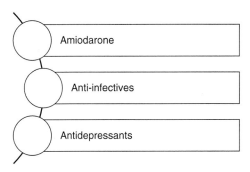

Figure 6-1. The three As of drug interactions with methadone.

Table 6-2

Selected Drug Interactions with Methadone (Enzyme Inducers and Inhibitors)[6]

Enzyme Inducers

Carbamazepine	The enzyme-inducing medication will *increase* the metabolism of methadone, resulting in a *decreased* methadone serum level. The dose of methadone may be insufficient, and the patient can experience increased pain.	Encourage use of rescue medication.
Efavirenz		
Fosamprenavir		
Nelfinavir		
Nevirapine		
Phenobarbital		
Phenytoin		
Rifampicin/rifampin/rifabutin		
Ritonavir		
St. John's Wort		
Spironolactone		

Enzyme Inhibitors

Amiodarone	The enzyme-inhibiting medication will slow the metabolism of methadone, resulting in an *increased* methadone serum level. The patient may become toxic from a methadone overdose.	Empirically reduce projected methadone dose by 25% or more and encourage use of rescue medication.
Amitriptyline		
Ciprofloxacin		
Citalopram		
Clarithromycin		
Desipramine		
Erythromycin		
Fluconazole		
Fluoxetine		
Fluvoxamine		
Itraconazole		
Ketoconazole		
Paroxetine		
Sertraline		

CANDIDATES FOR METHADONE THERAPY

So, for whom should methadone therapy be considered? Some proposed indications for methadone treatment include the following:

- Patients with true morphine allergy (or other pure mu-opioid agonists)
- Patients with significant renal impairment
- Presence of neuropathic pain
- Opioid-induced adverse effects (e.g., hallucinations)
- Pain refractory to other opioids or uncontrolled pain
- Cases where the cost of the opioid is an issue

- Patients who would benefit from an oral long-acting opioid, particularly those who require an oral solution
- Potentially any patient who requires opioid therapy, such as opioid-naïve patients

Patients for whom methadone may not be an appropriate therapeutic option include the following:

- Patients with a very limited prognosis (e.g., less than a week to live; patient may be a good candidate to use methadone in an adjunctive role that will be discussed later in this chapter)
- Numerous drugs in the medication regimen that interact with methadone, including those that prolong the QTc interval (if not contraindicated, at least requires closer oversight such as inpatient admission)
- Individuals with a history of syncope, arrhythmias, QTc prolongation
- Patients who live alone, have poor cognitive functioning, are unreliable, or are unable to comprehend instructions
- Patients with a history of unpredictable adherence to therapy (e.g., taking more or less opioid than prescribed)
- No practitioner available for continued methadone monitoring and dosage adjustment after hospital discharge
- Patients undergoing a definitive pain-relieving procedure (e.g., neurolytic block) that may result in a dramatic, sudden, opioid-sparing effect

Prior to starting methadone therapy, practitioners should follow published guidelines to evaluate the patient's QTc.[21]

METHADONE IN OPIOID-NAÏVE PATIENTS

Although there are mixed feelings about using methadone as a first-line opioid, there are some advantages to doing so. Methadone is the only opioid available as a solution that is inherently long-acting. For patients who cannot swallow tablets or capsules or have a feeding tube, methadone oral solution is an attractive option. Methadone can even be used as an initial opioid in older, frail patients at a very low dose (e.g., 1 mg a day), with close observation after initiation of therapy for potential accumulation and adverse effects.

The dosage recommendation for opioid-nontolerant (naïve) patients per the prescribing information for Dolophine® Hydrochloride (Roxane Laboratories) is 2.5 mg every 8 to 12 hours, slowly titrated to effect.[22] In 2014, the American Pain Society (APS), in conjunction with the College on Problems of Drug Dependence, in collaboration with the Heart Rhythm Society, published *Methadone Safety Guidelines*.[21] In this document, they did not explicitly recommend a starting dose of methadone in opioid-naïve patients, but for adults receiving up to 40 to 60 mg a day of morphine or the equivalent, the guidelines recommend starting methadone at 2.5 mg three times a day (tid) (for children they recommend 100 mcg/kg with a maximum of 5 mg/dose every 6 to 8 hours).[21]

Soon after the APS guidelines were published, a group of hospice and palliative care (HPC) experts convened to interpret the guidelines in caring for HPC patients.

This group considered patients receiving up to 40 to 60 mg oral morphine per day in the opioid-naïve group, and recommended a starting dose of 2 to 7.5 mg oral methadone per day for adults.[23] The intent was to explicitly allow for selecting a very low starting dose (e.g., 1 mg by mouth twice daily) and not automatically starting at 2.5 mg tid. **_Let's look at a typical case example._**

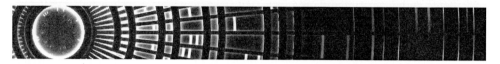

CASE 6.1
• •
Starting Methadone in an Opioid-Naïve Patient

FA is an 89-year-old man admitted to the hospital with a terminal diagnosis of failure to thrive, and he's complaining of general aches and pains. FA is still ambulatory but somewhat frail. He has a recent history of a bleeding ulcer; therefore, his primary care provider (PCP) does not want to begin NSAID therapy. FA has not responded with any degree of signifi-cance to acetaminophen, and his description of the pain is not suggestive of neuropathic pain. The PCP would like to start methadone. FA is not taking any other medications known to interact with methadone. *What dose would you recommend?*

The HPC expert group's recommended starting dose is 2 to 7.5 mg per day in divided doses. Given FA's frail state, it would be reasonable to begin with 1 mg twice daily (using the oral solution), or even 2.5 mg by mouth at bedtime (half of a 5-mg tablet). The PCP may or may not choose to provide rescue medication for FA. Some practitioners would be even more conservative and start at 1 mg a day (which is a little more drug than licking the label on the bottle)—perhaps even dosing in the morning for better observation during the dayshift. **_Let's take a look at another case._**

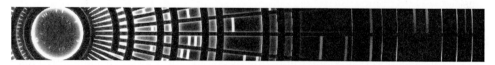

CASE 6.2
• •
Starting Methadone in an Opioid-Naïve Patient

BL is a 54-year-old woman with a 20-year history of type 2 diabetes mellitus. She has complained of painful diabetic neuropathy in her feet for the past 5 years. Unsurprisingly, the pain did not respond to acetaminophen or NSAIDs. Her physician tried gabapentin, but the patient complained of excessive somnolence and dizziness. She tried duloxetine (Cymbalta) but complained of excessive nausea. Her physician would like to start metha-done and asks your help in suggesting a starting dose. BL is not taking any other opioids and is not receiving any medications known to interact with methadone. *What do you recommend?*

BL is considerably younger than the patient we discussed in Case 6.1; therefore, we can safely recommend methadone 2.5 mg by mouth every 12 hours. Also, it would be acceptable to go right to 2.5 mg by mouth every 8 hours. Many times, especially early in therapy, we find that patients do better with a shorter dosing interval such as every 8 hours. When they achieve steady-state, they can receive their total daily dose (TDD) divided into two equal amounts (every 12 hours). Cancer pain patients have been shown to require 2.4 doses of methadone per day to achieve good pain control (e.g., which we can interpret to mean that half of this population take their methadone every 12 hours, and the other half take it every 8 hours).[24]

Monitoring the Methadone Regimen in Opioid-Naïve Patients

As we discussed at the beginning of this chapter, I promised you "edge-of-the-seat" excitement with methadone. One of the more interesting facts about methadone is its duration of analgesic action. Single doses of methadone are effective for about 4 to 8 hours. With chronic dosing, as steady-state approaches, the duration of action lengthens. As we discussed earlier, the elimination half-life is considerably longer than the half-life of analgesia. Because of this discrepancy, it takes days to achieve the full analgesic effect of methadone (see Figure 6-2). What are the implications of these findings? First, we must carefully explain to the patient that it takes several days to achieve the full analgesic effect of methadone (several days to achieve steady-state serum levels). Second, it is vital that healthcare professionals, patients, families, and caregivers work together closely to monitor the patient's response to methadone while on the road to steady-state. *Let's take a closer look at this important implication.*

Oral Methadone Dosage Formulations

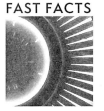 **FAST FACTS** Oral methadone is available as a 5- and 10-mg tablet (which may be cut in half). There is also a 40-mg soluble tablet, which is only available to substance abuse treatment programs. There are three different concentrations of methadone oral solution including 5 mg/5 mL, 10 mg/5 mL, and the oral concentrated solution 10 mg/mL. It is important to counsel patients, families, and caregivers carefully about accurate dosing and administration of all oral solutions, especially the concentrated 10-mg/mL solution.

You don't just start a patient on methadone (either as their first opioid, or converted from a different opioid) and walk away. The prescribing information states, "While serious, life-threatening, or fatal respiratory depression can occur at any time during the use of Dolophine, the risk is greatest during the initiation of therapy or following a dose increase. The peak respiratory depressant effect of methadone occurs later, and persists longer than the peak analgesic effect, especially during the initial dosing period. Closely monitor patients for respiratory depression when initiating therapy with Dolophine and following dose increases."[22]

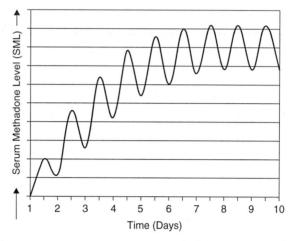

Figure 6-2. Methadone serum concentration increases gradually over 5 or more days while continuing the same daily dose.

Source: Adapted from Payte JT. Opioid agonist treatment of addiction. Slide presentation at: ASAM Review Course in Addiction Medicine; 2002. Used with permission.

What is important, however, is understanding that a patient doesn't go from sitting in their easy chair watching a rerun of *Law and Order* to cessation of breathing. What happens in between? Specifically, CNS depression, namely drowsiness, occurs first. Families, caregivers, and healthcare providers need to know to monitor the patient's level of arousal. We want patients to be able to wake up easily if they doze off when their name is called or if given a firm shake. Patients should also stay awake when others are interacting with them, and don't immediately fall asleep when the interaction is concluded.

Signs of methadone overdose from acute intoxication include evident euphoria, ataxia, and slurred speech. Late signs include unconsciousness, loud snoring, and brown pulmonary edema secretions from the mouth or nose.[25] Although these symptoms are associated with a 5- to 6-hour period after an acute ingestion of methadone, we can use this information to suggest a monitoring plan for the initiation of methadone when used for pain management.

Specifically, to prevent more serious toxicity, it is important to monitor the following during methadone initiation and titration:

- Excessive drowsiness/level of arousal
- Slowed respiration or periods of apnea, more rapid respiration, shallow breathing, Cheyne Stokes breathing
- Slurring of speech
- Loud snoring
- Pinpoint pupil size

Because patients are hopefully not taking one large dose (as in an acute overdose situation), it is important to monitor for these signs and symptoms of toxicity over a 5- to 7-day period after initiation of methadone therapy or a dosage change.

The vigilance with which we monitor the patient depends partially on the clinical situation. For ambulatory outpatients who are otherwise in good physical condition and are being started on a low dose of methadone, it is probably sufficient to educate the patient and family members who live in the home about what to keep an eye out for and monitor, and when to contact the healthcare provider. For example, ask the spouse to purposefully assess the patient's level of arousal/drowsiness twice a day (or more frequently if there are concerns). For patients with more advanced illness (e.g., hospice patients), some programs have the nurse call or visit the patient every day for the first 5 days, systematically assessing for signs and symptoms of methadone toxicity. Thorough education of the patient and family will help significantly, such as not missing or taking extra doses of methadone.

Another important consideration is understanding the variables that increase the risk for methadone toxicity:

- Starting at too high a dose
- Increasing the dose too quickly
- Forgetting to consider the influence of interacting medications (particularly those that inhibit methadone metabolism)
- Co-administration of medications such as benzodiazepines, alcohol, cocaine, cannabis, and other opioids. Co-administration of benzodiazepines with methadone has actually been shown to cause sleep apnea.[26]

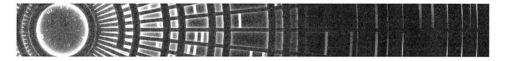

CASE 6.3
Importance of Determining Previous Total Daily Opioid Dose

Let's consider a case from this author's practice. A hospice nurse called for advice on an elderly patient experiencing significant pain. After discussing the case, we agreed that switching the patient from her current regimen of short-acting morphine to methadone was a good plan. I calculated the TDD of oral morphine, did the calculation, and made a recommendation that was accepted and implemented on day 1. The morning of day 2, the nurse case manager called me to tell me I was a rock star—the patient was tearfully grateful with her level of pain control. (*Note:* Today, I get very nervous when I'm a rock star on day 2—when this happens it generally means I'm in big trouble down the road. Back when this actually happened I probably grinned like a fool and said, "Thank you, thank you very much." Oh, to be young again!) On day 3, the nurse called to say all was well, but the patient was sleeping a bit more than normal. In retrospect, we should have intervened at this point. On day 4, the nurse called to say that the woman was increasingly sedated and "acting like a drunk monkey." I couldn't believe I had miscalculated so badly! Assailed by personal self-doubt, I instructed the nurse to hold the methadone for 24 hours, then resume at a significantly lower dose. The patient made it through day 5, and on day 6, the nurse called to say the patient was back to a good state of pain control and she was awake.

Then she told me that the patient's son confessed that he actually had never given his mother all the morphine he'd originally claimed; he didn't want the nurse to think he was a bad son!

What are the morals of this story? First, be alert when you have saved the universe on day 2 of methadone therapy. Second, don't believe the patient or family when they say, "I swear, she's been getting that liquid morphine stuff EVERY 2 hours around the clock!" Third, be vigilant in monitoring your patient to prevent an outcome no one wants! I don't want *you* saying one day, "My bad!"

Breakthrough Pain Management in Methadone-Treated Patients

There are two schools of thought as to whether to use methadone for breakthrough pain in patients getting methadone for their baseline pain: yes and no. Some propose utilizing dosing strategies (particularly with conversion from other opioids) that recommend using methadone around-the-clock and letting patients use their "prn" (as needed) methadone as a way to self-titrate to pain relief. Most practitioners do *not* use methadone for rescue dosing. If we use morphine, oxycodone, oxymorphone, or hydromorphone instead, we have a much greater comfort level knowing that the rescue opioid is not affecting the time to steady-state of methadone, or absolute methadone steady-state serum concentration (e.g., when using methadone as the around-the-clock opioid). Let's say you decide to go with morphine for breakthrough pain. If this is an opioid-naïve patient, you would choose an appropriate dose such as morphine 2.5 to 5 mg po every 2, 3, or 4 hours as needed, and so forth.

If you chose to use methadone for breakthrough pain, you could use 10% to 15% of the scheduled methadone TDD, and offer it every 3 hours for additional pain.[27] Make sure to ask the patient to maintain a pain diary documenting use of the methadone. Remember that this is NOT a preferred practice due to the risk of accumulation and unintentional methadone overdose.

Titrating the Methadone in Opioid-Naïve Patients

Methadone has been shown to be a safe and effective opioid for cancer and noncancer pain, often used as a second-line opioid option.[28-31] Reddy and colleagues evaluated overall survival of patients switching to methadone versus other strong opioids and found no difference.[32] There have been mixed reports evaluating mortality among patients receiving methadone as compared to sustained-release morphine.[33,34] However, methadone has been implicated in a growing and disproportionately high rate of opioid-induced deaths in recent years.[35] Part of this may be due to the nonprescribed use of methadone, but choosing overly aggressive starting doses of methadone and inappropriate titration strategies (in terms of milligram amount increases and how quickly the dose is escalated) may also be partially responsible.

The speed with which we titrate (increase) methadone depends to some extent on the patient's clinical situation and how closely the patient can be monitored. For outpatients, methadone should be titrated cautiously, based on patient response, signs of toxicity, and our knowledge of time to steady-state. Most practitioners adhere to the recommendation that the dose of methadone should not be increased until the patient has received 5 to 7 days of the same dose.[36] The APS guidelines recommend initial dose increases of no more than 5 mg/day every 5 to 7 days. When the methadone TDD exceeds 30 to 40 mg/day, the dose increase should be no more than 10 mg/day every 5 to 7 days.[21] The HPC expert panel agreed with these recommendations.[23] As discussed earlier, a daily phone call or visit to the patient is highly recommended during the titration period. Any card-carrying hospice nurse will tell you it's no coincidence that both "Monday" and "methadone" begin with "M"—this gives the nurse the workweek to assess for potential toxicity!

In situations where opioid-naïve patients are in a controlled, monitored environment, methadone may be started at a higher dose (e.g., 2.5 mg by mouth every 6 or 8 hours) and increased more aggressively. Shir and colleagues describe their experience using epidural and oral methadone in hospitalized patients for severe pain.[37] For opioid-naïve adult patients, the initial dose of methadone did not exceed 5 to 10 mg two or three times daily, and the dose was increased in increments of 20% to 30%. They reported no incidents of respiratory depression or severe mental obtundation, although minor side effects (e.g., mild-to-moderate mental obtundation, itching, nausea, urinary retention) were reported in 13% of patients. This is a fairly aggressive titration schedule, and it is important to know that these hospitalized patients were generally titrated off methadone prior to discharge. If this wasn't the case, it would be very important to monitor the patient for 4 to 5 days *after* the last dosage change (e.g., monitor until you are at or close to steady-state) before discharging the patient.

METHADONE PUBLIC HEALTH ADVISORY

In November 2006, the FDA issued a public health advisory titled, "Methadone Use for Pain Control May Result in Death and Life-threatening Changes in Breathing and Heart Beat."[38] They described patient deaths from the use of methadone in both opioid-naïve patients and those converted to methadone. This public health advisory actually led to a change in the product labeling of methadone.

Specific speaking points included the following:[38]

- **Patients should take methadone exactly as prescribed.** Taking more methadone than prescribed can cause breathing to slow or stop and can cause death. A patient who does not experience good pain relief with the prescribed dose of methadone should talk to his or her doctor.

- **Patients taking methadone should not start or stop taking other medicines or dietary supplements without talking to their healthcare provider.** Taking other medicines or dietary supplements may cause less pain relief. They may also cause a toxic buildup of methadone in the body leading to dangerous changes in breathing or heart beat that may cause death.

- **Healthcare professionals and patients should be aware of the signs of methadone overdose.** Signs of methadone overdose include trouble breathing or shallow breathing; extreme tiredness or sleepiness; blurred vision; inability to think, talk, or walk normally; and feeling faint, dizzy, or confused. If these signs occur, patients should get medical attention right away.

Earlier in this chapter, we discussed the need to monitor the patient closely for over-sedation and respiratory depression. The other important message in this FDA Public Health Advisory is the admonition to be mindful of methadone's ability to cause QTc (e.g., QT interval corrected for heart rate) interval prolongation. Prolongation of the QTc is a surrogate marker for the risk of developing a potentially fatal ventricular arrhythmia called *torsades de pointes* (TdP). Although QTc interval prolongation can occur in hospitalized patients or outpatients, it is thought that hospitalized patients may be at greater risk due to renal and cardiac disease and electrolyte abnormalities.[39] Trinkley points out both modifiable and nonmodifiable risk factors for drug-induced TdP including hypokalemia, drug-drug

(Continued)

METHADONE PUBLIC HEALTH ADVISORY (Continued)

interactions, hypomagnesemia (all modifiable), female sex, advancing age, genetic predisposition, heart failure, bradycardia, and QTc interval prolongation (less or not at all modifiable).[39]

Despite the causal relationship observed between methadone and QTc interval prolongation, the clinical significance and risk stratification is not entirely clear. Ehret and colleagues evaluated QTc interval prolongation in former and current IV drug users admitted to the hospital over a 5-year period; half of the subjects were receiving methadone maintenance therapy and half were not.[40] The QTc interval in healthy cardiac tissue is 400 milliseconds (ms) or less. International regulatory guidelines suggest a gender-independent threshold for QTc (QT corrected for heart rate) prolongation of 450 ms and a QTc interval greater than 500 ms as the threshold for significant arrhythmia risk.[41] The study by Ehret showed that 16.2% of patients receiving methadone had a QTc of 500 ms or longer on at least one electrocardiogram (ECG), whereas all patients in the control group had a QTc of less than 500 ms.[40]

Bart and colleagues evaluated the mean QTc interval in methadone maintenance patients, both while taking, and while off, methadone.[42] The mean QTc interval was significantly higher while patients were on methadone (436 ms) versus off methadone (423 ms), but the authors concluded this dose-related effect was not clinically significant.[42] Reddy and associates evaluated the impact of methadone on the QTc interval of 100 advanced cancer patients.[43] Twenty-eight percent of the patients had QTc interval prolongation at baseline (QTc >430 ms in men, >450 ms in women). Only one of 64 patients had a clinically significant increase in the QTc interval 2 weeks into therapy; no patients had an increase at weeks 4 and 8. The median dose of methadone was 23 mg at 2 weeks, and no patients exceeded 100 mg of methadone per day. Their conclusion was that QTc prolongation was rare in patients with advanced cancer at methadone doses <100 mg/day.[43] Juba and colleagues screened over 900 pain and palliative care

patients receiving methadone to determine predictors of QTc prolongation (defined as a QTc interval >470 ms for men or >480 ms for women, or a QTc interval increase by >60 ms from baseline).[44] Their conclusion was that QTc prolongation was predicted by history of heart failure, peptic ulcer disease, rheumatologic disorders, use of medications known to prolong QTc, malignancy, hypocalcemia, and methadone doses in excess of 45 mg a day.[33]

Guidance from the FDA provides the following:

Drugs that prolong the mean QT/QTc interval by around 5 ms or less do not appear to cause TdP. Whether this signifies that no increased risk exists for these compounds or simply that the increased risk has been too small to detect is not clear. The data on drugs that prolong the mean QT/QTc interval by more than around 5 and less than 20 ms are inconclusive, but some of these compounds have been associated with proarrhythmic risk. Drugs that prolong the mean QT/QTc interval by >20 ms have a substantially increased likelihood of being proarrhythmic, and might have clinical arrhythmic events captured during drug development.[45]

It is also important to be mindful of other medications that can prolong the QTc interval. A comprehensive review of drug-related QT interval prolongation by Crouch and colleagues describes "torsadogenic" drugs and categorizes them as definite, probable, and proposed.[46]

Medication categories that contain drugs that definitely prolong the QT interval include antiarrhythmics, antidepressants (primarily tricyclics), some antihistamines (now off market in the United States), anti-infectives, antipsychotics, chemotherapy agents, cardiovascular nonantiarrhythmics, and gastrointestinal agents.

This is an important reference for pain management practitioners to have readily available. You can access it online at: http://www.medscape.com/view-article/458868_print. Another useful website is www.crediblemed.org.[47]

Recommendations for Cardiac Safety Monitoring with Methadone

FAST FACTS

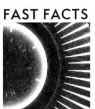

The APS made recommendations for electrocardiogram (ECG) monitoring baseline (before starting methadone) and for follow-up monitoring.[21]

Their recommendations are as follows:

Baseline Electrocardiogram	
Recommendation	**Follow-Up Action**
Obtain an ECG prior to initiation of methadone in patients with: ▶ Risk factors for QTc interval prolongation ▶ Any prior ECG demonstrating a QIc >450 ms ▶ A history suggestive of prior ventricular arrhythmia An ECG obtained within the previous 3 months with a QTc <450 ms in a patient with no new risk factors for QTc interval prolongation can be used for the baseline assessment. Consider obtaining an ECG prior to initiation of methadone in patients not known to be at higher risk for QTc interval prolongation. An ECG obtained within the previous year with a QTc <450 ms in patients without new risk factors for QTc interval prolongation can be used for the baseline assessment. ***Risk factors for QTc interval prolongation per the APS guidelines include:*** ▶ Electrolyte abnormalities such as hypokalemia or hypomagnesemia ▶ Impaired liver function ▶ Structural heart disease (e.g., congenital heart defects or a history of endocarditis or heart failure) ▶ Genetic predisposition such as congenital prolonged QT syndrome or familial history of prolonged QT syndrome ▶ Use of drugs with QTc-prolong properties	▶ The panel recommends *against* the use of methadone in patients with a baseline QTc interval >500 ms. ▶ The panel recommends considering an alternate opioid in patients with a baseline QTc interval ≥450 ms but <500 ms. If the decision is to use methadone in these cases, practitioners should attempt to identify and correct reversible causes of QTc interval prolongation.

(Continued)

Recommendations for Cardiac Safety Monitoring with Methadone (*Continued*)

Follow-Up Electrocardiograms	
Recommendation	**Follow-Up Action**
The panel recommends a follow-up ECG 2–4 weeks after beginning methadone therapy, and with each significant dose increase in the following situations: ▶ Patients with risk factors for QTc interval prolongation ▶ Any prior ECG demonstrating a QTc >450 ms ▶ History of syncope The panel recommends all patients receive a follow-up ECG when the methadone TDD reaches 30–40 mg, and again at 100 mg/day. The panel recommends a follow-up ECG for patients receiving methadone with new risk factors for QTc prolongation, or signs or symptoms suggestive of arrhythmia.	▶ The panel recommends clinicians switch from methadone to an alternate opioid, or immediately reduce the methadone dose, when a follow-up ECG discloses a QTc interval ≥500 ms. ▶ Clinicians should also identify and rectify any reversible causes of QTc interval prolongation and repeat ECG after the methadone dose has been decreased. ▶ The panel recommends clinicians consider switching from methadone to a different opioid in patients with a QTc interval ≥450 ms but <500 ms, or reducing the methadone dose. ▶ Clinicians should also identify and rectify any reversible causes of QTc interval prolongation and repeat ECG after the methadone dose has been decreased. ▶ Should methadone be continued, the panel recommends clinicians discuss the potential risks of continuing methadone with patients.

ECG = electrocardiogram; ms = milliseconds; TDD = total daily dose

The HPC expert group also discussed the role of ECG monitoring for HCP patients where methadone is being considered or taken by patients. The consensus was that the patient's clinical situation and prognosis should guide the clinicians. For example, if the patient is actively seeking disease-modifying therapies, then the APS guidelines should be followed. If the patient has chosen supportive care only, practitioners may choose to relax the ECG monitoring requirement and remain alert for risk factors, correcting those that are amenable to such.[23]

CONVERTING TO METHADONE FROM OTHER OPIOIDS (E.G., OPIOID-TOLERANT PATIENTS)

The majority of patients probably come to methadone as a second-line therapy, having converted from a different opioid such as morphine, oxycodone, hydromorphone, or hydrocodone. ***The $64,000 question is**—how can we best convert a patient from a different opioid to methadone, achieve pain relief as quickly as possible, while not increasing the risk of immediate or delayed toxicity?* If you walk outside on a clear night and look up, you will probably see a lot of stars—count them, because that's how many proposed conversion charts we have for methadone!

One thing is very, very, VERY clear—the conversion from other opioids such as morphine to methadone is NOT a linear conversion. What do we mean by this? If you look at the equianalgesic conversion table we've been using in previous chapters, you see recommendations such as: oxycodone 20 mg oral ≈ morphine 25 mg oral. We can quibble and say the oral oxycodone:morphine ratio is 15:15, or 15:30, and we can argue whether this is a bidirectional equivalency, but one clear implication is that it's linear. In other words, if you buy the fact that oxycodone 20 mg oral ≈ morphine 25 mg oral, then you also accept that oxycodone 200 mg oral ≈ morphine 250 mg oral. In other words— it's linear. This is **absolutely not** the case when converting to methadone. The higher the dose of the original opioid, the more potent the methadone is. There are numerous suggested ways to switch to methadone, and the morphine:methadone equivalency ranges from 3:1 to 40:1 or more! Remember, *more potent* doesn't mean *more effective*— **potency** *refers to an equivalent dose to achieve equivalent pain control.*

Why is this? Why does methadone become more powerful with increasing prior exposure to other opioids? Bruera suggests three possible reasons for this observation.[48] First, the molecular structure and chemical characteristics of methadone may alter binding to the opioid receptors, possibly resulting in less cross-tolerance to methadone (making the patient more sensitive to the effects of methadone than you would have suspected). Second, we discussed earlier in this chapter how methadone has additional mechanisms of action. Antagonism at the NMDA receptor may significantly reverse opioid tolerance, which can dramatically enhance the patient's response to methadone. Third, Bruera hypothesizes that more traditional opioids such as morphine and hydromorphone are metabolized to pharmacologically active products that may have a *proalgesic* effect (refers to a *pain-producing effect* such as seen with metabolites including morphine-3-glucuronide, normorphine, etc.). Whether it is due to one or more of these reasons, or other reasons, clearly the morphine to methadone conversion is not linear.

So what are the steps in converting from other opioids to methadone? Of course, you follow all the steps discussed earlier in this text, as follows:

- **Step 1**—Globally assess the patient (e.g., PQRSTU—precipitating and palliating events, previous treatment, quality, region/radiation, severity, temporal, how does the pain affect you [U]) to determine if the uncontrolled pain is secondary to worsening of existing pain or development of a new type of pain.

- **Step 2**—Determine the TDD of the current opioid. This should include all long-acting and breakthrough opioid doses.

- **Step 3**—In this case, we have already decided we are going to switch to methadone. If the patient was not already on oral morphine, the first part of Step 3 is to convert the patient's current opioid regimen to an equivalent dose of oral morphine. Then, using one of the many proposed methadone conversion methods, calculate the TDD of methadone.

- **Step 4**—Individualize the dosage based on assessment information gathered in Step 1 and ensure adequate access to breakthrough medication. It is important to determine if the patient is taking any other medications that may induce or inhibit the metabolism of methadone (this may affect your decision about the total daily methadone dose). In this step, you will also have to decide which opioid to use to treat breakthrough pain (methadone or another opioid), the dose, and dosing frequency. The last decision in Step 4 is whether to do a *rapid switch* (also known as a *stop-start*) or a gradual titration from the patient's current opioid regimen to methadone.

- **Step 5**—Finally, it is critical that you exercise very close patient follow-up and continued reassessment. Encourage the patient to use his or her rescue opioid while the methadone accumulates, and monitor the patient to make sure the accumulating methadone dose is not a toxic dose for the patient.

Let's look at a case to illustrate the process of switching to methadone!

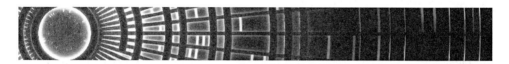

CASE 6.4
. . . .
Switching to Oral Methadone

> AO is a 64-year-old man with chronic low back pain. He is taking Kadian 80 mg by mouth every 12 hours with morphine immediate release 20 mg every 4 hours as needed for break-through pain (he uses on average one dose per day). He is not a surgical candidate, and his physician would like to switch him to methadone in hopes of achieving better pain control. AO is not taking any medications known to interact with methadone.

Step 1—Globally Assess the Patient (e.g., PQRSTU)

Of course we always start with complete analysis of the pain complaint. For patients with pain of mixed pathogenesis (e.g., nociceptive and neuropathic), methadone may be a preferred opioid. AO describes pain in his sacral area, with an occasional shooting pain down his leg and numbness in that extremity after standing a while. The physician hopes that switching to methadone will eliminate the need to add an adjuvant agent to the regimen, keeping things simpler for the patient.

Step 2—Determine Total Daily Dose of Opioid

Calculate the TDD of the patient's current opioid including long-acting tablets or capsules, and an average of their rescue opioid, particularly those doses used for spontaneous and nonvolitional incident pain. AO is taking Kadian 80 mg by mouth every

12 hours (160 mg TDD oral morphine) plus morphine immediate 20 mg for rescue (using about one dose a day for a total of 20 mg). His TDD of oral morphine is 180 mg.

Step 3—Convert to Daily Oral Morphine Equivalent Dose, Then Convert to Methadone

If the patient is already taking oral morphine, your work is almost done. If not, you need to do the mathematical calculations we discussed earlier in this text to determine the daily oral morphine equivalent dose. Be sure to consider both long- and short-acting opioids the patient is receiving (average the use of rescue opioid the patient takes). The patient may be taking more than one opioid—convert all opioids to the total daily oral morphine equivalent dose. Importantly, as we discussed with fentanyl, you *do not* reduce the total daily oral morphine equivalent dose for lack of complete cross-tolerance. This is taken into consideration when we convert the daily oral morphine to methadone. In the case of AO, he is already taking oral morphine, so we don't need to do any calculation.

Okay—now the tricky part—the actual conversion from oral morphine (or oral morphine equivalent) to methadone. There are a great number of ways to convert to methadone—just as there is more than one way to skin a cat or pluck a chicken! Differences between proposed methods include various models of how/when to discontinue the original opioid regimen and how/when to start methadone, different proposed equi-analgesic ratios between oral morphine and oral methadone, whether a loading dose of methadone should be administered to achieve pseudo-steady-state, whether to use a scheduled methadone regimen, or a self-titrated "as needed" dosing scheme, and differences in recommended dosing intervals. *Ay yi yi!!*

Okay, okay, I know what you're thinking. Actually I know what you're saying—"I can't believe I bought this book. You would think the answer to methadone conversion calculations would be in the book—but no, she gives us 18 possible ways to do it. I might as well pick up a dart and throw it!" I share your pain. But it's not just me—I promise! Weschules and Bain conducted an exhaustive—exhaustive AND exhausting (I had to take a nap after reading it)—review of opioid conversion ratios used with methadone for treatment of pain.[49] They reviewed 22 clinical studies (none of which was deemed to be of high quality) and 19 case reports or series, which included 730 patients. Ratios used to convert patients from morphine to methadone ranged from 4:1 to 37.5:1. And after this mind-boggling review, what was their bottom line? And I quote,

> There was no evidence to support the superiority of one method of rotation to methadone over another. Patients may be successfully rotated to methadone despite discrepancies between rotation ratios initially used and those associated with stabilization. Further research is needed to identify patient-level factors that may explain the wide variance in successful methadone rotations.[49]

I was particularly impressed with a passage in their discussion, as follows:

> One important distinction that needs to be made is between methadone rotations as a *care process* as opposed to a *dose calculation*. It may be less important to determine an exact opioid ratio when performing a methadone conversion than it is to assure that the patient is an appropriate candidate for methadone conversion, the switch is carried out over a time period consistent with the therapeutic goals, and that the patient is monitored closely by medical staff throughout the process.[49]

Brings a tear to your eye, doesn't it? This is *exactly* what we've been saying throughout this book—***Do the math based on the very best the literature has to offer, tempered with common sense clinical judgment, and monitor your patient like nobody's business!***

McLean and Twomey have provided an excellent review of these "care processes" used in switching to methadone.[50] Table 6-3 shows their summarization of the main methods of rotation to methadone.

McLean and Twomey compared the outcomes of two primary methods of switching to methadone: ***the stop-and-go method*** (which includes the *rapid conversion* method and the *ad libitum* method) and the ***3-day switch method***.

Table 6-3
Summary of Main Methods of Rotation to Methadone

Rotation Method	Description
3DS	• Day 1—30% of original opioid replaced with an equianalgesic dose of methadone given in three daily divided doses. • Days 2 and 3—dose of methadone is increased by 30% and dose of original opioid reduced by 30% each day.
RC stop and go	• Original opioid is discontinued. • Daily methadone dose is calculated according to evidence-based conversion ratios and given in three regular divided daily doses. • Regular methadone dose titrated to achieve effective analgesia. • It has been argued that a higher priming dose of methadone (20%–30% higher than as calculated using published conversion ratios) may be required initially.
AL stop and go	• Original opioid is discontinued. • A fixed dose of methadone that is one-tenth of the actual or calculated morphine equivalent oral daily dose up to a maximum of 30 mg is calculated. • The fixed dose is taken orally as required but not more frequently than three hourly (every 3 hours). • On day 6, the methadone requirement of the previous two days is noted and converted into a regular every 12-hour regime.
German model	• Original opioid is discontinued. • Methadone is prescribed at a dose of 5–10 mg orally every 4 hours and every 1 hour as needed. • On days 2–3, the dose of methadone is titrated up by 30% until analgesia is achieved. After 72 hours, methadone dosing is changed to an every 8-hour and every 3-hour as-needed regime as the same dose as prescribed on days 2–3. Methadone dose is titrated up until analgesia is achieved.
Outpatient titration	• Original opioid continued at same dose. • Methadone commenced at 5 mg orally every 4 hours and increased by 5 mg/dose every 3 days until improved analgesia is noted. • Original opioid then reduced by one-third, and the methadone dose increased according to breakthrough requirements. The original opioid dose is reduced, and the methadone dose increased accordingly over a variable period.

3DS = 3 day switch; RC = rapid conversion; AL = ad libitum (as needed)

Source: Reprinted from McLean S, Twomey F. Methods of rotation from another strong opioid to methadone for the management of cancer pain: A systematic review of the available evidence. *J Pain Symptom Manage.* 2015;50:248-259. ©2015, with permission of Elsevier.

The ***rapid switch stop-and-go***, as described in Table 6-3, includes stopping the original opioid and starting methadone with the next dose. The methadone dose is calculated from some evidence-based equianalgesic conversion (more on this later). Some have argued that a "loading dose" or "priming dose" of methadone (up to 30% higher than the calculated dose) should be administered initially. ***Ad libitum***, the other stop-and-go method, involves stopping the original opioid, and offering the patient one-tenth of the total daily morphine equivalent as needed (in other words, they used a 10:1 oral morphine:oral methadone conversion), but no more frequently than every 3 hours.

The 3-day switch method includes a calculated methadone conversion as described in the stop-and-go method, but the implementation is rolled out over 3 days. On day 1 of the switch, the original opioid dose is reduced by 30%, and 30% of the calculated methadone TDD is started. On days 2 and 3, the original opioid regimen is further reduced by 30%, and the methadone dose is increased on each day by 30%.

The other two methods McLean and Twomey very briefly discuss are the German model, which is somewhat complicated (see Table 6-3) and an outpatient titration approach that was in one publication. The actual decision—an operationalization of the rotation to methadone—is Step 4 (okay, maybe Step 3.5 because you consider both the dosage and the roll-out simultaneously).

Before we examine the conclusions of McLean and Twomey, let's discuss these *equianalgesic ratios* used in all the methods. As we discussed earlier, although there are many proposed ratios from morphine to methadone, there is one common theme—the higher the daily oral morphine equivalent dose, the more potent methadone is. This is *not* a linear relationship; *the more morphine equivalent the patient was on, the lower the percentage of methadone needed to give an equianalgesic effect.*

So, what is the magic number? First, it's a moving target—it depends on the daily oral morphine dose (or equivalent). The ratio tends to range from 3:1 to 40:1 (oral morphine:oral methadone).

Let's look at some of the commonly used ratio conversion charts.

Ripamonti, 1998[51]						
Morphine dose (mg/day)	30–90	90–300	Greater than 300			
Morphine: methadone EDR	4:1	6:1	8:1			
Mercadante, 2001[52]						
Morphine dose (mg/day)	30–90	90–300	>300			
Morphine: methadone EDR	4:1	8:1	12:1			
Ayonrinde, 2000[53]						
Morphine dose (mg/day)	Less than 100	101–300	301–600	601–800	801–1,000	1,001 or more
Morphine: methadone EDR	3:1	5:1	10:1	12:1	15:1	20:1

EDR = equianalgesic dose ratio

How do you use these charts? Let's look at applying each of these methods to the case of AO.

- Using the Ripamonti method, when the daily oral morphine dose is between 90 and 300 mg, you apply a 6:1 ratio (morphine:methadone). Therefore, applying a 6:1 (morphine:methadone) ratio to 180 mg per day of oral morphine would be approximately 180/6, or <u>30 mg oral methadone per day.</u>

- Using the Mercadante method, in the same dosage range, you apply an 8:1 ratio (180/8), giving you <u>22.5 mg oral methadone per day.</u>

- With the Ayonrinde method, it's a 5:1 ratio (180/5), <u>or 36 mg per day of oral methadone.</u>

- The Fast Facts published by Palliative Care Network of Wisconsin recommends the Ayonrinde method; however, after calculating the TDD of oral methadone they recommend reducing this dose by 50% to 75% (making this a fourth method!).[54] In this case, we would take our 36-mg oral methadone per day and reduce it by 50% to 75% to <u>9 to 18 mg oral methadone per day.</u>

- What does the manufacturer of Dolophine hydrochloride (methadone hydrochloride) recommend as a conversion, as recently updated in their prescribing information and approved by the FDA (yes, this would be the fifth method!)?[22] *Their recommended oral morphine to oral methadone conversion for chronic administration is as follows:*

Total Daily Baseline ORAL Morphine Dose	Estimated Daily ORAL Methadone Requirement as Percent of Total Daily Morphine Dose
Less than 100 mg	20% to 30%
100 to 300 mg	10% to 20%
300 to 600 mg	8% to 12%
600 mg to 1,000 mg	5% to 10%
Greater than 1,000 mg	Less than 5%

Using the case of AO, receiving 180 mg of oral morphine per day, the estimated daily oral methadone requirement would be 10% to 20% of the total daily morphine dose, or <u>18 to 36 mg per day.</u> So, looking at these very popular methods, this gives us a range from 9 to 36 mg of oral methadone per day—nothing like a fourfold difference to make you scratch your head!

- Just to make you crazy, let me lay one more simplified methadone conversion on you! Dr. William Plonk combined the above and other methods to derive a linear regression equation for dosing conversion (yes, by golly, this makes six, and I promise I'm going easy on you!).[55] *His final equation is as follows:*

$$\textit{Estimated oral methadone per day } (mg) = \frac{\left[\text{oral morphine equivalents per day (mg)}\right] + 15}{15}$$

Using AO, above, 180-mg oral morphine per day calculates to [(180/15) + 15] = <u>27 mg per day oral methadone.</u> This is in the ballpark of the answers we calculated using the other methods. This model is accurate up to 600 mg/day oral morphine.

- What do the APS guidelines recommend for conversion from other opioids to methadone? Basically they say "pick whichever method y'all like, but after you calculate your answer, reduce it by 75% to 90%" (of course, I'm paraphrasing here). They further state that regardless of the calculated dose, do not start methadone at greater than 30 to 40 mg per day.[21] So if you use the APS recommendations, the answer for AO would be 10% to 25% of ANY of the calculated doses above.

Before I share with you (finally) the method I use, let's discuss the one published comparison between the 3-day switch method and the rapid conversion method.[56] In this trial, 42 patients were randomized to either the stop-and-go strategy, or the 3-day switch. *The morphine:methadone equianalgesic dose was calculated as follows:*

Oral Morphine Equivalent Total Daily Dose	Oral Morphine:Oral Methadone Conversion
30–90 mg	4:1
91–300 mg	6:1
301 600 mg	8:1
601–1,000 mg	10:1
>1,000 mg	12:1

Pain intensity, adverse effects, and serious adverse events were tracked for 14 days after switching. The mean oral morphine equivalent dose was 900 mg in the stop-and-go group and 1,330 mg in the 3-day switch group prior to conversion to methadone.

Although there was no difference between the two groups in pain intensity on day 3, overall there was a trend of more pain, significantly more dropouts, and three serious adverse events (two deaths and one severe sedation) in the stop-and-go group. The authors concluded that the stop-and-go approach should not replace the 3-day switch approach.[56] The 3-day switch method (and the ad libitum [as needed]) methods require fairly intense education of patients, families, and nursing staff (because they are the parties most likely operationalizing this plan) as they require meticulous attention to patient response and dosing.

If it would please the jury, I would like to point out a few facts about the methods used in this study. The morphine to methadone conversion did not take into consideration any patient-specific variables, such as age. Nor was there a limit to the maximum starting dose of methadone; the starting dose ranged from 1/4 to 1/12 of the total daily oral morphine equivalent dose. This means in the stop-and-go group, these patients started out on day 1 at 90-mg oral methadone a day (900 mg; 10:1 oral morphine:oral methadone conversion). The 3-day switch group started at 110 mg (1,330 mg; 12:1 oral morphine:oral methadone conversion), but at about 35 mg on day 1, about 70 mg on day 2, then the full 110 mg on day 3 (as the previous opioid regimen was being cross-tapered down).

So why do you think the APS guidelines recommended not starting the methadone regimen at no greater than 30 to 40 mg per day, regardless of your calculated dose? Probably for the three reasons Bruera suggested the morphine:methadone relationship is not linear (methadone may have slight binding differences at the opioid receptor, methadone has additional mechanisms of action, simply switching from an opioid with proalgesic metabolites is a positive therapeutic intervention).[48] Chatham and colleagues reported on a series of 10 cases of patients on high oral morphine dose equivalents, and their conversion to oral morphine.[57] Ten patients were receiving between 1,200-mg and 10,940-mg oral morphine equivalent prior to conversion to oral methadone. As shown in Table 6-4, 9 of the 10 patients were switched to methadone 10 mg by mouth every 8 hours (1 switched to 5 mg by mouth every 6 hours and 1 switched to 15 mg by mouth every 8 hours). Eight of the 10 were stabilized (defined as the patient requiring no dose modifications for 5 consecutive days) at 10 mg by mouth every 8 hours (one stabilized at 20 mg by mouth every 8 hours and one stabilized by 15 mg by mouth every 8 hours).

The authors concluded that a fixed maximum methadone dose of 30 mg/day resulted in clinically meaningful pain relief without causing adverse effects for the majority of patients.[57]

But wait—back at the ranch—what DID McLean and Twomey conclude from their evaluation of methadone conversion care processes? Basically they agreed that there is no slam-dunk method based on the available literature. Both 3-day switch and the ad libitum methods seemed to be effective, but the data were low quality. They observed that the rapid conversion stop-and-go didn't seem to give any advantage over the 3-day switch.[50]

*****Ok, you've been waiting a long time for this—method number 8—used by this author and endorsed by the HPC expert group.*****

The 3-day switch may be useful but should definitely be limited to inpatient use where practitioners highly knowledgeable about opioid conversion practices can

Table 6-4

Dose Ratios Between High-Dose Oral Morphine or Equivalents and Oral Methadone[57]

Patient #	Oral MED	Initial Methadone Dose	Stabilized Methadone Dose
1	1,200 mg	5 mg po q6h	10 mg po q8h
2	1,220 mg	15 mg po q8h	20 mg po q8h
3	1,371 mg	10 mg po q8h	10 mg po q8h
4	1,495 mg	10 mg po q8h	15 mg po q8h
5	1,900 mg	10 mg po q8h	10 mg po q8h
6	2,440 mg	10 mg po q8h	10 mg po q8h
7	2,578 mg	10 mg po q8h	10 mg po q8h
8	7,500 mg	10 mg po q8h	10 mg po q8h
9	8,316 mg	10 mg po q8h	10 mg po q8h
10	10,904 mg	10 mg po q8h	10 mg po q8h

h = hour; MED = morphine equivalent dose; po = by mouth; q = every closely monitor the patient. *For the vast majority of conversions, we consider the age of the patient, use a simplified equianalgesic ratio conversion, and have a maximum daily dose, as follows:*

Oral Morphine Equivalent per Day	Oral Morphine:Oral Methadone Ratio
<60 mg	Refer to opioid-naïve dosing
60–199 mg OME and patient ≤65 years of age	10:1*
≥200 mg OME and/or patient >65 years of age	20:1*

*Not to exceed 30–40 mg per day regardless of previous opioid dose.[23]
OME = oral morphine equivalent

Based on this approach, the patient is 64 years old and he's receiving 180-mg oral morphine equivalent per day, so it would be a 10:1 conversion, or 18 mg per day. One limitation of this method is the discontinuous nature of the conversion. At 199-mg oral morphine per day, the conversion is 10:1 (oral morphine:oral methadone), but ONE milligram more (200 mg or more per day) warrants a 20:1 (oral morphine:oral methadone) conversion. Just like assessing the age if ±1 to 2 years of 65 years, I would also consider the clinical situation if the total daily oral morphine dose was 190 to 210 mg (in addition to their age) and decide to use the 10:1 or 20:1 (oral morphine:oral methadone) conversion. AO is a robust 64-year-old and he's taking less than 200-mg oral morphine per day, so let's be bold and increase to methadone 10 mg by mouth every 12 hours. This 20-mg dose is smack in the range of the other methods (9 to 36 mg per day). We'll discuss the rescue dose in the next step.

Step 4—Individualize the Dosage Regimen

With methadone, one of the most important steps is individualizing the dose based on interacting medications in the patient's medication regimen. As discussed earlier, we would reduce our calculated dose by 25% or more if the patient is taking an enzyme-inhibiting drug. Again, the prospective 25% decrease in oral methadone dose secondary to the anticipated drug interaction is only an estimate; the actual level of inhibition varies from drug to drug. If the patient is taking an enzyme-inducing medication, go with your calculated dose, but be liberal with the rescue medication. AO is not taking any medications that inhibit methadone metabolism so we have no need to reduce our calculated TDD of oral methadone.

Many methadone conversion models advocate using methadone not only for continuous pain control, but for rescue as well. Most pain experts prefer *not* to use methadone for breakthrough pain in addition to the standing dose of methadone.[58] If the patient takes rescue doses of methadone as needed, it may be more difficult to predict when you are finally at steady-state. *The more serious issue is the disparity in time to pain relief versus time to steady-state*—if a patient keeps taking rescue doses of methadone for unrelieved pain, by the time it reaches steady-state, it may be a potentially fatal dose.

Although there is not a shred of evidence to support this statement, most end-of-life practitioners will tell you that methadone doesn't seem to work as well as morphine in treating *dyspnea* (shortness of breath or an uncomfortable awareness of breathing). Therefore, if you are treating a patient with end-stage chronic obstructive pulmonary disease, lung cancer, or any other disease associated with dyspnea, it may be more prudent to use short-acting morphine for breakthrough pain OR dyspnea.

If you chose to use morphine or another short-acting opioid for breakthrough pain, follow the 10% to 15% of the TDD guideline we've discussed throughout the book. You would base the breakthrough dose on the total daily morphine equivalent you calculated back in Step 1. In the case of AO, his total daily oral morphine dose was 180 mg; therefore, you could suggest immediate-release morphine 18 to 27 mg every 2, 3, or 4 hours as needed for breakthrough pain. Twenty milligrams every 2 hours as needed for breakthrough pain seems like a reasonable dose (especially if you're using the morphine 20-mg/mL oral solution). It somehow seems a bit cleaner to use an opioid other than methadone if you have other variables influencing the situation such as converting from transdermal fentanyl in a cachectic patient where you're not sure how much benefit they were getting from the patch, or a patient with multiple comorbid conditions such as renal and/or hepatic impairment, or a patient on multiple interacting medications. Using a short-acting opioid such as morphine, oxycodone, oxymorphone, or hydromorphone for breakthrough introduces one less variable you have to worry about.

On the other hand, if you are switching to methadone because the patient had a poor outcome with morphine or another short-acting opioid (e.g., allergic reaction), it would certainly be acceptable to use methadone for breakthrough pain. We can still use our 10% to 15% of the TDD rule, but some practitioners may provide a bit larger dose while still on the way to methadone steady-state. For example, with AO, we could suggest an order such as methadone 10 mg by mouth every 12 hours, plus an additional 3 mg every 3 hours as needed for additional pain. If AO were in an excellent caregiving situation and experiencing significant pain, we could even consider methadone 5 mg every 3 hours as needed for additional pain if within the first few days of methadone therapy. Of course, we would ask AO to keep a pain diary and document use of rescue methadone, and we would expect to see less and less use of the rescue opioid as the days went by and he approached steady-state. If on day 7 of therapy we found that AO was taking his regularly scheduled methadone 10 mg by mouth every 12 hours, plus two extra doses of methadone 5 mg per day, we could change his regimen to methadone 15 mg by mouth every 12 hours, plus 5 mg every 3 hours for breakthrough pain. In this case, the rescue dose is slightly more than 15% of his TDD oral methadone (TDD is 30-mg oral methadone; 10% = 3 mg, 15% = 4.5 mg).

Again, the decision concerning how to implement the switch (stop-and-go or 3-day switch) is a Step 4 decision. *In my practice, I generally do the stop-and-go rapid conversion, unless one of the following situations exists:*

- The patient is on a high dose of morphine (e.g., greater than 400 to 600 mg total daily oral morphine dose).
- It's a complicated conversion calculation (e.g., converting from multiple opioids simultaneously).
- The patient is very cachectic, and we're converting from transdermal fentanyl.
- We need to build trust with the patient/family.

In very complicated cases, we will frequently admit the patient to an inpatient hospice unit to facilitate the conversion to methadone, where we can provide closer patient monitoring and better rescue for breakthrough pain crises. With the case of AO, I would stop the Kadian, begin the methadone 12 hours later, and continue the immediate-release morphine 20 mg every 2 hours as needed for breakthrough pain.

Step 5—Patient Monitoring

Your work is not over yet—not by a long shot! The *most* critical step is to monitor your patient very closely! We're even dragging AO's wife into the fray! We will ask AO's wife to observe AO several times a day for changes in his unstimulated respirations (depth, rhythm, and rate) over a full minute, difficulty in waking him up, snoring, and other signs of opioid overdose. We will either see or speak to AO daily over the next week.

TITRATING THE METHADONE REGIMEN

As we discussed previously, the patient probably will not achieve steady-state before 4 or more days. You can increase the methadone regimen by an absolute milligram amount, or you can calculate how much opioid they are using for breakthrough pain (methadone or another opioid), and adjust the standing methadone regimen accordingly. Well, we've talked methadone conversion calculations to death—*let's get our hands dirty and try a few more cases, shall we?*

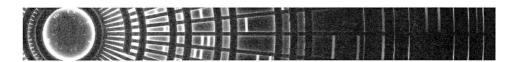

C A S E   6 . 5
• •
Switching to Oral Methadone: Comparing Different Methods

SM is a 63-year-old woman with significant osteoarthritis pain in both knees, both hips, and the sacral area of her spine. She has been referred to your pharmacotherapy service for evaluation and possible conversion to methadone because she describes occasional electric shooting pains down both legs. Her prescriber would like to keep her analgesic regimen as simple as possible. At present, SM is taking MS Contin 45 mg by mouth every 12 hours, plus immediate-release morphine 10 mg every 4 hours as needed (she generally takes three times a day).

You have done your history and physical and agree that converting to methadone is a good idea. Next step, calculate your total daily oral morphine dose—we don't need to calculate the daily oral morphine equivalent because the patient is already *on* morphine. She's getting MS Contin 45 mg by mouth every 12 hours (totals 90-mg oral morphine) plus three doses of the immediate-release morphine 10 mg (30 mg total) for a TDD of 120-mg oral morphine.

SM lives with her husband, who is very interested in her care; therefore, you are comfortable doing a rapid switch. Just for kicks, let's use some of the methods we described above to calculate an equivalent dose of methadone.

- **Ripamonti**—90- to 300-mg oral morphine is a 6:1 conversion; 120/6 = <u>20-mg oral methadone per day</u>

- **Mercadante**—90- to 300-mg oral morphine is an 8:1 conversion; 120/8 = <u>15-mg oral methadone per day</u>

- **Ayonrinde**—101- to 300-mg oral morphine is a 5:1 conversion; 120/5 = <u>24-mg oral methadone per day</u>

- **Fast Facts and Concepts**—Ayonrinde method and reduce by 50% to 75%; 24 mg × 0.75 (75% reduction) or 0.50 (50% reduction) = <u>6- to 12-mg oral methadone per day</u>

Looking at our results from the Ripamonti, Mercadante, Ayonrinde, and Fast Facts methods, the calculated dose is between 6- and 24-mg oral methadone a day. Using the HPC expert panel, the patient is 63-years-old and receiving 120-mg oral morphine per day, so it would be a 10:1 (oral morphine:oral methadone) conversion, or 12-mg oral methadone per day. Using methadone tablets, we could start at a dose of methadone 5 mg by mouth every 12 hours. The patient may actually require methadone 15 mg per day, so we can certainly increase to methadone 5 mg by mouth every 8 hours in 5 to 7 days. In the meantime, we can encourage the patient to use immediate-release morphine 15 mg every 2 hours (a little more than 10% of the 120 mg TDD oral morphine), or even increase that dose to 20 mg if appropriate.

It is important to educate SM and her husband that achieving good pain control with methadone is like climbing a set of stairs—it takes 4 or more days to "get to the top"—achieving steady-state. She should be encouraged to use her rescue opioid as needed, and *document* use of the immediate-release morphine. Mr. M needs to be instructed to systematically, explicitly assess (and document would be nice) SM's level of arousal. As described in the FDA Public Health Advisory, several times a day the husband should stop and purposefully check SM to take notice of any trouble or difficulty breathing (slowed breathing, periods of apnea, unstimulated respiratory rate over a full minute, possibly faster breathing, or shallow breathing), excessive tiredness or sleepiness, or snoring (unless SM routinely sucks the curtains off the wall while asleep!). He should question SM about changes in mentation (e.g., confusion), observe for gait imbalance, or signs of confusion. If Mr. M or Mrs. M suspects anything is amiss, they should contact you immediately.

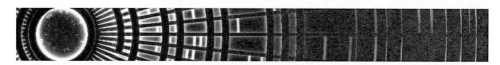

CASE 6.6
. . . .

Switching to Oral Methadone: What a Difference a Day Makes!

Let's look at the case of QG, a 67-year-old man with low back pain. He has been taking half of a Percocet tablet (5-mg oxycodone/325-mg acetaminophen) about four times a day with good success, but he complains about having to carry the Percocet tablets around with him, and it's an inconvenience having to cut them in half. He asks about a longer-lasting opioid. You think of OxyContin, but the lowest dosing regimen would be 10 mg by mouth every 12 hours, or 20-mg oxycodone per day. He is only using 10-mg oxycodone per day. Your assessment of his pain does not indicate an adjuvant medication would be of particular help.

Then you think of methadone—this can be dosed twice daily as well. *How do we come up with an equivalent dose of methadone to maintain pain control?*

Next, we have to determine the total daily oral morphine equivalents QG is receiving. He is taking 10 mg oxycodone per day. Using our 20 mg oral oxycodone ≈ 25 mg oral morphine, we see this is approximately 12.5 mg of oral morphine per day. Remember—we do *not* reduce this amount for lack of cross-tolerance; this is already taken into account when we convert to methadone.

His TDD is well under the 40- to 60-mg oral morphine equivalents, which fall in the "opioid-naïve" category using the HPC expert panel approach. Should his age (67 years) influence our decision about a methadone starting dose?

We have all seen patients over 65 years old who look and act 10 or more years younger, just as we have seen patients 60 years old who could pass for 80 physiologically. We know that when a patient goes to bed 64 years old and wakes up 65 years old the next day, he did not suffer a huge physiologic decline. We have to use common sense about this. I frequently ask nurses about patients whose age is *around* 65 years old, "Is he a *young* 67 or an *old* 67?" Hospice nurses TOTALLY get this—they give the patient the hairy eyeball (as if they are scrutinizing their innards) and make an informed decision. I trust their gut and dose the methadone accordingly!

So, for QG, he's only 67; you learn that he's in great shape other than the low back pain (he still works full time and exercises daily). Minimally, I would recommend methadone 2.5 mg by mouth once daily (perhaps in the a.m.), but it's very likely he'll do just fine on methadone 2.5 mg by mouth every 12 hours. You can still keep the Percocet tablets (one-half tablet every 4 hours as needed) for breakthrough pain (although QG wasn't too happy with the Percocet tablets to begin with; hopefully, he won't need a rescue opioid once he's at steady-state on methadone). And, of course, you would closely monitor your patient for therapeutic effectiveness and potential toxicity.

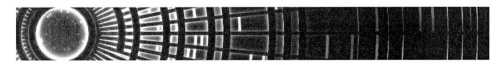

CASE 6.7
• •
Switching to Oral Methadone from Multiple Opioids

JK is a 54-year-old man referred to hospice care with a diagnosis of end-stage lung cancer. On admission to hospice, he is taking the following analgesics:

- Transdermal fentanyl 75 mcg/hr every 3 days

- OxyContin 20 mg by mouth every 12 hours

- Morphine 10 mg by mouth every 2 hours as needed (taking about five doses per day)

Despite this regimen, he rates his worst pain as an 8 (on a 0–10 scale; 0 = no pain, 10 = worst imaginable pain), his best as a 4, and his daily average as 5. Plus, it makes little sense clinically to have a patient take two long-acting opioid formulations (transdermal fentanyl and OxyContin). After a careful symptom analysis you decide that switching him to methadone is a good option. He is not receiving any medications known to interact with methadone. *How would you convert him to methadone?*

Next, we have to calculate the total daily morphine equivalent dose. Transdermal fentanyl 75 mcg/hr is approximately equivalent to 150-mg oral morphine (JK is not cachectic). OxyContin 20 mg by mouth every 12 hours equals 40-mg oxycodone per day, which is approximately equivalent to 50-mg oral morphine per day. Plus he's taking five doses of morphine solution 10 mg per dose which totals 50 mg. Altogether, he is receiving 250-mg oral morphine equivalent per day.

Using the HPC expert method, the patient is under 65 years of age, but he is receiving greater than 200-mg oral morphine equivalent per day, so we should use the 20:1 ratio (oral morphine:oral methadone), which is 12.5-mg methadone per day (260/10). Because he is still in pain, and he's actually quite a bit younger than 65 years old, we can increase to 15 mg per day and order methadone 5 mg by mouth every 8 hours. Because the patient has lung cancer and he experiences occasional shortness of breath, we will keep the morphine for breakthrough pain, but we will increase the dose to 30 mg, offered every 2 hours. Encourage use of a pain diary, monitor the patient, and adjust the methadone therapy as appropriate.

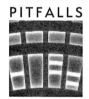

PITFALLS   Adjusting Oral Methadone Regimens

Because methadone has a long terminal half-life, it takes 4 or more days to achieve steady-state (range 4 to 14 days; let's say 5 days on average). Unless the patient is experiencing magnificent pain, do *not* increase the scheduled doses of methadone *before* 5 to 7 days; instead, use rescue opioids to treat additional pain. If you increase the scheduled methadone dose one or more times *before* the patient achieves steady-state (e.g., a stable blood concentration of methadone), by the time the *last* dosage increase achieves steady-state, it may be a toxic dose for the patient!

What about patients who lose the ability to swallow methadone tablets, and it's a situation where you'd rather not use a parenteral opioid (e.g., a home-based hospice patient close to death)? Does switching to the oral methadone intensol get the job done? Does the methadone dose need to be adjusted? Yes, and no! Twenty-five patients receiving oral methadone in the Toronto Grace Palliative Care unit were switched to the methadone 10-mg/mL oral solution at their same methadone dose.[59] The medication was instilled in the buccal cavity (area of oral cavity between the lower molars and buccal mucosa). The maximum volume was 1.5 mL; the TDD of methadone was divided into two or three doses (or four if necessary due to volume limitation). No increase in pain or adverse effects was noted, and there was no need to increase in the dose (in 22 of 24 patients; there was one dropout) or increased use of breakthrough analgesics.[59] Well done, Toronto! As you will read in Chapter 8, highly concentrated oral solutions can be administered to patients with difficulty swallowing, or even with an impaired level of consciousness. The patient's upper body should be propped up to about a 30-degree elevation, and up to 1 mL of solution instilled in the buccal cavity (although they used up to 1.5 mL in this study). Some of the drug will be absorbed transmucosally (the degree of transmucosal absorption depends on lipophilicity), but the rest eventually trickles down the throat and is absorbed orally—so, business as usual!

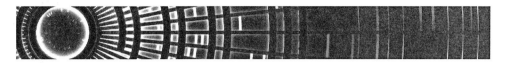

C A S E   6 . 8

Titrating Oral Methadone at Steady-State

AZ is a 48-year-old man with end-stage AIDS, referred to hospice. He was started on morphine around the clock, but it caused extreme itching, and he was switched to an equivalent dose of methadone, 5 mg by mouth every 12 hours. His physician also ordered the 5-mg methadone dose for breakthrough pain every 3 hours as needed. Let's take a look at AZ's pain diary:

Day	Scheduled Methadone Dose (by mouth every 12 hours)	# of Rescue Doses Methadone Taken for Spontaneous Pain	Average Pain Rating
1	Methadone 5 mg	4 doses	7
2	Methadone 5 mg	4 doses	5
3	Methadone 5 mg	3 doses	4
4	Methadone 5 mg	2 doses	3
5	Methadone 5 mg	2 doses	2–3
6	Methadone 5 mg	2 doses	2–3

You see AZ in your clinic on day 7. He is very content with his level of pain control. You have assessed his complaint of pain and feel that switching to methadone was still a good choice. *Do you leave his regimen as is, or make a change?*

You could make a good argument either way. Personally, I would increase his standing dose of methadone to 10 mg by mouth every 12 hours and reduce the breakthrough pain dose to 2.5 mg (because the patient is at steady-state now). Even though the two extra doses he's been using is not an unspeakable burden, I think it's worth a shot to maximize the standing dose, and hopefully alleviate the need for breakthrough doses at this time. If, however, you feel the patient is emotionally attached to regular use of the rescue opioid doses, you might be better off leaving well enough alone. Also, remember to review the other medications concomitantly prescribed and the adherence to taking them—antiretroviral therapy and antimicrobials commonly used in the management of opportunistic infections can significantly interact with methadone. The sudden withdrawal of an enzyme-inducer such as rifabutin can result in potentially toxic levels of methadone.

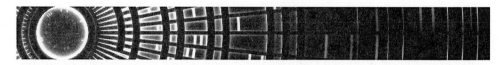

CASE 6.9

Switching to Oral Methadone: Taking the Slow Road

TH is a 28-year-old woman admitted to hospice with cervical cancer (this is a real case, but details have been altered). She comes to you on an IV basal hydromorphone infusion at 10 mg/hr with a 5-mg bolus every 15 minutes as needed (taking about six doses per day). She is a very angry young woman; she has twin daughters who are turning 3 years old soon, and she has several things she wants to accomplish before she dies. She wants to finish potty training the girls and transition them to a regular bed. She finds the hydromorphone infusion cumbersome as it limits her ability to accomplish her remaining goals. After assessing her pain complaint, you mention that you'd like to switch to oral methadone and she snaps at you, "My doctor tried that methadone stuff before. I was so loopy I was seeing two sets of twins. No way!" On closer questioning, you find that TH's physician started her on methadone 10 mg every 6 hours as her first opioid regimen, causing her to have an altered mental status, extreme tiredness, and weakness. You explain that this was probably too high of a dose at the time, which caused adverse effects. You explain that you'd like to revisit methadone as a therapeutic option, and you will carefully calculate the appropriate dose, with a slow and careful conversion process!

TH reluctantly agrees, but she wants to do it cautiously and carefully over a period of time, not as a rapid switch. She has a love-hate relationship with her hydromorphone infusion— it's a pain in the neck, but it does give her good pain control. You agree to do this slowly over a several-week period.

Next, let's determine the total daily oral morphine equivalent based on her current analgesic regimen. She's getting hydromorphone 10 mg/hr, which is 240-mg parenteral hydromorphone per day, plus six doses of 5-mg breakthrough (an additional 30-mg parenteral hydromorphone per day) for a total of 270-mg parenteral hydromorphone per day.

If we use the steady-state data described in Chapter 3 regarding conversion from IV hydromorphone to oral morphine, Reddy and colleagues found the conversion was 1:10 (IV hydromorphone → oral morphine).[60] If we use that conversion, the patient is receiving the equivalent of 2,700-mg oral morphine! Using our equianalgesic chart showing 2-mg IV hydromorphone ≈ 25-mg oral morphine, it calculates to 3,375-mg oral morphine! That's a WHOLE lotta morphine!

Despite receiving the equivalent of 2,700 to 3,375-mg oral morphine a day, the maximum dose of oral methadone would be 30 to 40 mg per the HPC expert panel guidelines. TH is distrustful of a complete and rapid switch, so we will complete this conversion slowly. It would be great if TH was willing to go inpatient for this switch, but of course she says "no dice." Also, I would consider the utility of obtaining a baseline ECG, and determine if she is receiving other medications that prolong the QTc interval, or inhibit the metabolism of methadone.

OK, here's the plan. On day 1 of week 1, we reduce the hydromorphone infusion to 5 mg/hr and keep the bolus at 5 mg. Simultaneously, we start methadone 5 mg by mouth every 8 hours. *So how did we come up with those numbers?* We have empirically halved the hydromorphone infusion (from 10 mg/hr to 5 mg/hr). Therefore, it would be reasonable to replace this with about one-half of the calculated total oral methadone dose (30[to 40]-mg oral methadone per day). We will encourage TH to use the breakthrough dose liberally as needed. On day 1 of week 2, if TH continues to have good pain control (once she's at steady-state), we will discontinue the hydromorphone continuous infusion, but keep the IV hydromorphone bolus in place, and increase the methadone to 10 mg by mouth every 8 hours. Assuming all goes well, on day 1 of week 3, we will discontinue the hydromorphone bolus and switch to an appropriate dose of oral morphine or hydromorphone for breakthrough pain.

Yes, this was a fairly long process, but TH was very fearful of giving up the hydromorphone pump, and she was leery of methadone. This slow process over several weeks allowed us to successfully transition her while allowing her to stay home with her family. Of course, if we had admitted her to our inpatient hospice unit, we could have done the transition more quickly. TH was admitted to our residential hospice facility a few days before her death. I had the honor of meeting her in person the day before she died, during her girls' third birthday party at our facility. Of note, TH accomplished all her goals prior to her death.

USING METHADONE AS AN ADJUNCTIVE ANALGESIC

Often we are in a clinical situation where we would like to take advantage of the unique characteristics of methadone, but are disinclined to attempt a complete switch to methadone. This may include times when a patient will die before they are likely to achieve methadone steady-state or perhaps a situation where we just want a little extra "kick" to boost the current opioid regimen. There is a slim body of evidence supporting the use of methadone adjunctively to an opioid regimen—this means using a small dose of methadone on top of the patient's current opioid regimen.

Because there is evidence implicating the NMDA receptor in the development of opioid-induced hyperalgesia, opioid tolerance, and opioid-resistant neuropathic pain, the addition of low-dose methadone may be beneficial.[61] Wallace and colleagues evaluated the impact of adding methadone to another opioid regimen in 20 cancer pain patients.[62] Their primary outcome measure was a decrease in pain score of 2 or more points from the time of methadone addition to the opioid regimen, to a 1-month follow-up assessment. Fifteen patients had a decrease of two or more points at one month or the closest assessment appointment to that time (pain score decreased from 7.7 ± 1.8 to 5.2 ± 2.4). The mean daily morphine dose was 338 ± 217.8 mg at the time of methadone initiation, and 332 ± 191 mg at the time of evaluation. The mean methadone dose was 4.4 ± 1.4 mg/day at inception, and 15.5 ± 5.9 mg/day at follow-up. Seventeen of the 20 patients tolerated the methadone well.

Courtemanche and colleagues reported on methadone use as a coanalgesic in palliative care cancer patients.[63] They followed a cohort of 146 cancer patients receiving methadone adjunctively; approximately 50% were considered significant responders

(≥30% reduction in pain intensity). The median time to significant response was 7 days (which is consistent with achieving steady-state). The median oral morphine equivalent dose was 120 mg per day, and the median oral methadone dose was 3 mg per day. This study, however, has been criticized due to missing data and its retrospective nature.

In this author's practice, occasionally if a patient is very close to death and we anticipate death prior to achieving steady-state with methadone, we will attempt adding low-dose methadone (e.g., 2.5 mg once or twice daily), although data supporting this approach is not exactly thick on the ground.

TITRATING/CONVERTING OFF METHADONE

Cue the orchestra—"To Dream the Impossible Dream." Okay, it's not that bad, but I am reminded of a line from a Stephen King book, "You can't get there from here!" There is only a very small amount of literature (mostly case reports) that evaluates the methadone-to-morphine conversion. Between this scanty literature and personal correspondence with other pain practitioners, it seems a 1:3 conversion (oral methadone:oral morphine, going TO oral morphine) is probably a safe bet, although it could very well be a higher ratio (e.g., 1:5 or 6).[49,64]

Walker and colleagues evaluated the conversion ratio from methadone (oral and IV) to different opioids.[65] Data from 29 patients were evaluated; the mean dose ratio for oral methadone to oral morphine equivalent daily dose (MEDD) was 1:4.7, and for IV methadone to MEDD was 1:13.5 (a surprising finding given methadone's high oral bioavailability). The authors acknowledged a number of limitations to this study, such as its retrospective nature, low number of subjects, homogeneity in the study population, lack of control for a host of potentially confounding factors, and limited data available related to pain scores. Their final conclusion was that pending additional study, it would be judicious to rotate patients off methadone using a more conservative ratio than what they found in this study, and rely on rescue opioid to maintain pain control. *In my practice, I multiply the total daily methadone dose by 3, and use that as my initial total daily oral morphine dose.*

Glue and colleagues evaluated switching 27 patients from methadone opioid substitution therapy (in other words, it was not for pain management) to oral morphine.[66] They used an initial conversion of total daily oral methadone dose × 4 = total daily oral morphine dose, but found for most patients they eventually required a fivefold increase. Bear in mind, their objective was to prevent withdrawal symptoms, not to maintain pain control.

Obviously, frequent monitoring for opioid withdrawal symptoms, pain ratings, and oversedation is critically important. Also, as the methadone serum concentration falls, additional morphine may be required. In some cases, it may not be possible to completely titrate a patient off methadone and switch them to another opioid completely. However, in such patients, a dosage reduction of methadone and titration of the newly substituted opioid may resolve methadone-related adverse events (if this was the reason for the switch) and still provide adequate pain relief.

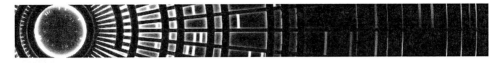

CASE 6.10

Switching Off Oral Methadone to Oral Morphine

GW is a 62-year-old woman with a history of osteoarthritis in both knees and hips. Her pain was not adequately controlled with nonopioids, and her prescriber started her on methadone 2.5 mg by mouth twice daily. Over several weeks, GW was titrated up to 7.5 mg methadone by mouth twice daily. She does not have any opioids available for breakthrough pain. Her pain is improved, but GW continues to complain of a "hung-over" feeling that she has experienced the entire time she's been taking methadone. Today, in clinic she tells you that she wants to stop taking the methadone. You do not want her to stop opioid therapy cold turkey, and she reluctantly agrees to switch to oral morphine. *What dose, and how do we go about this?*

GW's TDD of oral methadone is 15 mg. If we use the conversion ratio described above by Walker and colleagues, it would be 15 × 4.7, or 70.5-mg oral morphine per day. However, based on the researcher's own advice, it would probably be more prudent to use a lower conversion, such as 3:1 (morphine:methadone), which would be 45-mg oral morphine per day. A reasonable plan would be to advise GW to stop the methadone once she got her prescription filled for morphine, and 12 hours after her last methadone dose, begin morphine sulfate 7.5 mg every 4 hours. Also, you can suggest she take morphine 5 mg by mouth every 2 hours as needed for additional pain. I would anticipate that she will probably not need the rescue opioid in the first few days after stopping the methadone (because it takes days for the methadone concentration to fall), but she may need these extra morphine doses to achieve pain control. In about a week, you can make a better assessment of how much morphine GW actually needs per day to keep her comfortable, and you may choose to switch to a long-acting oral morphine product at that time.

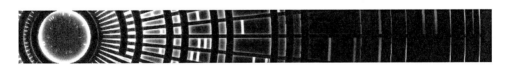

CASE 6.11

Switching Off Oral Methadone to IV Morphine

CR is a 58-year-old woman with end-stage cervical cancer. She is at home on hospice care, and her pain is managed with methadone 10 mg by mouth every 8 hours. For break-through, she is using oral morphine solution, 10 mg for moderate pain every 2 hours as needed, or 20 mg for severe pain every 2 hours as needed. Despite consistently taking an extra 100-mg oral morphine per day on top of the methadone, her pain is not at all well controlled. A decision was made to transfer CR to the inpatient hospice unit for conversion to IV morphine. Once her pain is controlled, a decision can be made about whether to switch her back to methadone. *How do we decide the starting dose of morphine?*

The patient is receiving methadone 10 mg by mouth every 8 hours, which is 30 mg a day. If we multiple by 3, that is approximately equivalent to 90-mg oral morphine. Add in the 100-mg oral morphine she is taking for breakthrough pain, we can approximate her total daily oral morphine dose to be 190 mg. Using our 10:25 (IV morphine:oral morphine) ratio, this is about 76 mg of parenteral morphine a day, or 3.17 mg/hr by continuous infusion. It would be reasonable to stop the methadone, start CR on a morphine infusion at 3 mg/hr, provide a bolus of 2.0 mg every 15 minutes as needed for additional pain, and order a clinician (nurse) bolus of 5-mg IV morphine hourly. You will learn more about titrating parenteral infusions in Chapter 7—trust me when I say we can increase the hourly infusion once we approach steady-state (about 12 or more hours)—but we can increase the patient-controlled analgesia (PCA) bolus or clinician bolus hourly as needed.

PARENTERAL METHADONE

Required reading for any practitioner even *thinking* about working with parenteral methadone is Shaiova and colleagues' consensus guideline document.[67] Parenteral methadone may be given by IV or sub-Q PCA, continuous and/or intermittent bolus infusion. Subcutaneous administration is a bit more challenging because it may cause local erythema and induration in some patients. Strategies to limit this local reaction include rotating the infusion site every 1 to 2 days, limiting the volume (less than 2 to 3 mL/hr), adding dexamethasone 1 to 2 mg/day to the infusate, or if irritation occurs, injecting hyaluronidase into the infusion site.[67]

Converting from Oral to Parenteral Methadone

The consensus guidelines recommend if the patient is not already on oral methadone, convert the patient's current opioid regimen to oral methadone using one of the methods described in this chapter. The TDD of parenteral methadone is then calculated as 50% of the total daily oral methadone dose (actual or as calculated from a different opioid regimen). The TDD parenteral methadone can then be divided by 24 to determine an hourly infusion rate, or divided into intermittent doses to be administered every 6 to 8 hours.

Patient-controlled analgesia is recommended as the preferred method for the administration of parenteral methadone in the consensus guidelines.[67]

Some specific recommendations include the following:

- Calculate a conservative initial basal rate based on current opioid use. Do not increase the basal rate for the first 12 hours after starting IV PCA therapy because both analgesic and sedative properties increase at the 12-hour mark (with infusion initiation or dose increase).
- A patient-demand bolus dose should be available, equivalent to the hourly infusion rate during the titration phase, offered every 15 to 30 minutes.
- Clinician-activated boluses should be available (a dose given by the healthcare provider), usually at twice the hourly infusion rate, and may be given hourly.

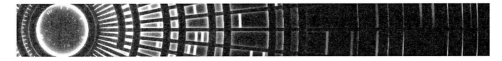

CASE 6.12

• •

Switching from Oral to IV Methadone

BL is a 42-year-old man with end-stage HIV disease. He has been admitted to the hospital with esophagitis, leaving him unable to swallow his MS Contin tablets. Also, he has significant neuropathic pain that is only partially controlled with his current oral morphine regimen. The prescriber has asked for your assistance in transitioning BL to an IV PCA infusion of methadone. Let's take a look at our five-step process as we make this switch.

STEP 1—Assess the patient's pain. You review the physician's admission note and talk briefly with BL who confirms that he has considerable pain in his throat, leaving him unable to swallow anything, and he has complaints of widespread pain that indeed have a neuropathic component. He is rating his pain as an 8 or 9 (on a 0–10 scale; 0 = no pain, 10 = worst imaginable pain).

STEP 2—Determine BL's TDD of opioid use. At present, he is taking MS Contin 120 mg by mouth every 12 hours plus morphine sulfate immediate release (MSIR) 30 mg every 4 hours as needed (using about four doses per day for spontaneous pain). This gives us a grand total of 240 mg plus 120 mg, or 360-mg TDD oral morphine.

STEP 3—Convert this TDD oral morphine to TDD oral methadone. The patient is less than 65 years of age, but on more than 200 mg of oral morphine a day, so using our HPC expert panel guidance, a 20:1 (morphine:methadone) conversion would be appropriate. Using this method, we calculate a TDD oral methadone of 18 mg (360/20). The last part of this step is to convert the TDD oral methadone to a TDD parenteral methadone. Using the 2:1 guideline described above, 18-mg TDD oral methadone would be 9-mg TDD parenteral methadone (18/2).

STEP 4—Individualize the dose for this patient. He is not taking any medications that are known or suspected to interact with methadone, and this is very important given his past medical history (HIV medications and anti-infectives frequently interact with methadone). The other aspect of individualization is to understand that BL is in significant pain right now; therefore, it would be appropriate to increase his dose a bit. Nine milligrams of parenteral methadone calculates to 0.375 mg/hr of IV methadone. Given his current pain complaint, it would be reasonable to increase the PCA continuous infusion to 0.5 mg/hr. We will also set the PCA demand dose at 0.5 mg every 15 minutes, and the clinician-activated bolus as 1 mg, available hourly. BL will likely require a 1-mg bolus as soon as we switch him to the PCA methadone infusion. We should stay with the continuous infusion at 0.5 mg/hr for at least 12 hours; at that time we may adjust the dose as indicated clinically.

STEP 5—The most important step of all—Monitor BL closely for both pain relief and methadone overdose. The clinician should be prepared to administer the clinician-activated bolus hourly as needed, and BL should be monitored for oversedation, respiratory difficulties, confusion, or other methadone-related toxicities; should such occur the PCA dose may need to be reduced.

CONVERTING FROM PARENTERAL TO ORAL METHADONE

The ratio for converting methadone from the oral to parenteral route has been cited as 2:1 by the guidelines described above as well as others.[67-70] Conversely, the recommended ratio for converting from parenteral to oral methadone is 1:2.[69] However, this is inconsistent with our knowledge of the oral bioavailability of methadone, which is 70% to 80% on average (range of 36% to 100%).[5] A 1:2 (parenteral:oral methadone) conversion implies an oral methadone bioavailability of 50%; if in fact this is a low estimate and the oral bioavailability is *higher*, we may be causing neurocognitive adverse effects such as sedation and confusion when switching from parenteral to oral methadone. González-Barboteo and colleagues evaluated conversions from parenteral to oral methadone in eight cancer patients with good pain control (patients were switched to oral methadone for each administration).[71] Their results showed the most accurate conversion ratio to maintain pain control and minimize adverse effects was an oral:parenteral methadone ratio of 1:0.7. Practically, one would multiply the TDD parenteral methadone by 1.3 to determine the TDD of oral methadone. Mathematically, this is consistent with the average bioavailability of methadone (70% to 80%). The researchers acknowledged the limitation of the small number of patients they reported on; but, darn it, their results just *make sense*! González-Barboteo and colleagues use a *stop-and-go approach* in their parenteral to oral conversion: the first dose of oral methadone is given at the discontinuation of the continuous IV or sub-Q infusion. Let's look at a case using the conversion ratio suggested by this research.

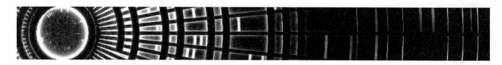

C A S E   6 . 1 2   *(Continues)*
. . . .

Switching from IV to Oral Methadone

One week after admission, BL's pain is very well controlled on an IV PCA methadone infusion at 3 mg/hr with a 3-mg bolus, which he has only used twice in the past 12 hours. He is able to swallow oral solutions and soft foods, and would very much like to be discharged home on oral methadone solution. Let's work out the math for this switch-a-roo.

BL is getting 3 mg/hr of IV methadone; this makes his TDD of parenteral methadone 72 mg (or 78 mg including the two boluses). Using the guideline proposed by González-Barboteo and colleagues, we multiply the TDD parenteral methadone by 1.3, which gives us 93.6-mg TDD oral methadone. When we stop BL's PCA infusion, we can immediately begin methadone 30 mg by mouth every 8 hours, administering the first dose when we discontinue the infusion. We can also offer methadone 15 mg by mouth every 4 hours as needed for additional pain, and, of course, we will monitor our patient carefully during this transition.

The parenteral methadone consensus guidelines offer additional guidance in converting from other IV opioids to IV methadone with PCA. For example, a patient receiving morphine 10 mg/hr by continuous infusion would be switched to a basal IV infusion of methadone at 1 mg/hr, with 1 mg every 15 minutes as needed. Hydromorphone 1.5 mg/hr continuous IV infusion would be equivalent to methadone 0.3 mg/hr with 0.3 mg every 15 minutes as needed, and fentanyl 250 mcg/hr would be methadone 1.25 mg/hr with 1.25 mg every 15 minutes as needed. A clinician bolus of 5 mg (likely hourly) could be made available and used at nurse discretion. The guidelines further recommend reducing these suggested doses by 25% to 50% if the original opioid dose was very high (e.g., morphine 50 mg/hr).[67]

The consensus guidelines are clear in pointing out that the risk of methadone-induced QTc prolongation is significantly greater with parenteral methadone than with oral methadone. This increased risk in QTc prolongation association with parenteral methadone is thought to be due to the preservative chlorobutanol in the IV preparation; therefore, preservative-free methadone may be more appropriate for patients at high risk (although this formulation is considerably more expensive and difficult to obtain). They recommend close monitoring in patients with risk factors such as unexplained syncope (in the patient or a family member), seizures or congenital deafness, history of abnormal serum potassium or magnesium levels, renal impairment, advanced age, female gender, cardiovascular disease, bradycardia, heart failure, hypotension, myocardial ischemia, hypothermia, and pituitary insufficiency.[67] These are in addition to the recommendation for close monitoring when there is concurrent administration with a medication known to inhibit methadone metabolism. The consensus guidelines recommend a screening ECG prior to starting parenteral methadone, after 24 hours of therapy, after 4 days of therapy, when methadone dose is significantly increased, and with any change in patient's condition that increases risk for QT prolongation. They also recommend monitoring electrolytes in patients receiving parenteral methadone.

In this amazing chapter, we have talked about everything worth discussing regarding the incredibly versatile yet demanding opioid, methadone.

As with the chapters that preceded this one, the important things with conversion calculations involving methadone are:

- Understand the pharmacokinetics of the drug.
- Use evidence-based medicine as best we can.
- Above all, be guided by common sense and close monitoring of our patients.

PRACTICE PROBLEMS

P6.1: Starting Oral Methadone in an Opioid-Naïve Patient

KG is a 72-year-old woman with a 1-year history of postherpetic neuralgia. She has tried several adjuvant analgesics with minimal success; therefore, you decide to start methadone. She is not taking any other opioids. Her medications at this time include:

- Lisinopril 20 mg by mouth once daily
- Hydrochlorothiazide 25 mg by mouth once daily
- Sertraline 50 mg by mouth once daily
- Multivitamin with iron one tablet by mouth daily

What is your recommendation for starting methadone in this patient?

P6.2: Starting and Titrating Oral Methadone in an Opioid-Naïve Patient

BM is a 50-year-old man with a history of low back pain. The patient has had recent imaging studies, and no surgical intervention is indicated at this time. He describes the pain as an achy-type feeling, which worsens with bending, stooping, or lifting more than 20 pounds. He rates the constant pain as 6 out of 10 (on a 0–10 scale; 0 = no pain, 10 = worst imaginable pain), increasing to an 8 or 9 with exacerbating activities. He states that when he stands for more than 15 minutes his left leg goes numb, and he frequently experiences shooting pain down his left leg as well. BM's physician has him on pregabalin 100 mg every 8 hours; he had tried duloxetine 60 mg by mouth once daily, but the patient complained of nausea and discontinued therapy. BM's physician would like to begin methadone therapy. BM is receiving no drugs known to interact with methadone.

What starting dose of methadone would you recommend? BM's physician does *not* want to give BM an opioid for breakthrough pain due to suspected abuse of Percocet (oxycodone/acetaminophen) years earlier.

If BM's pain is not entirely controlled on the methadone dose you recommend, when would you increase the dose, and to what dose? What should you monitor while titrating BM for potential methadone-induced side effects?

P6.3: Switching to Oral Methadone; What to Do with an Interacting Drug?

GH is a 42-year-old man who suffered an accident while working at a construction site. There was a cave-in, and he was crushed under an I-beam, requiring reconstruction of his left hip. This has left him with residual pain for which he takes MS Contin 60 mg by mouth every 12 hours plus immediate-release morphine 20 mg every 4 hours as needed (and he takes about six doses per day). This regimen, in addition to the pregabalin (Lyrica) he is already taking, has not successfully controlled his pain. GH is also taking sertraline (Zoloft) 100 mg a day for depression. You decide to switch him to methadone. Perform the calculation using all the methods described. Once you decide on a TDD of methadone, recommend a dosing strategy for both the *rapid-switch* method and the *slow conversion* method. That should keep you off the streets for a while!

P6.4: Switching from Transdermal Fentanyl to Oral Methadone

JR is a 64-year-old man admitted to hospice with a terminal diagnosis of pancreatic cancer. His analgesic regimen on admission is transdermal fentanyl 200 mcg/hr and oxycodone 20 mg every 4 hours as needed for breakthrough pain (taking about six doses per day). Convert to methadone using the HPC method as a rapid switch. Patient is not receiving any medications known to interact with methadone. JR's pain is fairly well controlled on this regimen, but transdermal fentanyl is not on your formulary. He is slim, but not cachectic.

P6.5: Adding Methadone as an Adjunctive Analgesic

VH is a 58-year-old woman with end-stage breast cancer receiving home hospice care. She is currently receiving long-acting oral morphine 90 mg by mouth every 12 hours and oral morphine solution 20 mg every 2 hours as needed for additional pain (taking about five doses per day). The hospice nurse believes VH is within 3 to 4 days of death, but does NOT feel the patient's pain is well controlled. The patient is becoming less lucid, and is now flinching and pulling away when touched. VH's husband refuses to transfer VH to the inpatient hospice unit. *What role can methadone play in the case of VH?*

P6.6: Switching Off Oral Methadone to Another Oral Opioid

AH is a 34-year-old woman with HIV-related neuropathy, receiving pregabalin 100 mg three times daily. Oral hydromorphone was eventually added to her regimen after her pain progressed, and the patient did not tolerate antidepressant agents known to reduce neuropathic pain. AH's pain never responded adequately to the hydromorphone so her prescriber transitioned her to methadone, currently at 15 mg three times daily. Unfortunately, AH's prescriber suspects that the methadone is responsible for the edema AH has been experiencing, and, in fact, worsening as the methadone dose has been increased. The prescriber asks your advice on transitioning AH to morphine. What do you suggest? AH is taking no other medications that are likely to interact with methadone.

P6.7: Switching from Oral to IV Methadone

PV is a 68-year-old man with end-stage lung cancer, receiving hospice care at home. He is receiving oral methadone 20 mg every 12 hours, with methadone 5 mg every 3 hours for breakthrough pain. His pain has been increasing in intensity over the past week, with PV using six doses per day of his breakthrough methadone in addition to the two scheduled doses. The physician suspected bone metastases and naproxen 500 mg by mouth every 12 hours was added, with marginal success. PV is now requesting euthanasia; because you are unable to honor this request, you counter with an offer to move PV to an inpatient facility, switch him to parenteral methadone, and titrate to relief. You are unwilling to do this switch in the home environment because PV is debilitated and he has an unreliable caregiver situation. You further agree that if you are successful at managing PV's pain, you will transition him back to oral methadone so he can return to his home. PV agrees with this plan and is admitted to a hospice bed in your local hospital. *How do you transition PV to a PCA methadone infusion?*

P6.8: Switching from IV to Oral Methadone

One week later, PV, our patient from Case 6.7 has been stabilized for several days now on a methadone IV PCA infusion at 2.5 mg/hr with a demand bolus of 2.5 mg, which he uses about once per 8-hour shift. He is very happy with his level of pain control, no longer requesting euthanasia, and would like to return home on oral methadone therapy. A repeat ECG shows you are still on firm ground (his QTc is still below 450 ms). *What dose of oral methadone do you recommend for discharge?*

Could I Get That to Go, Please? Bottom Line It for Me . . .

▶ As my friend and colleague Dr. Doug Gourlay from Canada says, "Buprenorphine can take a joke, but methadone has no sense of humor!" Methadone is an amazing multimechanistic opioid that demands careful attention to detail, dosing, monitoring, and dosage adjustment.

▶ You should perform a risk assessment prior to starting methadone therapy. Follow published recommendations for ECG monitoring, and correct factors that predispose to QTc interval prolongation as able.

▶ When patient is taking an enzyme-inhibiting medication, reduce calculated methadone dose by 25%. Start by asking about amiodarone, anti-infective agents, or antidepressants, and use a more comprehensive drug database as needed.

▶ You should start opioid-naïve patients on no more than 2 to 7.5 mg oral methadone per day (in two or three divided doses). Do not increase by more than 5 mg/day and no more often than every 5 to 7 days.

▶ There are many recommendations for converting to methadone from other opioids. First, you must decide if you want to do a 3-day switch or a stop-and-go approach.

▶ *This author prefers a stop-and-go approach, using the following conversion:*

  ▶ Up to 60 mg per day oral morphine equivalent—default to opioid-naïve dosing

  ▶ 60 to 199 mg per day oral morphine equivalent and patient <65 years old—10:1 (oral morphine:oral methadone) conversion

  ▶ ≥200 mg per day oral morphine equivalent and/or patient ≥65 years old—20:1 (oral morphine:oral methadone) conversion

  ▶ Regardless of previous opioid use, do not start oral methadone at greater than 30 to 40 mg per day.

  ▶ Increase oral methadone by 5 mg/day no sooner than every 5 to 7 days. When the total daily dose exceeds 30 to 40 mg, practitioners may increase by up to 10 mg/day but still no sooner than every 5 to 7 days.

▶ Practitioners, patients, and family members must work together to monitor the patient's response to methadone therapy.

▶ Methadone may be used as an adjunctive analgesic, instead of switching completely to methadone.

▶ Parenteral methadone is available; practitioners should read and follow the published consensus guidelines for using parenteral methadone.

REFERENCES

1. Sandoval JA, Furlan AD, Mailis-Gagnon A. Oral methadone for chronic noncancer pain. A systematic literature review of reasons for administration, prescription patterns, effectiveness and side effects. *Clin J Pain.* 2005;21:503-512.

2. Foster DJR, Somogyi AA, Dyer KR, et al. Steady-state pharmacokinetics of (R)- and (S)-methadone in methadone maintenance patients. *Br J Clin Pharmacol.* 2000;50:427-440.

3. Rajan J, Scott-Warren J. The clinical use of methadone in cancer and chronic pain medicine. *BJA Education.* 2016;16(3):102-106.

4. Eap CB, Buclin T, Baumann P. Interindividual variability of the clinical pharmacokinetics of methadone. Implications for the treatment of opioid dependence. *Clin Pharmacokinet.* 2002;41:1153-1193.

5. Lugo RA, Satterfield KL, Kern SE. Pharmacokinetics of methadone. *J Pain Palliat Care Pharmacother.* 2005;19:13-24.

6. Dale O, Sheffels P, Kharasch ED. Bioavailability of rectal and oral methadone in healthy subjects. *Br J Clin Pharmacol.* 2004;58(2):156-162.

7. Chang Y, Fang WB, Lin S-N, et al. Stereo-selective metabolism of methadone by human liver microsomes and cDNA-expressed cytochrome P450s: a reconciliation. *Basic Clin Pharmacol Toxicol.* 2011;108(1):55-62. http://doi.org/10.1111/j.1742-7843.2010.00628.x. Accessed July 3, 2018.

8. Gerber JG, Rhodes RJ, Gal J. Stereoselective metabolism of methadone N-demethylation by cytochrome P4502B6 and 2C19. *Chirality.* 2004; 16(1): 36-44. http://doi.org/10.1002/chir.10303. Accessed July 3, 2018.

9. Greenblatt DJ. Drug interactions with methadone: Time to revise the product label. *Clin Pharmacol Drug Dev.* 2014;3(4):249-251.

10. Kharasch ED, Regina KJ, Blood J, et al. Methadone pharmacogenetics: CYP2B6 polymorphisms determine plasma concentrations, clearance, and metabolism. *Anesthesiology.* 2015;123(5):1142-1153. http://doi.org/10.1097/ALN.0000000000000867. Accessed July 3, 2018.

11. Kharasch ED, Stubbert K. Role of cytochrome P4502B6 in methadone metabolism and clearance. *J Clin Pharmacol.* 2013;53(3):305-313.

12. Carlquist JF, Moody DE, Knight S, et al. A possible mechanistic link between the CYP2C19 genotype, the methadone metabolite ethylidne-1,5-dimethyl-3m3-diphenylpyrrolidine (EDDP), and methadone-induced corrected QT interval prolongation in a pilot study. *Mol Diagn Ther.* 2015;19(2):131-138.

13. Baselt RC, Casarett LJ. Urinary excretion of methadone in man. *Clin Pharmacol Ther.* 1972;13:64-70.

14. Weschules DJ, Bain KT, Richeimer S. Actual and potential drug interactions associated with methadone. *Pain Med.* 2008;9:315-344.

15. Ferrari A, Coccia CP, Bertolini A, et al. Methadone: metabolism, pharmacokinetics and interactions. *Pharmacol Res.* 2004;50:551-559.

16. Zanger UM, Klein K. Pharmacogenetics of cytochrome P450 2B6 (CYP2B6): advances on polymorphisms, mechanisms, and clinical relevance. *Front Genet.* 2013;4:24.

17. Somogyi AA, Barratt DT, Ali RL, et al. Pharmacogenomics of methadone maintenance treatment. *Pharmacogenomics.* 2014;15:1007-1027.

18. Fricke-Galindo I, Cespedes-Garro C, Rodrigues-Soares F, et al. Interethnic variation of CYP2C19 alleles, 'predicted' phenotypes and 'measured' metabolic phenotypes across world populations. *Pharmacogenomics J.* 2016;16:113-123.

19. Gadel S, Friedel C, Kharasch ED. Differences in methadone metabolism by CYP2B6 variants. *Drug Metab Dispos.* 2015;43:994-1001.

20. Flockhart DA. Drug Interactions: Cytochrome P450 Drug Interaction Table. Indiana University School of Medicine; 2007. http://medicine.iupui.edu/clinpharm/ddis/clinical-table/. Accessed May 6, 2018.

21. Chou R, Cruciani RA, Fiellin DA, et al. Methadone safety guidelines: a clinical practice guideline from the American Pain Society and College on Problems of Drug Dependence, in collaboration with the Heart Rhythm Society. *J Pain.* 2014;15(4):321-337.

22. Dolophine® Hydrochloride (Boehringer-Ingelheim) Prescribing Information. http://docs.boehringer-ingelheim.com/Prescribing%20Information/PIs/Roxane/Dolophine/Dolophine%20Tablets.pdf, Accessed May 6, 2018.

23. McPherson ML. Methadone safety guidelines for hospice and palliative care. *AAHPM Quarterly.* 2016;17(2):8-9.

24. Mercadante S, Sapio M, Serretta R, et al. Patient-controlled analgesia with oral methadone in cancer pain: preliminary report. *Ann Oncol.* 1996;7:613-617.

25. Caplehorn JR, Drummer OH, Cyrne A, et al. Fatal methadone toxicity: signs and circumstances, and the role of benzodiazepines. *Aust N Z J Public Health.* 2002;26:358-363.

26. Webster LR, Choi Y, Desai H, et al. Sleep-disordered breathing and chronic opioid therapy. *Pain Med.* 2008;9:425-432.

27. Palat G, Shary S. Practical guide for using methadone in pain and palliative care practice. *Ind J Palliat Care.* 2018;24(Suppl 1):S21-S29.

28. Porta-Sales J, Garzon-Rodriguez C, Villavicencio-Chavez C, et al. Efficacy and safety of methadone as a second-line opioid for cancer pain in an outpatient clinic: a prospective open-label study. *Oncologist.* 2016;21:981-987.

29. Rhondali W, Termellat F, Ledoux M, et al. Methadone rotation for cancer patients with refractory pain in a palliative care unit: An observational study. *J Palliat Med.* 2013;16(110):1382-1387.

30. Good P, Afsharimani B, Movva R, et al. Therapeutic challenges in cancer pain management: a systemic review of methadone. *J Pain Palliat Care Pharmacother.* 2014;28:197-205.

31. Mercadante S, Porzio G, Ferrera P, et al. Sustained-release oral morphine versus transdermal fentanyl and oral methadone in cancer pain management. *Eur J Pain.* 2008;12:1040-1046.

32. Reddy A, Schuler US, de la Cruz M, et al. Overall survival among cancer patients undergoing opioid rotation to methadone compared to other opioids. *J Palliat Med.* 2017;20:656-661.

33. Krebs EE, Becker WC, Zerzan J, et al. Comparative mortality among Department of Veterans Affairs patients prescribed methadone or long-acting morphine for chronic pain. *Pain.* 2011;152:1789-1795.

34. Ray WA, Chung CP, Murray KT, et al. Out-of-hospital mortality among patients receiving methadone for noncancer pain. *JAMA Intern Med.* 2015;175(3):420-427.

35. Centers for Disease Control and Prevention. Vital signs: Risk for overdose from methadone used for pain relief—United States, 1999–2010. *MMWR Morb Mortal Wkly Rep.* 2012;61:493-497.

36. Toombs JD, Kral LA. Methadone treatment for pain states. *Am Family Physicians.* 2005;71:1353-1358.

37. Shir Y, Rosen G, Zeldin A, et al. Methadone is safe for treating hospitalized patients with severe pain. *Can J Anesth.* 2001;48:1109-1113.

38. FDA Public Health Advisory. Methadone use for pain control may result in death and life-threatening changes in breathing and heart beat. November 27, 2006, updated July 2007. http://www.methadone.org/downloads/documents/fda_comsumer_updates_2006_methadone_pain_control_death_changes_breathing_heart_beat_nov_.pdf. Accessed May 6, 2018.

39. Trinkley EK, Page RL, Lien H, et al. QT interval prolongation and the risk for torsades de pointes: essential for clinicians. *Curr Med Res Opin.* 2013;29(12):1719-1726.

40. Ehret GB, Voide C, Gex-Fabry M, et al. Drug-induced long QT syndrome in injection drug users receiving methadone. *Arch Intern Med.* 2006;166:1280-1287.

41. Bednar MM, Harrigan EP, Ruskin JN. Torsades de pointes associated with nonantiarrhythmic drugs and observations on gender and QTc. *Am J Cardiol.* 2002;89:1316-1319.

42. Bart G, Wyman Z, Wang Q, et al. Methadone and the QTc interval: Paucity of clinically significant factors in a retrospective cohort. *J Addict Med.* 2017;11(6):489-493.

43. Reddy S, Hui D, El Osta B, et al. The effect of oral methadone on the QTc interval in advanced cancer patients: a prospective pilot study. *J Palliat Med.* 2010;13(1):33-38.

44. Juba K, Khadem TM, Hutchinson D, et al. Methadone and corrected QT prolongation in pain and palliative care patients: a case-control study. *J Palliat Med.* 2017;20(7):722-728.

45. U.S. Food and Drug Administration. *Guidance for Industry: E14 Clinical Evaluation of QT/QTc Interval Prolongation and Proarrhythmic Potential for Non-Antiarrhythmic Drugs.* Rockville, MD: Center for Drug Evaluation and Research; 2005. https://www.fda.gov/downloads/Drugs/GuidanceComplianceRegulatoryInformation/Guidances/UCM073153.pdf. Accessed May 6, 2018.

46. Crouch MA, Limon L, Cassano AT. Clinical relevance and management of drug-related QT interval prolongation. *Pharmacotherapy.* 2003;23:881-908. http://www.medscape.com/viewarticle/458868_print. Accessed July 3, 2018.

47. Woosley RL, Heise CW, Romero KA. QTDrugs List. https://crediblemeds.org/. Accessed May 7, 2018.

48. Bruera E, Sweeney C. Methadone use in cancer patients in pain: a review. *J Palliat Med.* 2002;5:127-138.

49. Weschules DJ, Bain KT. A systematic review of opioid conversion ratios used with methadone for the treatment of pain. *Pain Med.* 2008;9:595-612.

50. McLean S, Twomey F. Methods of rotation from another strong opioid to methadone for the management of cancer pain: a systematic review of the available evidence. *J Pain Symptom Manage.* 2015;50:248-259.

51. Ripamonti C, Groff L, Brunelli C, et al. Switching from morphine to oral methadone in treating cancer pain: what is the equianalgesic dose ratio? *J Clin Oncol.* 1998;16:3216-3221.

52. Mercadante S, Casuccia A, Fulfaro F, et al. Switching from morphine to methadone to improve analgesia and tolerability in cancer patients: a prospective study. *J Clin Oncol.* 2001;19:2898-2904.

53. Ayonrinde OT, Bridge DT. The rediscovery of methadone for cancer pain management. *Med J Aust.* 2000;173:536-540.

54. Gazelle G, Fine PG. *Fast Facts and Concepts #75: Methadone for the treatment of Pain.* 3rd ed. Appleton, WI: Palliative Care Network of Wisconsin; 2015. https://www.mypcnow.org/blank-tryqt. Accessed May 6, 2018.

55. Plonk WM. Simplified methadone conversion. *J Palliat Med.* 2005;8(3):478-479.

56. Moksnes K, Dale O, Rosland JH, et al. How to switch from morphine or oxycodone to methadone in cancer patients? A randomized clinical phase II trial. *Eur J Cancer.* 2011;47:2463-2470.

57. Chatham MS, Dodds Ashley ES, Svengsouk JS, et al. Dose ratios between high dose oral morphine or equivalents and oral methadone. *J Palliat Med.* 2013;16(8):947-950.

58. Lipman AG. Methadone: a double-edged sword. *J Pain Palliat Care Pharmacother.* 2005;19:3-4.

59. Spaner D. Effectiveness of the buccal mucosa route for methadone administration at the end of life. *J Palliat Med.* 2014;17(11):1262-1265.

60. Reddy A, Vidal M, Stephen S, et al. The conversion ratio from intravenous hydromorphone to oral opioids in cancer patients. *J Pain Symptom Manage.* 2017;54:280-288.

61. Mao J, Price DD, Mayer DJ. Mechanisms of hyperalgesia and morphine tolerance: A current view of their possible interactions. *Pain.* 1995;62:259-274.

62. Wallace E, Ridley J, Bryson J, et al. Addition of methadone to another opioid in the management of moderate to severe cancer pain: A case series. *J Palliat Med.* 2013;16(3):305-309.

63. Courtemanche F, Dao D, Gagne F, et al. Methadone as a coanalgesic for palliative care cancer patients. *J Palliat Med.* 2016;19(9):1-7.

64. Peng PWH, Tumber PS, Gourlay D. Review article: perioperative pain management of patients on methadone therapy. *Can J Anesth.* 2005;52:513-523.

65. Walker PW, Palla S, Pei B, et al. Switching from methadone to a different opioid: what is the equianalgesic dose ratio? *J Palliat Med.* 2008;11:1103-1108.

66. Glue P, Cape G, Tunnicliff D, et al. Switching opioid-dependent patients from methadone to morphine: Safety, tolerability, and methadone pharmacokinetics. *J Clin Pharmacol.* 2016;56(8):960-965.

67. Shaiova L, Berger A, Blinderman C, et al. Consensus guidelines on parenteral methadone use in pain and palliative care. *Palliat Support Care.* 2008;6:165-176.

68. Davis MP, Walsh D. Methadone for relief of cancer pain: a review of pharmacokinetics, pharmacodynamics, drug interactions, and protocols of administration. *Support Care Cancer.* 2001;9:73-83.

69. Gagnon C. The use of methadone in the care of the dying. *Eur J Palliat Care.* 1997;4:152-158.

70. Inturrisi CE. Clinical pharmacology of opioids for pain. *Clin J Pain.* 2002;18:S3-S13.

71. González-Barboteo J, Porta-Sales J, Sanchez D, et al. Conversion from parenteral to oral methadone. *J Pain Palliat Care Pharmacother.* 2008;22:200-205.

SOLUTIONS TO PRACTICE PROBLEMS

P6.1: KG is opioid naïve; therefore, 2- to 7.5-mg methadone per day by mouth is the dosage range we're considering. KG is also taking Zoloft (sertraline), a selective serotonin reuptake inhibitor, which is known to inhibit the metabolism of methadone. Based on this, it would be prudent to start KG on methadone 2.5 mg by mouth at bedtime and use an alternate opioid for rescue as needed such as morphine 5 mg or oxycodone 2.5 mg every 4 hours as needed. Once KG achieves steady-state (e.g., 1 week to 10 days) we can safely increase the methadone if necessary. An alternate strategy would be to order methadone 2.5 mg by mouth at bedtime and methadone 2.5 mg by mouth every 3 hours as needed for pain (although this approach will require great care and attention in monitoring due to the increased risk). This will allow for good pain control through self-titration while not risking an overdose due to the drug interaction with sertraline.

P6.2: Because BM is a relatively young patient with no comorbid conditions, we can start methadone at 2.5 mg by mouth every 12 hours or even every 8 hours. We would educate the patient and his wife to look for feelings of faintness, dizziness, confusion, trouble breathing or shallow breathing, loud snoring, extreme tiredness or sleepiness, blurred vision, and difficulty thinking, walking, or talking.

BM should also maintain a diary tracking his pain ratings (on a 0–10 scale; 0 = no pain, 10 = worst imaginable pain) per day, including the best, the worst, and the average. He should comment on his ability to perform activities, and the presence or absence of symptoms such as numbness and radiating or shooting pain. If his pain is not controlled after a week, you could recommend increasing to 5 mg by mouth every 12 hours. One week later, if necessary, increase to 7.5 mg by mouth every 12 hours, 1 week later to 10 mg by mouth every 12 hours, and so forth. And during all this, don't forget the bowels!

P6.3:

STEP 1—Assess GH's pain and you feel that switching to methadone is preferable to adding another adjuvant analgesic at this time.

STEP 2—Calculate the total daily morphine dose GH is receiving. Between his MS Contin (120 mg per day) and immediate-release morphine (120 mg per day), he is receiving 240-mg oral morphine per day.

STEP 3—Convert the TDD oral morphine to a TDD oral methadone. Looking at our different methods, we get the following potential methadone doses:

- *Ripamonti:* 90 to 300 mg per day oral morphine is a 6:1 conversion: calculated total daily oral methadone dose is 40 mg
- *Mercadante:* 90 to 300 mg per day oral morphine is 8:1 conversion: calculated total daily oral methadone dose is 30 mg
- *Ayonrinde:* 101 to 300 mg per day oral morphine is 5:1 conversion: calculated total daily oral methadone dose is 48 mg
- *Fast Facts:* Ayonrinde reduced by 50% to 75%: calculated total daily oral methadone dose is 12 to 24 mg
- *HPC Expert Group:* Patient less than 65 years old and on greater than 200-mg oral morphine per day is a 20:1 conversion: calculated total daily oral methadone dose is 12 mg

So our calculated range is 12- to 48-mg oral methadone per day.

STEP 4—Remember two things: This patient is receiving sertraline (Zoloft) a known enzyme inhibitor and his pain isn't well controlled. Let's take the 12-mg oral methadone TDD we calculated with the HPC Expert Group method, but NOT reduce by 25% for the drug interaction, to allow for a greater effect for the uncontrolled pain. Our dose, therefore, would be methadone 6 mg by mouth every 12 hours (you'd have to use the oral solution; if the patient didn't want to do this, we could start with methadone 5 mg by mouth every 12 hours using tablets). To keep things simpler, let's keep the morphine for breakthrough pain; 10% to 15% of 240-mg total daily oral morphine is 24 to 36 mg, therefore, let's go with immediate-release morphine 30 mg by mouth every 2 hours as needed for breakthrough pain.

The second part of your mission was to recommend a *rapid switch* and a *slow conversion* plan. For the rapid switch, you would discontinue the MS Contin, and begin oral methadone 5 (or 6) mg 12 hours after the last dose of MS Contin (methadone 5 mg by mouth every 12 hours). Increase the MS immediate-release (IR) from 20 to 30 mg immediately and advise patient he can take it as frequently as every 2 hours as needed.

STEP 5—Monitor your patient like a maniacal stalker!

If you want to slow things down, smell the roses, enjoy the experience; you can do it over 3 days. On day 1, reduce the MS Contin to 30 mg by mouth every 12 hours (you have to choose between MS Contin 45 mg by mouth every 12 hours and MS Contin 30 mg by mouth every 12 hours because that's the way the tablets come) and start methadone 2 mg by mouth every 12 hours. Also, I would increase the MSIR to 30 mg every 2 hours as needed for breakthrough pain at this point. On day 2, reduce the MS Contin to 15 mg by mouth every 12 hours (of course, this means you'll have to get the 15-mg tablets) and increase methadone dose to 4 mg by mouth every 12 hours. Continue using MSIR 30 mg by mouth every 2 hours as needed for pain. On day 3, discontinue the MS Contin, increase the methadone to 6 mg by mouth every 12 hours, and either continue the MSIR 30 mg by mouth every 2 hours as needed for pain or switch to methadone 2.5 mg by mouth every 3 hours as needed for breakthrough pain. Most practitioners would prefer to do this type of slow switch in an acute-care facility due to the increased risk for respiratory depression.

P6.4: You have assessed JR's pain and have no reason to suspect neuropathic or bone pain; therefore, no adjuvant analgesics are necessary at this time. The first step is to calculate the total daily oral morphine equivalent for JR. He is on transdermal fentanyl 200 mcg/hr, which is approximately equivalent to 400-mg oral morphine. He is taking six doses per day of oxycodone 20 mg, which is 120-mg oral oxycodone. Using our oxycodone:morphine ratio of 20:25, 120-mg oral oxycodone is equivalent to 150-mg oral morphine. This gives us a grand total of 550-mg oral morphine total daily equivalent for JR.

The patient is less than 65 years old, but receiving more than 200-mg oral morphine equivalent per day; therefore, the recommended ratio is 20:1, or 27.5 mg per day of oral methadone. Using a rapid-switch transition, after we're sure the methadone has been delivered to JR's home (this is an important logistical point!), we instruct him to remove the transdermal fentanyl (TDF) patch, and begin methadone 10 mg by mouth every 8 hours approximately 12 hours after the TDF was removed. We have increased the oxycodone oral solution to 40 mg, and have instructed the patient to use his rescue opioid every 2 hours as needed for breakthrough pain. But before we sign off on this case, how did we get that dose of oxycodone for breakthrough? The patient was on the equivalent of 550 mg TDD oral morphine, which is about a TDD of 440-mg oral oxycodone. Using our 10% to 15% rescue analgesia guideline, oxycodone 40-mg oral solution every 2 hours seems reasonable.

P6.5: VH is close to death, has poorly controlled pain, and may possibly be exhibiting opioid-induced hyperalgesia. One option would be to add oral methadone solution to reduce any hyperalgesia, and assist with pain control. We could add methadone oral solution (and it's always best to use a whole number dose for ease of measurement) 2 or 3 mg every 12 hours, on top of the long-acting morphine and oral morphine solution for breakthrough. The methadone in this case would be scheduled, not as needed. If VH survives 5 to 7 days, it may be appropriate to increase the dose of methadone based on response.

P6.6: You agree with the prescriber's assessment of AH; her TDD of methadone is 45 mg (15 mg by mouth every 8 hours). Using the 1:3 (oral methadone:oral morphine) conversion, you calculate an oral morphine TDD of 135 mg. You suggest using the immediate-release morphine for the time being, at 20-mg oral morphine every 4 hours, starting 12 hours after the last methadone dose. You also recommend an additional 10 mg of oral morphine every 2 hours as needed for additional pain. After 5 to 7 days on this regimen, the prescriber can evaluate AH's response to therapy, increase or decrease the TDD oral morphine, and switch to long-acting oral morphine if appropriate.

P6.7: You agree with the prescriber's plan and meet with PV to assess his pain. Just to be safe, you recommend getting an ECG to make sure PV's QTc interval is not excessively long. Remember, parenteral methadone is even more likely to prolong the QTc than oral methadone. You get the ECG and all is well (430 ms). What a relief!

Your next step is to calculate PV's TDD of oral methadone. He is taking 20 mg every 12 hours scheduled (40 mg a day) plus six doses per day according to his diary of the 5-mg rescue methadone (5 × 6 doses = 30 mg per day) for a TDD of 70-mg oral methadone. According to the parenteral methadone consensus guidelines, we give 50% of this as parenteral methadone, or 35 mg (70/2). We divide this by 24 to determine our hourly infusion rate, which calculates to 1.46 mg/hr (35/24)—you recommend beginning IV methadone at 1.5 mg/hr, with a 1.5 mg bolus every 15 minutes and a 3-mg clinician-activated bolus hourly. You would wait 12 hours before adjusting the infusion rate so as to avoid dose-stacking and potential toxicity, and, of course, you recommend a fairly aggressive monitoring plan.

P6.8: Congratulations on doing such a terrific job controlling PV's pain on the IV methadone PCA infusion! Let's get busy switching him to oral methadone! He is receiving 2.5 mg/hr by continuous infusion, and approximately three extra doses of 2.5 mg per day for breakthrough pain. This gives us a TDD of 67.5-mg parenteral methadone. Using our guideline to multiply the TDD IV methadone by 1.3, we get a TDD of oral methadone of 87.75 mg. For ease of administration, you recommend methadone 30 mg by mouth every 8 hours. You can also offer methadone 10 mg by mouth every 3 hours for additional pain. Ask PV to continue his pain diary, and pay close attention to his response to therapy during this transition. Good job!

CHAPTER 7

Patient-Controlled Analgesia and Neuraxial Opioid Therapy

INTRODUCTION

In this chapter, we will explore more advanced methods of treating pain—specifically, PCA and neuraxial (epidural, IT) opioid administration. Much of neuraxial opioid administration comes under the purview of a specialist such as an anesthesiologist, but practitioners "in the trenches" often inherit patients receiving these therapies and need an understanding of them.

PATIENT-CONTROLLED ANALGESIA

Patient-controlled analgesia is a precise and convenient method of providing opioid therapy to patients with moderate-to-severe acute or chronic pain. The convenience aspect is the patient's ability to decide when he or she needs a dose of opioid, without having to rely on the nurse to administer it. A PCA system uses a computerized pump that has a syringe, cartridge, or infusion bag that contains the opioid, which may be secured (locked) inside the pump. The PCA pump can be configured in different ways (with or without a continuous infusion of opioid), but it generally has the capability for a patient to self-administer a small dose of opioid frequently. When we say a *small dose*, this means relative to an "every 4 hours" dose.[1]

OBJECTIVES

After reading this chapter and completing all practice problems, the participant will be able to:

1. Calculate, monitor, and adjust patient-controlled analgesia (PCA) opioid therapy for acute and chronic pain management, with and without a continuous opioid infusion.

2. Convert a patient between parenteral PCA therapy and an oral opioid regimen.

3. Using the limited evidence available, recommend a conservative strategy to convert a patient between epidural or intrathecal (IT) opioid therapy and other opioid regimens.

There are several features that you need to be familiar with regarding PCA pumps. Pump nomenclature differs among manufacturers, but all have the capability for the following:

- The pump needs to be programmed for the drug concentration in the cartridge, syringe, or infusion bag. In other words, we tell the pump what volume is available for infusion or bolus dosing, and the concentration of the opioid solution (e.g., mg/mL).

- We must also program the rate of the continuous opioid infusion, if applicable; the PCA bolus dose (the amount of drug the patient receives when the bolus button is pushed); the delay interval, also known as the lockout period (the period of time during which no additional bolus doses will be administered despite the patient pushing the demand bolus dose button); and the 1- or 4-hour limit (the total amount of opioid the patient can receive in 1 or 4 hour(s) by PCA bolus plus basal infusion).

- We can also retrieve historical information from the PCA pump, including the number of PCA bolus attempts the patient has made, the number of PCA bolus doses given, the volume given, and the volume remaining in the syringe, cartridge, or infusion bag.

Wow—that sounds complicated! While it's not rocket science, it can get confusing, and PCA pump therapy is an error-prone, high-risk source of medication errors.

PCA therapy is usually administered via intravenous (IV) infusion, but it can be administered via subcutaneous (sub-Q) or epidural routes, as well. Let's first consider the use of PCA therapy post-operatively using the sub-Q or IV route of administration.[1]

PATIENT-CONTROLLED ANALGESIA POST-OPERATIVELY

Although PCA therapy has been shown to be beneficial for acute pain (postoperatively and other) and chronic pain (cancer and noncancer), we must ensure the patient is an acceptable candidate. Patients must have sufficient cognitive functioning to use the infusion pump. For example, children who are 7 years or older are likely to be successful with PCA therapy, and in some cases, children as young as 5 years old are appropriate candidates.[2] Advanced age is not a contraindication if the patient has adequate cognitive functioning. Patients who do not understand how to activate the PCA demand bolus would not be good candidates. Patients with comorbid conditions that increase the risk of respiratory depression may not be good candidates, such as those with obstructive sleep apnea and/or obesity. Some institutions use the *STOP-BANG* questionnaire (which evaluates several patient variables including snoring, tired, observed (apnea during sleep), blood pressure, BMI (body mass index), age, neck circumference, and gender).[3] Risk assessment may help respiratory therapists and pulmonologists determine precautions such as breathing assistance.[4] Chronic obstructive pulmonary disease, hypoxemia, head injury, or respiratory failure are also risk factors for therapeutic misadventure with PCA therapy.[1,2,4] Underlying renal or hepatic impairment may result in opioid accumulation, increasing the risk of respiratory depression.

Most patients who receive PCA therapy postoperatively are opioid-naïve. In opioid-naïve persons, generally practitioners use standardized dosing unless there is a compelling clinical reason to use a different dosing strategy. For example, standard orders are typically for 1 mg of morphine or its equivalent (0.2 mg hydromorphone or 20 mcg fentanyl) every 10 minutes (8 minutes for fentanyl) (see Table 7-1).[2,5,6] These doses should be reduced for frail or elderly patients, patients with less than severe pain, or patients at high risk for respiratory depression. When beginning PCA therapy in the immediate postoperative period, the patient will likely be in pain. In this case, the clinician (e.g., recovery room nurse or anesthesiologist) would administer one or more loading doses (a *clinician loading dose*) of the opioid to get the patient comfortable. This may be given every 10 minutes

Table 7-1
Starting IV PCA Prescription Ranges for Opioid-Naïve Adults

Drug	Typical Concentration	Loading/ Clinician Dose*	Starting PCA Dose[†]	Usual Lockout[‡]	Range Lockout	Approx. Time to Onset of Action	Approx. Time to Peak Effect	Approx. Duration of Effect
Morphine	1 mg/mL	2.5 mg	1.0 mg	10 min	5–10 min	2–4 min	15–20 min	≈ 2 hr
Hydromorphone	0.2 mg/mL	0.4 mg	0.2 mg	10 min	5–10 min	2–3 min	10–15 min	≈ 2 hr
Fentanyl	10–20 mcg/mL	25 mcg	20 mcg	8 min	5–8 min	1–2 min	5 min	1–2 hr

IV = intravenous; PCA = patient-controlled analgesia

*Repeat as necessary; administered and response monitored by clinician. May be repeated every 10 minutes up to three to five times or until pain controlled (e.g., a 50% reduction in pain).

[†]Reduce usual starting PCA dose by 50% for frail or elderly patients.

[‡]Increase lockout for frail, elderly, or patients at high risk of opioid-related respiratory depression.

Source: Adapted from *Principles of Analgesic Use in the Treatment of Acute Pain and Cancer Pain.* 7th ed. Glenview, IL: American Pain Society; 2016; Pasero C, McCaffery M. *Pain Assessment and Pharmacologic Management.* St. Louis, MO: Elsevier Mosby; 2011; Strassels SA, McNicol E, Ruleman R. Postoperative pain management: A practice review, part 1. *Am J Health-Syst Pharm.* 2005;62:1904-1916.

until the pain is reduced by at least 50%, or up to three to five times as indicated by hospital policy. Strassels and colleagues recommend that the clinician dose be increased by 50% if the patient has not achieved pain relief within 1 hour. If pain relief has not been achieved in another hour, they recommend considering a reduction in the dosing interval.[6]

Let's consider a variety of scenarios regarding level of pain control, and the development of adverse effects with IV or sub-Q PCA therapy (see Table 7-2).

Table 7-2
Improvement of Pain Control and Reduction of Adverse Effects Associated with IV or Sub-Q PCA Analgesia[5]

Clinical Situation	Proposed Interventions
Patient has insufficient or no pain relief, and no adverse effects.	Verify infusion system is patent and functional; verify pump is assembled, loaded, and programmed correctly. Confirm lockout interval is appropriate. Administer a clinician loading dose. Increase PCA bolus dose by 25%–100%.
Patient has insufficient or no pain relief, but experiences adverse effects.	Treat adverse effects. Add or increase nonopioid or adjuvant analgesic (be careful of bleeding risk with NSAIDs on postoperative patients). Decrease opioid dose cautiously by 25%. Rotate to a different opioid (reduce calculated dose for cross-tolerance).
Patient has pain relief, but experiences adverse effects.	Treat adverse effects. Reduce opioid dose by 25%–50%, possibly more with excessive sedation and/or respiratory depression. Rotate to a different opioid (reduce calculated dose for cross-tolerance).
Patient has pain relief with adverse effects after PCA bolus dose administration (e.g., excessive sedation).	Treat adverse effects. Give smaller doses more often (e.g., decrease the PCA bolus dose by 25%–50% and shorten the lockout interval). Rotate to a different opioid (reduce calculated dose for cross-tolerance).
Patient has pain relief except during periods of activity.	Remind patient to use PCA bolus prior to activity (10–15 minutes beforehand) and to continue to self-administer during activity.
The maximum programmed amount of opioid used (in 1- or 4-hour block).	In patient still in pain, administer clinician-loading dose. Verify hourly or 4-hourly limit was calculated correctly, PCA pump is programmed correctly and functioning, and IV line is patent. Determine amount of pain relief obtained; if <50%, increase programmed 4-hourly limit by 100%. If pain relief >50% but less than optimal, increase programmed 4-hourly limit by 50%.
Patient is somnolent and difficult to arouse, or is experiencing respiratory depression.	In an opioid-naïve patient, discontinue opioid. If patient is opioid-tolerant, reduce opioid dose by 75% (do not stop opioid as this may precipitate opioid withdrawal in opioid-tolerant patients). Consider use of low-dose naloxone if necessary (titrate to respiratory rate of 8–10 breaths/minute and recovery of cognition; do not titrate to reversal of analgesia). Add nonsedating nonopioid analgesic after resolution of sedation. When adverse effects resolve, resume opioid at approximately 50% of previous dose.

Table 7-2

Improvement of Pain Control and Reduction of Adverse Effects Associated with IV or Sub-Q PCA Analgesia[5] (continued)

Clinical Situation	Proposed Interventions
There are a disproportionate number of injections and attempts (injection/attempt ratio).	Determine if someone other than the patient is pressing the demand button (proxy dosing); this practice is not safe, unless PCA via authorized agent is being used.
	Determine if patient fully understands use of the demand button; re-educate if appropriate.
	If patient gets one injection with less than two to three attempts and is not in pain, do nothing.
	If patient gets one injection with less than two to three attempts and patient has pain, administer clinician-loading dose(s) and increase PCA bolus dose by 25%–100%.
	If patient gets one injection delivered with more than three attempts, and has no pain and tolerable and manageable adverse effects, administer supplemental clinician-loading dose(s) and remind the patient to use the PCA bolus dose (remind them to self-dose before pain is uncontrolled) Ask the patient to redose after evaluating response to initial dose by waiting long enough (e.g., the length of the lockout period) to evaluate the dose effect before pressing the button again.

IV = intravenous; PCA = pain-controlled analgesia; sub-Q = subcutaneous

Source: Adapted with permission from Pasero C, McCaffery M. *Pain Assessment and Pharmacologic Management.* St. Louis, MO: Elsevier Mosby; 2011.

Let's do a case or two!

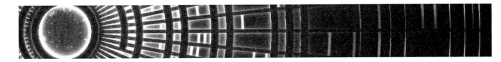

CASE 7.1

Your Mama Told You Not to Get a Motorcycle!

BT is a 32-year-old man who was involved in a motor vehicle accident. He was riding his motorcycle, and an unexpected pile-up accident caused him to flip off the back of the car in front of him. He flew 50 feet in the air, landed hard on his ankle, and skidded for about 30 more feet. He has broken several bones and peeled off a considerable amount of skin. He was brought to Shock Trauma at your institution, and he is now in the postanesthesia care unit (PACU) postoperatively from having several rods placed in his ankle. The surgical team has asked that you write the orders for BT's IV PCA with morphine. What order do you write? BT was opioid-naïve on admission.

You consult your IV PCA dosing chart, and order morphine at 1 mg/mL, with a PCA demand dose of 1 mg every 10 minutes as needed. You also write for a clinician bolus (loading dose) of 2.5 mg every 10 minutes up to five doses, until pain is reduced by 50%. The PACU nurse hunts you down about 40 minutes later to say she's given four doses of 2.5 mg and the patient is still complaining of pain that is at a 10 (on a 0–10 scale; 0 = no pain, 10 = worst imaginable pain). You and the nurse together verify the infusion system is patent and functional, and the PCA pump is programmed correctly. The patient is moaning in significant pain. What do you do now?

At this point, you increase the clinician-loading dose to 4 mg, and increase the PCA bolus dose to 2 mg. After two additional clinician loading doses (another 8 mg), the patient reports his pain is now a 6 and tolerable. You educate him about using the PCA bolus button as often as he needs it. The nurse in the PACU will continue to follow the patient for another hour or so, at which point he'll be transferred to the floor.

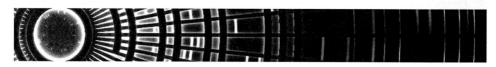

CASE 7.2
The Perils of Proxy!

VP is a 58-year-old woman who was recently diagnosed with colon cancer. She was admitted for tumor resection and is receiving hydromorphone by IV PCA pump. Her prescription order is 0.2 mg every 10 minutes, and a clinician-loading dose of 0.4 mg every 30 minutes for uncontrolled pain to be administered by the nurse. She is in her hospital room 8 hours after surgery. When the nurse checks on VP, she sees that the patient is asleep, is snoring loudly, has a respiratory rate of six breaths per minute, and her breathing is irregular and erratic. With vigorous shaking, the nurse is able to awaken her, but she falls right back asleep. Her oxygen saturation (O_2) is 88%, which increases to 96% with oxygen at 2 L per nasal cannula. Mr. P is visiting his wife. The nurse asks if VP has been hitting her PCA bolus button. He admits that VP has been asleep so he has continued to hit the button so VP won't awaken in pain. *What do you do now?*

This is known as *PCA by proxy*, meaning the PCA demand bolus button has been activated by someone other than the patient such as a family member, a friend, or even a clinician, more times than not at times when the patient is *not* in need! This practice is obviously strongly discouraged! The beauty of *patient*-controlled analgesia is that the *patient* takes a dose, and if pain-free, frequently falls asleep. While sleeping, the patient is unable to hit the demand button, preventing further doses from being administered. Obviously Mr. P needs to be educated about how he has put Mrs. P's life in jeopardy. Your action at this time is to hold the hydromorphone, and consider the use of naloxone, particularly if the clinical situation worsens.

The American Society for Pain Management Nursing has issued a position statement and clinical practice guidelines for *authorized agent controlled analgesia*. In this case, the authorized agent refers to a competent individual who is authorized by a prescriber to activate the PCA demand dose for a patient incapable of doing so.[7] The guidelines are clear that this is NOT an endorsement of PCA by proxy where unauthorized individuals activate PCA for a patient. Rather, the authorized agent must be screened and educated, as well as able to perform diligent patient assessment and medication management.

Back to the case of the hypersomnolent VP—the nurse should stop the pump, have someone else immediately notify the prescriber, stay with the patient, keep her aroused (remind her to take deep breaths every 5 seconds), and administer oxygen and naloxone as appropriate. And we need to take Mr. P out behind the woodshed!

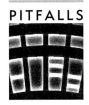

PITFALLS **PCAs Are Error-Prone!**

In addition to PCA by proxy, the Institute for Safe Medication Practices has provided a list of additional causes of errors with PCA, including improper patient selection, inadequate monitoring, inadequate patient education, drug product mix-ups, practice-related problems, device design flaws, inadequate staff training, and prescription errors.[8] It is obvious that PCA therapy has great potential for therapeutic misadventure and extensive education is called for with prescribing, administering, and monitoring therapy.

Adding a Continuous Infusion to the PCA in Opioid-Naïve Patients

A continuous infusion of opioid is generally *not* used in opioid-naïve patients. Most practitioners prefer that the patient rely on the bolus dose option to avoid inadvertently overdosing. The primary safeguard with PCA therapy is the need for the patient to be awake to self-administer a dose of opioid. By providing a continuous infusion of opioid, we have lost the safeguard of patient alertness (and the infusion keeps chug-a-lugging along regardless of the patient's level of sedation). If you choose to give a continuous infusion, it is especially important not to start it until at least 8 hours after surgery to allow for resolution of the residual effects from anesthesia.[6] If, however, the patient is free of adverse effects, and is consistently using the PCA bolus such that sleeping would be difficult, some practitioners would consider giving a portion of the opioid requirement by continuous infusion. Two examples are Strassels and Pasero. Strassels recommends averaging the analgesic dose administered during the previous two 8-hour shifts and providing half that amount by continuous infusion. Of course, the bolus option would remain in place in addition to that.[6] Pasero recommends an even lower dose, enough to take the edge off so the patient doesn't have to ride the bolus button all night long. Pasero also stresses that absolutely essential to this practice is close monitoring by nursing staff of respiratory status and sedation. If careful monitoring of sedation and respiratory status is not available, Pasero recommends not using a continuous infusion in opioid-naïve patients.[5]

Other practitioners take exception to the concept of continuous infusion, because it has been noted that continuous infusion PCA does not necessarily improve pain control, may increase the risk of adverse effects including respiratory depression, and patients may end up receiving more opioid than they otherwise would have.[9] *Let's look at an example of incorporating a continuous infusion into PCA.*

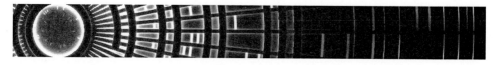

CASE 7.3
∙ ∙

Adding Continuous Infusion to the PCA in an Opioid-Naïve Patient

CG is a 32-year-old woman status-post C-section at 6 a.m. this morning. She had been in hard labor for 14 hours prior to the surgical intervention, and she has been quite vocal about the pain and suffering she's been through. CG has been on a PCA pump since surgery, receiving morphine 1 mg every 10 minutes, and ringing the call button ceaselessly, crying "I can't stand the pain, and I'm exhausted. How am I going to get any rest when I have to keep hitting this button! Can't you DO something?" The nurse taking care of CG threatens to hurt you if you don't address this situation. So, you decide to start a continuous infusion during the night so CG can get a little rest (not to mention the nurse!).

Over the first 8 hours, she used 30 mg IV morphine; over the second 8 hours, she used 22 mg IV morphine. You could average these, or just go with the amount used during the second 8-hour shift. The amount used in the second 8 hours is probably more reflective of steady-state blood levels of the opioid, and her pain may already be lessening. Twenty-two milligrams of IV morphine over 8 hours is 2.75 mg/hr; half of this is 1.375 mg/hr. To be safe, let's round down to 1 mg/hr of IV morphine as a continuous infusion and leave the 1 mg every 10 minutes order on top of that. Don't forget to leave explicit instructions for exemplary nursing care and close observation of CG during the night so she will not experience a serious adverse drug reaction (especially respiratory depression) secondary to adding the continuous infusion. So much for the nurse getting some well-deserved rest!

Switching from Parenteral to Oral Opioid Therapy

As acute pain begins to subside, the pain stabilizes, and the patient is able to tolerate oral medications, it is appropriate to consider calculating an oral opioid regimen to transition from the PCA pump (with or without the continuous infusion). *Because most acute pain patients receiving IV PCA therapy do not receive a continuous infusion, let's look at a more typical case.*

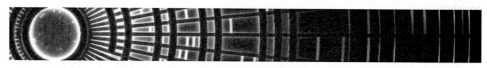

CASE 7.4
∙ ∙

Switching from Parenteral to Oral Opioid Therapy

FO is a 71-year-old man who had a below-the-knee amputation several days ago. He has been on an IV PCA morphine pump since surgery. You do a pain assessment and rule out neuropathic or phantom limb pain. His current regimen is 2 mg every 10 minutes. Over the past 24 hours, he has used on average one or two boluses per hour (a total of 32 boluses, or 64 mg, in 24 hours). His physician anticipates FO will continue to experience moderate pain after discharge, so he would like to transition FO to oral long-acting oxycodone. What would be an equivalent dose to what FO has received via IV PCA over the past 24 hours?

FO has received 32 boluses of 2 mg morphine over the past 24 hours, for a total daily dose (TDD) of 64 mg IV morphine. Let's set up an equation to convert this to oral oxycodone.

$$\frac{\text{"X" mg TDD oral oxycodone}}{\text{64 mg TDD parenteral morphine}} = \frac{\text{20 mg equianalgesic factor of oral oxycodone}}{\text{10 mg equianalgesic factor of parenteral morphine}}$$

$(10) \times (X) = (64) \times (20)$

$10X = 1{,}280$

$X = 128$ mg oral oxycodone

Because we are switching from one opioid to another, let's reduce this by 25% to 50% (because of incomplete cross-tolerance), which would be 64 to 96 mg TDD oral oxycodone. OxyContin is available as a 30-mg tablet; therefore, an appropriate around-the-clock order would be OxyContin 30 mg by mouth every 12 hours. Next, you need to determine what dose of immediate-release oxycodone to order for breakthrough pain. On one hand, FO tells us a 2-mg dose of IV morphine did a very fine job relieving his pain (which is equivalent to 4 mg of oral oxycodone). On the other hand, 10% to 20% of our TDD of scheduled oxycodone (TDD is 60 mg) is 6 to 12 mg (which rounds nicely to 5 or 10 mg, or even 15 mg). Therefore, you could initially recommend oxycodone 5 mg by mouth every 2 hours (or every 3 or every 4 hours) as needed for breakthrough pain and increase to 10 mg, if needed. Even though the prescriber requested you calculate the dose of a long-acting opioid, current guidance suggests using a short-acting opioid postoperatively. In this case, we could recommend oxycodone 10 mg by mouth every 4 hours around the clock, with oxycodone 5 mg by mouth every 2 hours as needed. It would be preferable NOT to have both the IV PCA demand bolus AND oral breakthrough opioid both available. FO can swallow, so let's just go with the oral opioid.

PATIENT-CONTROLLED ANALGESIA IN PATIENTS WITH ADVANCED ILLNESS

PCA can be used very successfully by opioid-naïve and -tolerant patients with advanced illness. We frequently turn to parenteral opioid therapy when pain is rapidly escalating, when patients can't swallow or don't have a feeding tube, when transdermal opioid therapy is not an option, or when the patient has a bowel obstruction. The same or similar PCA pumps are used for patients with advanced illness whether they are at home, in a facility, or in the hospital. The prescriber will still have to determine the PCA bolus dose, possibly a clinician-loading dose, a continuous infusion if appropriate, and sometimes an hourly (or 4-hourly) limit. The 1-hour limit may be omitted in palliative care due to the need for frequent dosage adjustments based on patient status (which may be rapidly changing). Just as with acute or post-operative pain, PCA therapy in this setting may be used to deliver morphine, hydromorphone, or fentanyl. Parenteral methadone is now also used more often for patients with advanced illness (see Chapter 6). Intravenous and sub-Q PCA remain the primary routes of PCA therapy, although it can be used for epidural, IT, or intracerebral ventricular administration.[7]

A word about sub-Q opioid infusions—morphine, hydromorphone, and fentanyl (or less commonly used opioids) are frequently given by this route. Methadone may also be given sub-Q, but may cause skin irritation (see Chapter 6). As discussed in earlier chapters, we consider sub-Q and IV doses to be equivalent (1 mg IV = 1 mg sub-Q). The big issue with a sub-Q infusion is the volume limitation—it is generally recommended that we not exceed 3 mL/hr because the subcutaneous tissue cannot absorb much more volume than that. Some practitioners actually prefer to limit sub-Q volume to less than 2 mL/hr. To exceed 3 mL/hr imperils your site of administration. When patients have high opioid requirements that result in larger volumes of drug that need to be administered, you might want to consider switching from morphine to hydromorphone because it is more potent and results in a smaller infusion volume. When administering PCA by the sub-Q route, it is recommended that the 25- or 27-gauge butterfly sub-Q needle be placed on the upper arm, shoulder, abdomen, or thigh. It is recommended that practitioners avoid placing the needle in the chest wall to prevent iatrogenic pneumothorax during needle insertion.[10] Generally speaking, a sub-Q site will last about a week unless a high volume is infused, or local skin irritation, itching, site bleeding, or infection occurs.

PCA Infusions in Opioid-Naïve Patients with Advanced Illness

When beginning PCA therapy in an opioid-naïve patient with advanced illness, you can choose to either begin solely with demand dosing, or start a low-dose opioid infusion. It is probably preferable to start with demand dosing (and clinician loading dose if needed), using dosages shown in Table 7-1. For very frail or elderly patients, consider reducing the dose by 50%. For example, you might want to start morphine PCA demand dosing in an older frail patient at 0.5 mg every 10 minutes (and possibly a clinician-loading dose of 1 mg every 10 minutes, as discussed previously). *One technique that has been published for determining the appropriate dose for your continuous infusion is to calculate the amount of opioid that was needed over the first 4 hours to achieve patient comfort.*[7] For example, if the patient received 9.2 mg over the first 4 hours, you can calculate an infusion rate of 9.2/4 = 2.3 mg/hr and then start your continuous infusion at 2 mg/hr. Because the patient is not yet at steady state, this may be an overestimation of what the patient requires continuously; therefore, you may choose to reduce this to 1 or 1.5 mg/hr, and use a PCA demand bolus dose to titrate to effect.

It is important to note that there is a difference between the role of the PCA demand bolus dose and the continuous infusion in patients with *acute pain* (e.g., postoperative pain) and *chronic pain*. The purpose of the continuous infusion with *acute pain* (if used at all) is to give the patient a "leg up" so they can sleep and not have to activate the PCA bolus button every 8 to 10 minutes or so. You do *not* use the continuous infusion in this case to eliminate the need for the PCA bolus. In *chronic pain* patients, however, the purpose of the continuous infusion (in a patient with persistent pain) is to minimize the need for the PCA bolus dose, but it is still there if the patient needs it. This is the same principle as using an oral long-acting opioid with an oral short-acting opioid for breakthrough pain.

Back to the discussion at hand—an opioid-naïve patient with an advanced illness— we've established a continuous infusion rate that we anticipate will meet the majority of the patient's opioid needs, but, of course, we also have the PCA bolus dose available. *How do we calculate that dose?* A good starting point is 50% of the hourly infusion.[11] This dose can be increased or decreased based on patient response. One reference suggests the bolus be 50% to 150% of the hourly infusion rate.[12] As we discussed in Chapter 4, occasionally a patient will experience incident pain that is significantly more painful than we anticipate. In this case, you may need a higher dose for the PCA bolus. For IV PCA, you can offer the PCA demand bolus dose every 10 to 15 minutes; for sub-Q PCA you may want to consider every 15 to 30 minutes. These lockout periods should also be tailored to meet patient needs. For example, with stable pain control, the "prn" (as needed) dosing interval could be extended to every 1 or 2 hours.

Titrating the PCA Infusion

An important safety point: When in doubt, be conservative with the continuous infusion and more liberal with the PCA bolus dose. *So, how quickly CAN we increase the continuous infusion? Let's consider the following Fast Fact!*

It's Not What You Know, It's How You Order It!

FAST FACTS 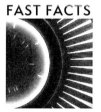 In a *PC Now Fast Facts*, Dr. David Weissman offers the following example of a typical opioid infusion titration order: "Morphine 2–10 mg/hour, titrate to pain relief."[13] *What's wrong with this order?* First, an order of this type leaves the hard work to the nurse—there is no guidance on how fast to titrate or how the dose should be incrementally increased (1 mg at a time, 2 mg at a time? Go right from 2 mg/hr to 10 mg/hr?). Plus, the only option for poorly controlled pain is to increase the continuous infusion. *Dr. Weissman suggests a better order would be:* "Morphine 2 mg/hour AND morphine 2 mg every 15 minutes for breakthrough pain (or 2 mg via PCA bolus). Nurse may dose escalate the 'as needed' dose to a maximum of 4 mg within 30 minutes for poorly controlled pain." He further suggests that the continuous opioid infusion rate be increased NO SOONER than 8 hours. How'd he come up with 8 hours I wonder? *Let's take a look.*

As we discussed above, the risk of a continuous opioid infusion as opposed to simply using as-needed demand PCA dosing, is that a continuous infusion does just that—continuously supplies opioid to the patient regardless of level of consciousness. *The same concept applies as we wrestle with HOW soon we can increase the dose of a continuous opioid infusion.* **The issues we are contending with are twofold:**

- We need to FULLY appreciate the clinical impact of the current continuous opioid infusion dose when it achieves steady-state serum levels (both therapeutic gain and potential toxicity) BEFORE we increase the dose (and make the situation worse, and that always seems to happen at 3 a.m. when no one is really paying close attention).

- We don't want the patient to suffer with pain while we are waiting for the magical moment of steady-state to make sure we haven't overdosed the patient.

We can address the second bullet point by allowing for generous bolus doses—both patient demand PCA boluses and clinician boluses. So, what's the deal with steady-state? A patient will achieve a *steady-state* serum concentration of a medication when the rate of medication entering the body is equal to the rate of medication leaving the body. The rate of the medication leaving the body is defined by the half-life of the medication. After one half-life of a medication, 50% of the medication in the body will have been eliminated. Let's assume we administer ONE IV dose of a medication, it achieves a peak serum concentration of 100 mcg/mL, and the medication has a half-life of 3 hours. *If we supply no additional doses, here's what would happen to the serum level of the drug:*

Half-Life	Time	Serum Concentration
0	0	100 mcg/mL
1	3 hr	50 mcg/mL
2	6 hr	25 mcg/mL
3	9 hr	12.5 mcg/mL
4	12 hr	6.25 mcg/mL
5	15 hr	3.125 mcg/mL
6	18 hr	1.5625 mcg/mL

We could keep this up, getting closer and closer to zero until the cows come home, but for all intents and purposes, clinically speaking, we consider 5 half-lives close enough to say the drug has been eliminated. In this case, it would take about 15 hours to eliminate the drug.

However, the plot thickens when a patient receives multiple doses, or a continuous infusion of a medication. You have drug entering the body and drug leaving the body, but it still takes about 5 half-lives to achieve steady-state (where rate in = rate out). Take a look at Figure 7-1.

With multiple doses administered sequentially, we see that the patient achieves 87.5% of the ultimate steady-state serum concentration after 3 half-lives of the drug, 93.75% after 4 half-lives, and 96.875% after 5 half-lives.

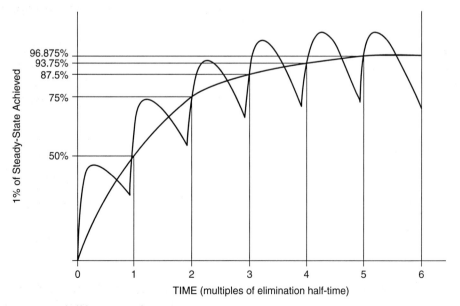

Figure 7-1. Five half-lives to steady-state.

So, when are we on firm ground to increase the continuous opioid infusion? Let's consider an example of morphine by PCA continuous infusion. Morphine is metabolized to two primary metabolites—morphine-3-glucuronide and morphine-6-glucuronide, both of which are pharmacologically active. The elimination of morphine from the body is dependent on both efficient hepatic and renal functions. With normal physiologic functioning, the elimination half-life of morphine is approximately 2 to 3 hours, but with reduced renal or hepatic function (e.g., cirrhosis), hepatic carcinoma, or terminal illness, the elimination half-life can be extended to 3 to 5 hours, or even longer than 9 hours.[14-19] *Let's take a look at what degree of steady-state is achieved with a continuous infusion of morphine, given a normal (2 hours), longer (5 hours), and significantly prolonged (8 hours) half-life.*

Half-life Number	% of Steady-State Achieved	2-hour Half-life	5-hour Half-life	8-hour Half-life
1	50	2	5	8
2	75	4	10	16
3	87.5	6	15	24
4	93.75	8	20	32
5	96.875	10	25	40

If a patient has a "normal" morphine half-life of elimination (2 hours), adjusting the continuous infusion at 8 hours is likely acceptable, because the drug is 93.75% of the way to steady-state. If they're really a red-hot mess at 6 hours, it's probably even okay to bump it up at that time (87.5% of the way to steady-state). Less than 6 hours is just asking for trouble. Again, with this scenario we are talking about someone in the pink of health! This conversation actually started by talking about patients with an advanced illness. As you can see from the 5-hour half-life column, it would be safer to wait closer to 24 hours before adjusting the continuous infusion. For patients with significantly prolonged morphine elimination, it may even take longer.

To summarize, Dr. Weissman recommended in his publication to not adjust the infusion prior to 8 hours (see above).[13] This author contends waiting closer to 12 hours if you do NOT suspect significant organ impairment, or possibly waiting a full 24 hours if you do suspect such. In any case, writing an order for the nurse to "titrate to comfort" is absolutely inappropriate.

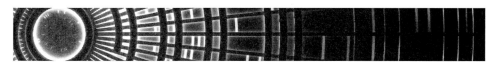

CASE 7.5
. . . .
PCA Continuous Infusion—Starting Doses

SW is a 60-year-old man residing in a long-term care facility admitted to hospice with a diagnosis of end-stage esophageal cancer. He has an order for Ultracet (tramadol 37.5 mg/ acetaminophen 325 mg) 1 tablet every 6 hours as needed for pain. He has tried a few in the past, but now refuses to take them because they "didn't do any darn good!" The Ultracet has also become a moot point because the patient can't swallow tablets or capsules. He is complaining of significant pain, which he rates as high as a 9 or 10 on average (on a 0–10 scale; 0 = no pain, 10 = worst imaginable pain). He has a central line that is still patent. You decide to start him on a PCA morphine pump and would like to start with only demand bolus dosing. Your original order is for 0.5 mg every 10 minutes as needed. An hour into therapy, he has taken six doses and his pain is only down to a 7. You increase the demand bolus dose to 1 mg and order a clinician-loading dose of 2 mg. Approximately 6 hours later, he has received two clinician-loading doses, is averaging about four doses per hour of the PCA demand bolus dose, and is fairly comfortable (he rates pain as a 4). After 18 hours, you review his opioid use—you see that he has taken on average three PCA demand bolus doses per hour over the past few hours. You would like to begin him on a morphine infusion. *What rate do you write for?*

SW is at, or close to, steady-state on his morphine PCA therapy. He has been getting about 3 mg/hr of IV morphine to achieve his current level of pain control; therefore, you could begin SW on an infusion at 3 mg/hr with a bolus of 1.5 mg every 10 minutes. You would continue to evaluate his pain control hourly for the next few hours (to determine if you need to adjust his PCA continuous infusion or bolus dose).

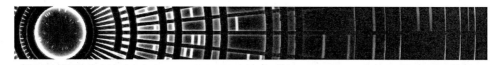

CASE 7.6
PCA Continuous Infusion—Starting Doses

Mr. Svenson is a 78-year-old man receiving home hospice care; he has an admitting diagnosis of end-stage hepatic carcinoma. He is receiving MS Contin 30 mg by mouth every 12 hours, with oral morphine solution 5 mg every 2 hours as needed. Over the past 48 hours, he has been experiencing greatly increased pain, and he has taken about eight doses per day of the rescue morphine. He is exhausted from lack of sleep and trying to get on top of this pain, so you decide to admit him to your inpatient hospice unit. On admission, he rates his pain as a 7 (on a 0–10 scale; 0 = no pain, 10 = worst imaginable pain), and you determine it seems to be opioid-responsive pain. Based on his TDD of oral morphine (100 mg), you calculate an equivalent total daily IV morphine dose of 40 mg, or 1.66 mg/hr. Because he is in significant pain, you decide to give him a 4-mg bolus of IV morphine and start his morphine infusion at 2 mg/hr with a 1-mg bolus every 15 minutes as needed, and a 2-mg hourly clinician bolus per nursing discretion. Although you see no mention of explicit renal or hepatic dysfunction in his record, he is 78 years old with hepatic carcinoma. Chances are excellent his morphine elimination half-life is greater than 2 hours.

Eighteen hours after admission, Mr. Svenson is still receiving the morphine IV infusion at 2 mg/hr. Over the past 6 hours, he has received three clinician boluses of 2 mg, and used his 1-mg demand dose about twice per hour. The boluses total 18 mg over the past 6 hours, or an additional 3-mg IV morphine (on top of his 2 mg/hr). He is currently rating his pain as a 4. Because the patient is likely over 90% of the way to steady-state, you can safely increase his continuous infusion to 4 or even 5 mg/hr morphine continuous infusion. You may also want to increase his bolus dose to 2.5 mg every 15 minutes and increase the clinician bolus to 5 mg. The important thing is that we got Mr. Svenson comfortable, but we did not significantly increase the risk of central nervous system or respiratory depression by titrating too quickly. Milk and cookies for everyone!

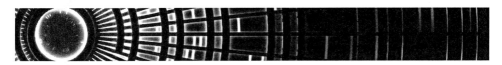

CASE 7.7

Converting from Multiple Opioids to PCA Therapy

HY is a 34-year-old woman with end-stage breast cancer, with widespread metastases including the bones and brain. She is admitted to hospice on the following medications: transdermal fentanyl 50 mcg/hr, MS Contin 60 mg by mouth every 12 hours, and hydromorphone 2 mg by mouth every 2 hours (taking about four times per day). She is also taking dexamethasone 8 mg by mouth every 12 hours. Despite this regimen, she rates her pain as 8 to 10 (on a 0–10 scale; 0 = no pain, 10 = worst imaginable pain) constantly, and off the chart with movement. HY is 5'3" and weighs 120 pounds (slim but not cachectic). You decide to convert her to IV PCA morphine (she has a peripherally inserted central catheter [PICC] line in place).

How do you convert HY to IV PCA morphine? First things first—this is a complicated conversion and is best done in a monitored environment. Just so you know, HY is just starting day 2 of her current 50 mcg/hr transdermal fentanyl (TDF) patch, and her last MS Contin dose was about 6 hours ago. To keep me out of jail, we'll be doing HY's conversion in our inpatient palliative care unit!

STEP 1—Determine the patient's current opioid regimen and calculate a conversion to IV morphine. Let's do this one opioid at a time:

1. TDF 50 mcg/hr ≈ 100-mg oral morphine TDD (using guideline 1 mcg/hr TDF ≈ 2 mg by mouth morphine)

2. MS Contin 60 mg by mouth every 12 hours = 120-mg oral morphine TDD

Adding together the oral morphine from the TDF and MS Contin, we get a total of 220-mg oral morphine TDD.

Let's convert that to IV morphine now.

$$\frac{\text{"X" mg IV morphine}}{\text{220-mg oral morphine}} = \frac{\text{10-mg IV morphine}}{\text{25-mg oral morphine}}$$

(X)(25) = (220)(10)

X = 2,200/25

X = 88-mg IV morphine per day

3. Hydromorphone 2 mg × 4 doses = 8-mg oral hydromorphone TDD

Let's set up our ratio:

$$\frac{\text{"X" mg TDD parenteral morphine}}{\text{8-mg TDD oral hydromorphone}} = \frac{\text{10-mg equianalgesic factor of parenteral morphine}}{\text{5-mg equianalgesic factor of oral hydromorphone}}$$

$(5) \times (X) = (10) \times (8)$

$5X = 80$

$X = 16\text{-mg TDD parenteral morphine}$

Now we need to combine all the parenteral morphine amounts we've calculated:

88-mg IV morphine (from TDF and MS Contin), plus

16-mg IV morphine (from hydromorphone)

Add these together and we get 104-mg IV morphine as her equianalgesic TDD. Wow, that's a lotta morphine! I sure hope she's lovin' some Senna!

STEP 2—*What do we do with the number we've just calculated?* We generally don't apply the 25% to 50% reduction rule with conversions involving TDF (see Chapter 5), and the MS Contin does not require dosage reduction (going from morphine to morphine), but maybe we should consider a slight reduction for the hydromorphone. On the other hand, she's complaining of pain that she rates from 8 to "off the chart." Therefore, let's take our number and run with it or even increase a bit. When we divide 104 by 24 (hours), we get 4.3 mg/hr. There's a lot to consider here—the patient is having pain, but she was only on day 2 of her TDF patch. Because she is experiencing severe pain, let's determine her continuous morphine infusion to be 5 mg/hr.

STEP 3—Because we're increasing her TDD of morphine, AND she's in pain, a clinician bolus would be appropriate at this point, anywhere from equal to or double the hourly infusion. We also need to consider that we're removing the TDF patch (which is pretty much as pseudo steady-state) so we do need to consider the depot fentanyl even as we remove the patch. However, recall that the patch only represents about one-third of our calculated IV morphine dose and the patient is in a lot of pain *now*. I think I need a Tylenol, how about you? Think like a Boy Scout—*safety first*. I vote we give her a 5-mg IV morphine bolus now, take off the TDF patch, begin the infusion at 3 mg/hr for the first 6 hours, and then kick it up to the calculated 5 mg/hr rate. We will also make a PCA bolus option available to her (see Step 4).

STEP 4—Speaking of the bolus calculation—the bolus is anywhere from 50% to 150% of the hourly infusion rate. Let's be conservative and go with a 2.5-mg bolus. Let's also order a clinician bolus of 5-mg IV morphine hourly as needed.

STEP 5—Now we get to pick a dosing interval for the PCA bolus. Because we're giving it IV and she's in pain, let's go with every 15 minutes.

STEP 6—Now we're going to assess HY like nobody's business. We have given the 5-mg IV morphine clinician-loading dose, we removed the TDF patch, we've started the continuous infusion at 3 mg/hr (for the first 6 hours), and HY has the PCA bolus option of 2.5 mg every 15 minutes. One hour later, HY is still telling you her pain is a 10. Be bold men—let's repeat the clinician bolus of 5 mg and increase her bolus dose to 4 mg every 10 minutes. We will continue to evaluate the effectiveness of the bolus dose and adjust every 30 to 60 minutes.

STEP 7—It has now been 18 hours since HY was admitted to the palliative care unit and she was switched to IV PCA morphine. Her continuous infusion was increased from 3 to 5 mg/hr about 12 hours ago (because we were comfortable that the depot fentanyl has dissipated); over the past 12 hours, she has received two clinician boluses at 5 mg and 20 PCA demand bolus doses at 4 mg. However, over the past 2 hours, she has only used two PCA bolus doses and she tells you she is comfortable. You could increase the continuous infusion at this time, but with the wearing off of the TDF and the MS Contin, and her apparently stability over the past 2 hours, I would probably hold the course at 5 mg/hr continuous IV infusion with 4 mg every 15 minutes as needed for breakthrough pain. You should plan to re-evaluate both the continuous infusion and PCA bolus dose in about 2 to 4 hours, and every shift thereafter. ***Importantly, you should only change one parameter at a time: the PCA demand bolus dose, the PCA demand dose lockout interval, or the continuous infusion dose.*** *I think I need to go take a little nap now!*

Converting from a PCA Infusion to Oral or Transdermal Opioid Therapy

There are many occasions where we need to convert a patient from a continuous infusion PCA to oral or transdermal therapy. We simply use the reverse process we used in converting from oral to the PCA infusion. There are, of course, some timing issues (e.g., when to start the oral long-acting or TDF relative to discontinuing the infusion), and the calculation of breakthrough doses to consider.

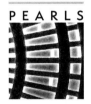

PEARLS **Switching from PCA to Oral Long-Acting Opioid Therapy**

When converting to an oral long-acting opioid from a PCA or continuous infusion, you must consider the lead time necessary for the new opioid to achieve adequate serum levels before stopping the parenteral infusion. For example, in Chapter 5 we discussed one protocol when switching to a TDF patch from parenteral fentanyl. In that protocol, 6 hours after application of the TDF patch, the continuous infusion was reduced 50%; then, at 12 hours after TDF patch application, it was discontinued. When switching to an oral long-acting opioid, it would be appropriate to administer the first dose 2 to 4 hours before discontinuing the parenteral opioid infusion.

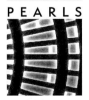

PEARLS **Incident Pain Is Not Incidental!**

We talked in Chapter 4 about not including opioid rescue doses that were administered for incident pain when doing conversion calculations. This is because incident pain, particularly that which is under the patient's control, varies significantly depending on the frequency of the precipitating events.

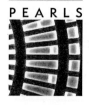

Timing Is Everything When Switching Off PCA Therapy

When converting a patient from PCA therapy (continuous plus demand), it is important not to convert the patient until pain is controlled. For example, it is important to achieve the correct continuous infusion rate, such that the patient requires only occasional PCA demand doses, otherwise we end up chasing the person's pain and having to start over.

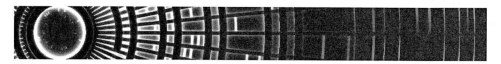

CASE 7.8
• •

Converting from Parenteral PCA Therapy to Oral or Transdermal Opioid Therapy

NA is a 62-year-old woman with cancer who had been admitted to the hospital for pain that was out of control. She now has good pain control and would like to go home. She is taking naproxen 500 mg by mouth every 12 hours, gabapentin 300 mg by mouth every 8 hours, and sub-Q PCA morphine running at 1.5 mg/hr, plus a 2-mg bolus she takes before her physical therapy. You have been asked to convert her to a long-acting opioid regimen.

First we calculate her TDD of opioid—she's getting 1.5 mg/hr × 24 hours = 36 mg sub-Q morphine TDD. Multiplying by 2.5 gives us the total daily oral morphine dose, or 90 mg. For long-acting morphine, our choices are Kadian 50 mg by mouth every 12 hours, MS Contin 45 mg by mouth every 12 hours, or OraMorph 30 mg by mouth every 8 hours. Which- ever you choose, the tablet or capsule should be administered about 2 to 3 hours prior to discontinuing the PCA infusion. You could give the tablet or capsule 3 hours before discon- tinuing the PCA infusion, but keep the PCA bolus dose in place for an additional period of time to ensure the patient doesn't experience additional pain. Alternately (and preferably), a dose of oral rescue morphine, such as oral morphine 15 mg by mouth every 2 hours as needed may be provided.

If you were going to switch NA to a TDF patch, 90 mg per day of oral morphine is approxi- mately equivalent to a 50-mcg/hr TDF patch. You would apply the patch; 6 hours later, reduce the continuous infusion to 0.7 mg/hr; and then discontinue the continuous infusion 12 hours after patch application. You can still have the immediate-release morphine 15 mg by mouth every 2 hours as needed available from the time of patch application.

So, why didn't we include the 2-mg PCA bolus the patient takes before therapy when we calculated our TDD of morphine? Because physical therapy is *volitional incident* pain! If she doesn't participate in therapy, there is no need to include that dose. If she does participate in therapy, she can use the immediate-release morphine 15 mg 30 to 60 minutes before her scheduled appointment time.

NEURAXIAL OPIOID THERAPY

Neuraxial, or intraspinal, opioid therapy refers to administering opioids into the spaces or potential spaces surrounding the spinal cord. This generally refers to epidural and intrathecal (IT; sometimes referred to as *spinal*) opioid administration. The bony vertebral column and three connective tissue layers known as the meninges protect the spinal cord. The meninges are known as the dura mater (the outermost layer closest to the skin), the arachnoid mater (the middle of the three layers), and the pia mater (the membrane closest to the spinal cord and brain).

The **epidural space** (also known as the *extra dural space*) is outside the dura mater, and contains blood vessels, nerve roots, fat, and connective tissue. There is a potential cavity between the dura and the arachnoid mater, referred to as the **subdural space**. The space between the arachnoid mater and the pia mater is the **subarachnoid space**, or the *IT or spinal space*. The *subarachnoid space* contains the cerebrospinal fluid that bathes the spinal cord. Therefore, we can provide opioid therapy either by the intraspinal route (inserting a needle into the subarachnoid space) or by the epidural route (injecting the opioid or threading a catheter into the space outside the dura mater; see Figure 7-2). Medications can be administered into the epidural or IT space as an injection or infusion, or by PCA. When medications are administered intraspinally, it is important to use only preservative-free solutions. At present, only morphine is approved by the Food and Drug Administration for IT use, although off-label use of neuraxial hydromorphone and fentanyl is quite common.

The Polyanalgesic Consensus Conference (PACC) by Deer and colleagues have provided a series of three articles that provide extensive guidance on trialing IT drug delivery infusion therapy, improving safety, mitigating risks, and infusion systems best practices and guidelines.[20–22] In the first article, appropriate candidates for IT are reviewed including both chronic noncancer pain and cancer pain.[20] In this document, they also discuss the importance of knowing the patient's previous exposure to opioids; patients on high-dose systemic opioid therapy before starting IT therapy have a higher

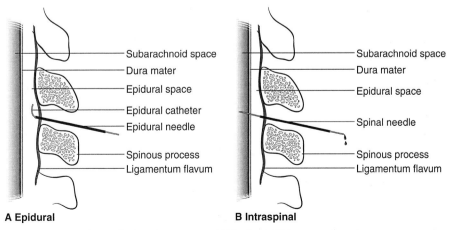

A Epidural **B Intraspinal**

Figure 7-2. Neuraxial opioid administration sites. (A) Epidural; (B) Intraspinal.

likelihood of therapeutic failure if only one medication is used for IT delivery.[20] In the second article in the series, the use of "trialing" IT prior to implanting an IT drug delivery system is discussed.[21] There are a variety of proposed trialing methods (e.g., single-shot, bolus, and catheter trialing techniques), but trialing provides the clinician and patient a preview of likely clinical response with longer-term infusion via implanted pump. Potential outcomes include pain relief (with or without side effects) or no relief (with or without side effects).

The guidelines acknowledge that a trial is not required or appropriate for all patients (e.g., such as a patient with advanced disease).[21] They provided recommendations for both trial dosing and long-term delivery of several commonly used opioids. For example, the recommended dose for IT bolus trialing of hydromorphone is 0.025 to 0.1 mg. They recommend that starting doses of medications in the opioid-naïve patient for outpatient bolus delivery do not exceed 0.04 mg hydromorphone, and that starting doses of continuous IT delivery should be half of the trial dose for opioid-based medications. Using our hydromorphone example, they recommend 0.01 to 0.15 mg/day as the recommended starting dosage range for IT long-term delivery.[20]

Converting Between Routes of Administration (Including Intraspinal) with the Same Opioid

Now we come to the tricky part—the discussions about conversion calculations that involve neuraxial opioid therapy (this won't take long!). A couple of fairly common examples that would necessitate conversion from epidural to IV opioid include a case where the epidural catheter is accidently pulled out or where the patient is not achieving satisfactory pain relief, and epidural catheter placement is questioned. In these cases, it would be appropriate to switch from the epidural to IV opioid, and possibly on to the oral opioid. Very few data provide guidance on switching between routes of administration (including epidural and IT) for any one opioid. ***One commonly referenced guide is the following:***[23]

- 300-mg oral morphine, equals
- 100-mg parenteral morphine, equals
- 10-mg epidural morphine, equals
- 1-mg IT morphine

Even though this conversion is seen *everywhere* in the neuraxial literature, it is not evidence based (it was based on modeling), and in my personal discussions with anesthesiologists, a recurring theme is "don't believe everything you read." One anesthesiologist commented that it's probably safe (e.g., conservative, and won't get you in trouble, but won't necessarily be 100% equivalent in terms of effective pain relief) to use this equivalency when going in the direction of oral to IT, but not the other way. As an example, in the late 1980s and early 1990s, a survey of experts showed a range of IV to epidural conversion ratios ranging from 10:1 to 10:2 to 10:5, but none have been validated in clinical trials or even garnered consensus.[24] A recent survey of pain specialists regarding conversion of high-dose IV to neuraxial opioids disclosed that over two-thirds of respondents agreed with the equivalencies mentioned above for morphine (100-mg parenteral morphine/24 hr ~ 10-mg epidural morphine/24 hr ~ 1 mg IT morphine/24 hr).[25] To a lesser extent, respondents also applied this model to hydromorphone and fentanyl, but the researchers concluded there was significant variability in opinions.

DuPen reported that his experience converting from IV morphine to epidural morphine indicated that the ratio was approximately 3:1 (this is an unpublished observation).[24] Unfortunately, we don't know if this information is bidirectional, or only applicable when going from IV to epidural. Kalso and colleagues also described the conversion of 10 cancer patients from epidural to sub-Q morphine.[26] The authors concluded the median epidural:sub-Q ratio was 1:3, but ranged from 1:1 to 1:10, and recommended individualization of conversion ratios.

DuPen states that he has found 90-mg oral morphine to be approximately equivalent to 1-mg of IT morphine.[24] He further advises that after doing the mathematical conversion, one should reduce the oral opioid administered by "no more than 50%," then titrate the dose down weekly by about one-third while at the same time increasing the IT dose by 10% to 15%.[24]

How do we deal with all these differences of opinion? At least everyone agrees that we begin at a low dose, titrate slowly, and always have rescue medication available. In fact, the PACC recommendations state, "The use of pretrialing systemic opioid dose conversions to derive an appropriate dose for IT opioid trialing is not recommended because of pretrial weaning of systemic opioids and differences in pharmacology between systemic and IT opioids."[20]

Let's look at an epidural to IV conversion and see if we go completely blind.

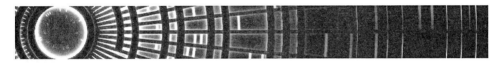

CASE 7.9
• •
Uh-oh! The Epidural Catheter Got Pulled Out. What Do I Do Now?

LK is a 62-year-old woman who has had severe chronic pain for years. She had an above-the-knee amputation 3 days ago. Her pain was well controlled on an epidural PCA infusion with a continuous infusion of 0.4 mg/hr of morphine and a 0.2-mg PCA bolus every 15 minutes. While in therapy today, LK's epidural catheter was accidently pulled out. LK cannot swallow solid dosage formulations, so you've been called to calculate an appropriate IV PCA prescription.

If we go with the 10-mg IV morphine ≈ 1 mg epidural morphine (10:1 ratio), then an appropriate basal infusion rate would be 4-mg IV morphine/hr. If we go with the 3-mg IV morphine ≈ 1 mg epidural morphine (3:1 ratio), the basal infusion rate would be 1.2-mg/hr IV morphine. The answer is probably somewhere between 1.2- and 4-mg/hr IV morphine. I would err on the conservative side, and go with 1.5 mg/hr, being generous with the IV PCA bolus dose. Using the 10:1 rule, an equivalent IV PCA bolus dose would be 2 mg; using the 3:1 it would be 0.6 mg, our bolus dose range is 0.6 to 2 mg. We could compromise and start LK on IV PCA with the continuous infusion running at 1.5 mg/hr, and the IV PCA bolus at 1.5 mg every 10 minutes. This allows us to be conservative, particularly since we don't know the exact conversion. Additionally, it will probably take hours for the epidural morphine to wear off. Meanwhile, we've given the patient a generous IV PCA bolus dose, which we can increase up or down every 30 to 60 minutes.

Converting Between Neuraxial Opioids

So, how's life treating you WAY out there on the limb? If you thought we were on thin ice calculating conversions to and from an intraspinal route of administration and another route using one opioid, we are completely without ice when we think about converting from one opioid to another by the same intraspinal route. According to PACC, there is no definitive evidence of a true conversion factor for calculating dose changes when switching from one IT opioid to another.[27] Panelists did comment that switching from a more lipophilic drug (sufentanil, fentanyl) to a less lipophilic drug (morphine, hydromorphone) carried a high risk for respiratory depression when using conventional equianalgesic dosing charts. The conclusion was to start a very low dose of the new opioid, titrating slowly while tapering down on the initial opioid.

Do you remember this case way back at the beginning of the book?

WE is a 54-year-old man with an end-stage malignancy referred to hospice. He has an implanted IT pump, which is delivering 1 mg of morphine per day. The hospice nurse calls you and wants to know what would be an appropriate dose of oral morphine to give the patient for breakthrough pain?

Unbelievably, this was the impetus for me to write this book. This was a real case and I had no clue how to answer the question (that sure burst my bubble!). I went home, pulled as much literature as I could find, and basically ended up with the conversion recommendations from that modeling study (1-mg IT morphine = 10-mg epidural morphine = 100-mg IV morphine = 300-mg oral morphine). Based on this, I advised the nurse to request an order for immediate-release morphine 40 mg every 2 hours as needed for breakthrough pain—my rationale was that 1-mg IT ≈ 300-mg oral morphine, and 20% of that was 60 mg (I decided to go big!). The nurse asked the physician for an order for immediate-release morphine 20 mg with a 20-mg repeat in an hour, every 4 hours as needed for breakthrough pain, and the 20-mg dose was more than enough. Was I wrong? (Never—I think everyone is entitled to my opinion!) This just points out the variability in doing this kind of calculation. Now that I'm older and wiser (and much better looking!), I probably would have gone with the 20-mg dose with no repeat— *safety first!*

Well, we've done some wild and crazy conversion calculations in this chapter! We started this book with a discussion of "safety first" and that principle is still extremely important with the calculations we describe in this chapter. ***Consideration of patient-related variables, and exemplary patient monitoring are the keys to success with difficult opioid conversion.***

PRACTICE PROBLEMS

P7.1: Determining an Initial PCA Dose

JB is a 62-year-old woman status-post total abdominal hysterectomy. She has just been moved to the recovery room and has been started on a morphine PCA pump. You have been asked to write the orders including a clinician-loading dose for the recovery room nurse to give at her discretion. The patient was opioid-naïve prior to surgery. *What parameters should the recovery room nurse and surgical floor nurse case manager follow to manage JB's pain?*

P7.2: Adjusting PCA Doses

GK is a 68-year-old man status-post total hip replacement. He was started on a hydromorphone PCA pump at 0.2 mg every 10 minutes, with a clinician bolus (loading dose) of 0.4 mg as needed. GK was transferred to the floor about 6 hours ago, and the nurse case manager has called you to assess GK. He is complaining of pain that he rates as 10 (on a 0–10 scale; 0 = no pain, 10 = worst imaginable pain). "This stuff doesn't work," he huffs, indicating the hydromorphone PCA pump. "I want the good stuff—I have the best health insurance money can buy!" And here you were holding out on GK giving him the mediocre stuff! When you check historical data on the PCA pump, you see that GK has made four bolus attempts over the last 6 hours, and received one dose. *How will you handle the case of GK and the second-rate* hydromorphone *PCA order?*

P7.3: Calculating a PCA Continuous Infusion Dose

LD is a 42-year-old man who has been admitted to the intensive care unit (ICU) after an automobile accident and emergency abdominal surgery. He was started on a fentanyl PCA pump, 20 mcg every 8 minutes, which was increased to 30 mcg every 8 minutes. Over the past 16 hours, he has received a total of thirty 20-mcg doses and eighty 30-mcg doses. His pain is about a 4 or 5 (on a 0–10 scale; 0 = no pain, 10 = worst imaginable pain) at this time, which he finds to be acceptable. LD insists that he wants to get this medication automatically overnight so he can sleep and not have to push the button. LD's physician asks that you calculate the dose of a continuous infusion that provides 50% of what he has been getting on average, but keep the hourly limit the same as if he were only getting the maximum allowed with the bolus option. *What do you recommend?*

P7.4: Converting from IV PCA to Oral Morphine

MJ is a 75-year-old woman status-post Whipple procedure 4 days ago. She has been receiving IV PCA morphine for the pain as morphine 1-mg IV every 10 minutes as needed. For the past 24 hours, she has received 34 doses with acceptable pain control. *What would be an equivalent oral morphine regimen to send her home on?*

P7.5: Converting from Oral to Sub-Q PCA Morphine

DT is a 60-year-old man with a history of widespread metastatic cancer, with no identified primary site. His pain has been controlled on MS Contin 30 mg by mouth every 12 hours with oral morphine 10 mg by mouth every 2 hours as needed for breakthrough pain until recently. Co-analgesics have been added with no success. A decision has been made to admit DT to the inpatient palliative care unit and convert him to a sub-Q PCA infusion. DT is admitted at 6 p.m.; he took his last dose of MS Contin at 8 a.m. that morning. He has been averaging six doses per day of the oral morphine 10 mg, and he has taken three doses since 8 a.m. this morning. DT rates his pain as a 6 on average (on a 0–10 scale; 0 = no pain, 10 = worst imaginable pain), but it can increase to 8 or more without provocation. *What prescription will you write for DT's sub-Q PCA morphine?*

P7.6: Converting from IV PCA Hydromorphone to Oral Oxycodone

GJ is a 62-year-old man who has a history of pancreatic cancer. He was admitted for a Whipple procedure, and his current oral opioid regimen was converted to a parenteral PCA regimen for ease of administering postoperative analgesia. It is now several days post-op, and GJ's pain is stable and he would like to go home. He is receiving hydromorphone 0.5 mg/hr by IV PCA, with a PCA bolus dose of 0.3 mg, which he uses about four times in a 12-hour period. He would like to resume taking OxyContin and OxyIR. *What dosage regimen do you recommend and how do you make this conversion?*

Could I Get That to Go, Please? Bottom Line It for Me . . .

▶ PCA may be used to treat acute or chronic pain, generally including a demand bolus dose, and potentially including a continuous infusion of opioid.

▶ The usual PCA demand bolus dose for acute pain in an opioid-naïve patient is 1 mg for morphine (every 10 minutes), 0.2 mg for hydromorphone (every 10 minutes), or 20 mcg for fentanyl (every 8 minutes).

▶ A patient's response to PCA demand bolus dosing requires careful consideration of the number of bolus attempts and patient response (therapeutic and toxic). Adjustment of the prescription is guided by these parameters (see Table 7-2).

▶ Family members and others should be strictly counseled NOT to give the patient's PCA demand bolus dose by proxy (meaning without the patient's consent). This does NOT include PCA demand bolus dosing performed by an authorized agent.

▶ A continuous infusion is rarely used for acute pain in opioid-naïve patients. If the situation warrants a continuous infusion, consider providing 30% to 50% of the patient's opioid requirement by continuous infusion (may be substantially less, however).

▶ In patients with an advanced illness, the continuous infusion will provide 75% or more of the opioid requirement. A demand bolus dose is also provided.

▶ The PCA demand bolus dose may be increased every 2 hours, but the continuous infusion should not be increased before 12 hours (with competent organ function) to 24 hours (with suspected renal or hepatic dysfunction).

▶ Neuraxial opioid therapy refers to administering opioids into the spaces or potential spaces surrounding the spinal cord. There is very little information to guide conversion calculations with neuraxial therapy.

REFERENCES

1. Stewart D. Pearls and pitfalls of patient-controlled analgesia. *US Pharm.* 2017;42(3):HS24-HS27.

2. *Principles of Analgesic Use in the Treatment of Acute Pain and Cancer Pain.* 7th ed. Glenview, IL: American Pain Society; 2016.

3. Official STOP-Bang Questionnaire. Toronto Western Hospital, University Health Network, University of Toronto; 2012. http://www.stopbang.ca/osa/screening.php. Accessed March 3, 2018.

4. Craft J. Patient-controlled analgesia: is it worth the painful prescribing process? *Proc (Bayl Univ Med Cent)*. 2010;23(4):434-438.

5. Pasero C, McCaffery M. *Pain Assessment and Pharmacologic Management*. St. Louis, MO; Elsevier Mosby; 2011.

6. Strassels SA, McNicol E, Ruleman R. Postoperative pain management: a practice review, part 1. *Am J Health-Syst Pharm*. 2005;62:1904-1916.

7. Cooney MF, Czarnecki M, Dunwoody C, et al. American Society for Pain Management Nursing position statement with clinical practice guidelines: authorized agent controlled analgesia. *Pain Manage Nursing*. 2013;14(3):176-181.

8. Institute for Safe Medication Practices. Acute ISMP Medication Safety Alert! Safety issues with patient-controlled analgesia. Part I—How errors occur; 2003. http://www.ismp.org/Newsletters/acutecare/articles/20030710.asp. Accessed February 25, 2018.

9. Hagle ME, Lehr VT, Brubakken K, et al. Respiratory depression in adult patients with intravenous patient-controlled analgesia. *Orthop Nurs*. 2004;23:18-27.

10. Weissman DE. Fast Facts and Concepts #28: Subcutaneous Opioid Infusions, 3rd ed. Appleton, WI: PC Now Palliative Care Network of Wisconsin; 2015. https://www.mypcnow.org/blank-d5l0b. Accessed March 3, 2018.

11. Prommer E. *Fast Facts and Concepts #92: Patient Controlled Analgesia in Palliative Care*. 3rd ed. Appleton, WI: PC Now Palliative Care Network of Wisconsin; 2015. https://www.mypcnow.org/blank-ypz41. Accessed March 3, 2018.

12. Weinstein E, Arnold R, Weissman DE. *Fast Facts and Concepts #54: Opioid Infusions in the Imminently Dying Patient*. 3rd ed. Appleton, WI: PC Now Palliative Care Network of Wisconsin; 2015. https://www.mypcnow.org/blank-mxj27. Accessed March 3, 2018.

13. Weissman DE. *Fast Facts and Concepts #72: Opioid Infusion Titration Orders*. 3rd ed. Appleton, WI: PC Now Palliative Care Network of Wisconsin; 2015. https://www.mypcnow.org/blank-wvb8b. Accessed March 3, 2018.

14. Conway BR, Fogarty DG, Nelson WE, et al. Opiate toxicity in patients with renal failure. *BMJ*. 2006;332:345-346.

15. Tegeder I, Lotsch J, Geisslinger G. Pharmacokinetics of opioids in liver disease. *Clin Pharmacokinet*. 1999;37(1):17-40.

16. Hasselstrom J, Eriksson S, Persson A, et al. The metabolism and bioavailability of morphine in patients with severe liver cirrhosis. *Br J Clin Pharmacol*. 1990;29:289-297.

17. De Gregori S, Minella CE, De Gregori M, et al. Clinical pharmacokinetics of morphine and its metabolites during morphine dose titration for chronic cancer pain. *Ther Drug Monit*. 2014;36(3):335-344.

18. Koth HIM, El-Kady SA, Emara SES, et al. Pharmacokinetics of controlled release morphine (MST) in patients with liver carcinoma. *Br J Anaesth*. 2005;94(1):95-99.

19. Franken LG, Masman AD, de Winter BC, et al. Pharmacokinetics of morphine, morphine-3-glucuronide and morphine-6-glucuronide in terminally ill adult patients. *Clin Pharmacokinet*. 2016;55:697-709.

20. Deer TR, Pope JE, Hayek SM, et al. The Polyanalgesic Consensus Conference (PACC): recommendations on intrathecal drug infusion systems best practices and guidelines. *Neuromodulation: Technology at the Neural Interface*. 2017;20:96-132.

21. Deer TR, Hayek SM, Pope JE, et al. The Polyanalgesic Consensus Conference (PACC): recommendations for trialing of intrathecal drug delivery infusion therapy. *Neuromodulation*. 2017;20:133-154.

22. Deer TR, Pope JE, Hayek SM, et al. The Polyanalgesic Consensus Conference (PACC): recommendations for intrathecal drug delivery: guidance for improving safety and mitigating risks. *Neuromodulation*. 2017;20:155-176.

23. Krames ES. Intraspinal opioid therapy for chronic nonmalignant pain: current practice and clinical guidelines. *J Pain Symptom Manage*. 1996;11:333-352.

24. DuPen SP, DuPen AR. Neuraxial analgesia by intrathecal drug delivery for chronic noncancer pain. *Medscape*. https://www.medscape.org/viewarticle/466349_2. Accessed March 4, 2018.

25. Gorlin AW, Rosenfeld DM, Maloney J, et al. Survey of pain specialists regarding conversion of high-dose intravenous to neuraxial opioids. *J Pain Research*. 2016;9:693-700.

26. Kalso E, Heiskanen T, Rantio M, et al. Epidural and subcutaneous morphine in the management of cancer pain: a double-blind cross-over study. *Pain.* 1996;67:443-449.

27. Deer T, Krames ES, Hassenbusch SJ, et al. Polyanalgesic Consensus Conference 2007: recommendations for the management of pain by intrathecal (intraspinal) drug delivery: report of an interdisciplinary expert panel. *Neuromodulation.* 2007;10:300-327.

SOLUTIONS TO PRACTICE PROBLEMS

P7.1: A reasonable order would be a 1-mg morphine PCA bolus dose every 10 minutes, with a loading dose (clinician bolus) of 2.5 mg every 10 minutes as needed, up to five doses, until the patient experiences a 50% reduction in pain. The recovery room and floor nursing staff should monitor JB's pain rating and her ability to perform activities such as moving about in bed, transferring, ambulating, going to the bathroom, and providing personal care. For toxicity, the nursing staff should monitor JB's respiratory rate, pupil size, level of arousal (difficulty arousing patient), snoring, excessive sleepiness, bowel habits (constipation), itching, nausea, and vomiting.

P7.2: Clearly GK missed a memo! He is both hitting the button too quickly for one episode of pain, and isn't hitting the PCA bolus button enough overall. As discussed in Table 7-2, if the patient has received one injection to more than three attempts and has no pain relief, the patient should be re-instructed on the idea and use of the PCA pump. GK should be given a clinician-loading dose now (0.4 mg) and taught to hit the PCA button *before* the pain gets ahead of him, and frequently to keep the pain at bay. He should also WAIT the full lockout period (10 minutes) to evaluate the effect of the dose before hitting the button again (clearly he hit the button four times in a row—one hit gave him a bolus, and the other three he was locked out). And reassure GK—hydromorphone is *quality* stuff!

P7.3: Over the past 16 hours, LD has received 30 × 20 mcg (600 mcg) plus 80 × 30 mcg (2,400 mcg) of fentanyl for a total of 3,000 mcg. This averages 187.5 mcg/hr. Half of this would be 93.8 mcg/hr. Therefore, you recommend a continuous infusion of 90 mcg/hr and keep the bolus of 30 mcg every 8 minutes, but with an hourly limit of 210 mcg (which would be if he took all seven boluses of 30 mcg during an hour).

P7.4: MJ received 34 doses × 1 mg/dose of IV morphine over the past 24 hours, for a TDD of IV morphine of 34 mg. Because the oral:parenteral morphine ratio is 2.5:1, this is equivalent to 85 mg of oral morphine per day. We're converting from morphine to morphine, so we do not have to reduce for lack of cross-tolerance; however, her pain should be improving each day. You could start MJ on short-acting oral morphine 10 mg by mouth every 4 hours as needed (total daily dose of 60 mg). You could continue the IV PCA demand bolus doses for some period of time, but it would be preferable to switch to oral morphine for breakthrough pain (e.g., morphine 5 mg by mouth every 2 hours as needed for additional pain). You could also use 5-mg morphine tablets and advise MJ that her pain should be noticeably improving every day, and she can reduce to 5-mg tablets in a day or two.

P7.5:

STEP 1—The first step in calculating DT's sub-Q PCA morphine is to determine the patient's total daily opioid regimen. He is taking MS Contin 30 mg twice a day plus six doses per day of oral morphine (10 mg each), for another 60 mg, or 120-mg TDD oral morphine. Oral morphine 120 mg per day is equivalent to 48-mg parenteral morphine per day.

STEP 2—Next, we have to decide whether to increase, decrease, or go with this number. DT's pain is not well controlled, and we don't have to worry about reducing for lack of complete cross-tolerance. If we go with the 48-mg parenteral morphine per day, this works out to 2 mg/hr. A 25% increase would be 2.5 mg/hr; therefore, that seems to be a reasonable starting dose for the continuous infusion. DT took his last MS Contin dose 10 hours ago, so we can begin the infusion at 2.5 mg/hr at this time.

STEP 3—Do we want to give DT a clinician bolus dose? Since he's in pain right now, that would be appropriate.

STEP 4—We calculate the bolus dose (50% to 150% of the hourly rate); therefore, we will go with 3 mg (he's in pain and we're not sure how much he's going to need).

STEP 5—Let's go with every 20 minutes sub-Q for the dosing interval for the bolus dose.

STEP 6—Assess the efficacy of the PCA bolus dose; if the patient is consistently demanding a bolus dose, increase this by 50% to 100%.

STEP 7—Re-evaluate appropriateness of continuous infusion once patient achieves steady-state.

P7.6: First, let's calculate GJ's TDD of IV hydromorphone. He's getting 0.5 mg/hr, which is 12 mg/day, plus 2.4 mg from his bolus doses (four boluses of 0.3 mg in 12 hours = 1.2 mg; multiply by 2 to get the 24-hour bolus dose utilization). This gives us a TDD of 14.4 mg parenteral hydromorphone.

Let's set up a conversion between parenteral hydromorphone and oral oxycodone:

$$\frac{\text{"X" mg TDD oral oxycodone}}{\text{14.4-mg parenteral hydromorphone}} = \frac{\text{20-mg equianalgesic factor of oral oxycodone}}{\text{2-mg equianalgesic factor of parenteral hydromorphone}}$$

$(20) \times (14.4) = (2) \times (X)$

$288 = 2X$

$X = 144$-mg oral oxycodone TDD

Because we are switching from one opioid to another and the patient's pain is well controlled, we will need to reduce this amount by 25% to 50%, to 72 to 108 mg of oral oxycodone per day. Because GJ was still using eight doses a day of her rescue opioid, let's err on the side of being a bit more aggressive with her standing opioid dose, and recommend OxyContin 45 mg by mouth every 12 hours with OxyIR 15 mg by mouth every 2 hours as needed for breakthrough pain. We can give the first dose of OxyContin about 3 hours before discontinuing the PCA opioid infusion.

CHAPTER 8

Calculating Doses from Oral Solutions and Suspensions

INTRODUCTION

Medications are available in a wide range of dosage formulations, suitable for various routes of administration (e.g., oral, rectal, parenteral, topical). Oral dosage forms may be solid (tablets or capsules), semisolid (troches, lozenges), or liquid (solutions, suspensions, or emulsions). This chapter is not about opioid *conversion* calculations specifically; rather it is to learn how to calculate an appropriate volume of an oral solution or suspension to give a specific prescribed dose. This may seem like a simple calculation, but done incorrectly, the results could be disastrous. Common liquid analgesics are shown in Appendix 8-A.

A **solution** is a homogeneous mixture (uniform in composition throughout) prepared by mixing two or more substances. The **solute** (the substance being added for dissolution, usually present in the smaller amount) may be a solid, liquid, or gas. The **solvent** (volume to which the solute is added) is a liquid, hence the reference to **oral solution.** Because one substance is completely dissolved in another, there is generally no need to shake the oral solution prior to administration, as there is with a **suspension.** A suspension is a mixture in which solid particles are suspended in a fluid. The particles are prone to settle on standing; therefore, the mixture must be shaken prior to administration.

Oral solutions *are used to treat patients with advanced illnesses for several reasons, including the following:*

- The dose of medication may be individualized to a greater degree than that allowed by dividing tablets or taking multiple tablets or capsules. This is especially important in managing small dose increments in upward or downward titration.

- The administration of certain medications at higher dosages would not be feasible due to pill burden (e.g., taking 18 tablets at a time).

- Most commonly, patients with advanced illnesses are often unable to swallow solid oral dosage formulations or may have a feeding tube in place. Also, some patients of all ages have an aversion or inability to swallow pills or capsules.

OBJECTIVES

After reading this chapter and completing all practice problems, the participant will be able to:

1. Define what is meant by a medication solution or suspension.

2. Explain why these dosage formulations are used in caring for patients with advanced illnesses, and how they should be administered.

3. Calculate the appropriate volume of a medication solution or suspension to administer a specific prescribed dose.

4. Verify the calculated volume of an oral solution or suspension intended to deliver a specific prescribed dose.

- Opioids and other medications may be administered as a concentrated oral solution in the sublingual or buccal cavity when the oral route is not available (e.g., bowel obstruction, difficulty swallowing, nausea or vomiting, reduced level of consciousness), or when parenteral or rectal routes of opioid administration are not desired or feasible.

Oral solutions may be administered by mouth to be swallowed or administered via a feeding tube. They may be administered by the **sublingual** (under the tongue) route or into the **buccal** cavity (cheek of the mouth) if the oral solution is sufficiently concentrated. Hikma makes a line of highly, or intensely, concentrated oral solutions (referred to as concentrates or Intensols) of medication that are dispensed with a calibrated dropper. Examples include alprazolam 1 mg/mL, dexamethasone 1 mg/mL, diazepam 5 mg/mL, lorazepam 2 mg/mL, methadone 10 mg/mL, morphine 20 mg/mL, oxycodone 20 mg/mL, and prednisone 5 mg/mL. Other pharmaceutical manufacturers offer some of these products in the same concentrations.

Some oral solutions are simply referred to as *liquids* while others are called *elixirs*, *concentrates*, *syrups*, or *drops*. Elixirs historically referred to oral solutions that contained alcohol and syrups used to contain sugar. Today, the terms do not hold these meanings. *Drops* generally refer to an oral solution in a dropper bottle and *concentrates* are concentrated solutions as discussed in the preceding paragraph.

PRINCIPLES

So, how do you go about calculating the appropriate volume of an oral solution to give a specific prescribed dose? Look at the following equation. On the left is the concentration of the oral solution in milligrams per milliliters. On the right is the desired dose in the numerator, and the unknown variable (X), the appropriate volume, in the denominator.

$$\frac{\text{concentration of oral solution in } \textbf{milligrams}}{\text{per } \textit{milliliters}} = \frac{\text{desired dose of medication in } \textbf{milligrams}}{\text{unknown (X) volume of medication in } \textit{milliliters}}$$

Note in the above equation that **milligrams** are in the numerator on both sides of the equation, and *milliliters* are in the denominator on both sides of the equation.

To determine the appropriate volume of medication to administer, cross-multiply and solve for the unknown (X), as shown in the following example.

CASE EXAMPLES

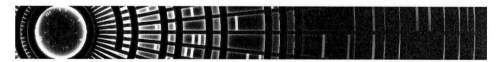

CASE 8.1

Calculating the Volume of an Oral Solution

Patient is an 82-year-old man with esophageal cancer. He had been receiving morphine extended-release tablets 15 mg by mouth every 12 hours with good pain control. His cancer has progressed, and now he struggles to swallow the morphine tablets. His prescriber would like to discontinue the morphine extended-release tablets and instead switch to morphine 5 mg by mouth every 4 hours around the clock using a 10 mg/5 mL morphine oral solution. *What volume should you administer?*

Set up your ratio as described above.

$$\frac{10 \text{ mg}}{5 \text{ mL}} = \frac{5 \text{ mg}}{\text{"X" mL}}$$

Cross-multiply:

$$10 \text{ mg} \times X \text{ mL} = 5 \text{ mg} \times 5 \text{ mL}$$

Solve for X by dividing both sides of the equation by 10 mg and canceling units that appear in both the numerator and denominator, as follows:

$$\frac{10 \text{ mg} \times X}{10 \text{ mg}} = \frac{5 \text{ mg} \times 5 \text{ mL}}{10 \text{ mg}}$$

$$\frac{\cancel{10 \text{ mg}} \times X}{\cancel{10 \text{ mg}}} = \frac{5 \cancel{\text{ mg}} \times 5 \text{ mL}}{10 \cancel{\text{ mg}}}$$

$$X = \frac{25 \text{ mL}}{10}$$

$$X = 2.5 \text{ mL}$$

You would administer 2.5 mL of the 10 mg/5 mL oral morphine solution to the patient every 4 hours.

How can you check your math? First, *think* about it. You are giving 5 mg from a 10 mg/5 mL solution. Five milligrams is one-half of the 10 mg in the numerator, so the volume should be ½ the 5 mL in the denominator. So, this passes the "it makes sense" test. As a check, however, you know that multiplication is the reverse of division, so multiply the volume you plan to administer by the oral solution concentration to make sure you end up with the intended dose, as follows:

$$2.5 \text{ mL} \times \frac{10 \text{ mg}}{5 \text{ mL}}$$

Solve by canceling units that appear in both the numerator and denominator as follows:

$$2.5 \cancel{\text{ mL}} \times \frac{10 \text{ mg}}{5 \cancel{\text{ mL}}} = \frac{2.5 \times 10 \text{ mg}}{5} = \frac{25 \text{ mg}}{5} = 5 \text{ mg}$$

This leaves an answer of 5 mg, the correct, intended dose.

Accurately Measuring a Dose of an Oral Solution

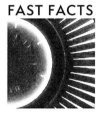

FAST FACTS What's the best way to accurately measure a dose of a medication in an oral solution? Many people associate a "teaspoonful" with a volume of 5 mL, and a "tablespoonful" with 15 mL. However, the household teaspoon is insufficiently accurate to reliably deliver 5 mL, just as a household tablespoon is unreliable for administering 15 mL when dosing accuracy is important. Alternate methods include the use of medicine cups, dosing spoons, droppers, and *oral* syringes. According to the U.S. Pharmacopeia's (USP) standards, an appropriate measuring device should deliver a dose with no more than a ±10% dosing error. Calibrated droppers and *oral* syringes are the best bet for minimizing dosing errors.

This calculation works the same way when administering a dose of a combination analgesic oral solution. For example, Roxicet is available as an oral solution, containing 5-mg oxycodone plus 325-mg acetaminophen per 5 mL. Generally, the calculation is based on the opioid component, not the nonopioid component. Therefore, in this case, the oxycodone dose is generally the more important component of the calculation. However, it is important to remember that patients with normal renal and hepatic function should not receive in excess of 4 grams of acetaminophen per day (less than 4 grams per day in patients with organ dysfunction, malnourished patients, or patients with a history of alcoholism). Let's look at an example.

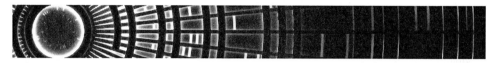

CASE 8.2
••
Calculating the Volume of a Combination Drug Solution

LS is a 62-year-old woman with end-stage breast cancer. She has intermittent fevers and abdominal pain. She has grown too weak to swallow her Percocet tablets (7.5-mg oxycodone/325-mg acetaminophen per tablet), so her prescriber would like to switch her to the oral solution. Generally, LS takes one tablet every 4 hours; knowing that Roxicet is available as a 5-mg oxycodone plus 325-mg acetaminophen per 5-mL solution, what would be an equivalent volume of Roxicet oral solution?

The more important component of LS's analgesic regimen is the oxycodone. If LS is taking 7.5-mg oxycodone every 4 hours, how much of the Roxicet oral solution should be administered?

Set up your ratio as described above, focusing on the opioid component of the solution.

$$\frac{5 \text{ mg oxycodone}}{5 \text{ mL Roxicet soln}} = \frac{7.5 \text{ mg oxycodone}}{\text{"X" mL Roxicet soln}}$$

Cross-multiply:

$$5 \text{ mg} \times X \text{ mL} = 7.5 \text{ mg} \times 5 \text{ mL}$$

Solve for X by dividing both sides of the equation by 5 mg and canceling units that appear in both the numerator and denominator, as follows:

$$\frac{\cancel{5 \text{ mg}} \times X}{\cancel{5 \text{ mg}}} = \frac{7.5 \cancel{\text{ mg}} \times 5 \text{ mL}}{5 \cancel{\text{ mg}}}$$

$$X = \frac{37.5 \text{ mL}}{5}$$

$$X = 7.5 \text{ mL}$$

You would administer 7.5 mL of the Roxicet solution (5-mg oxycodone and 325-mg acetaminophen per 5 mL).

However, you still have two tasks to perform before administering this dose.

First, check your math. Multiply the volume you intend to administer by the oral solution concentration, to make sure you end up with the correct oxycodone dose, as follows:

$$7.5 \text{ mL} \times \frac{5 \text{ mg}}{5 \text{ mL}}$$

Solve by canceling units that appear in both the numerator and denominator as follows:

$$7.5 \text{ mL} \times \frac{5 \text{ mg}}{5 \text{ mL}} = \frac{7.5 \times 5 \text{ mg}}{5} = \frac{37.5 \text{ mg}}{5} = 7.5 \text{ mg}$$

This leaves an answer of 7.5 mg, the correct prescribed dose.

But you're not done! Remember what we said about keeping an eye on the total daily acetaminophen dose. When you administer 7.5 mL of Roxicet solution, six times daily, what is the patient's total daily dose of acetaminophen, and is it less than 4 grams?

Let's check it out, as follows:

$$7.5 \text{ mL} \times \frac{325 \text{ mg acetaminophen}}{5 \text{ mL}}$$

Solve by canceling units that appear in both the numerator and denominator as follows:

$$7.5 \text{ mL} \times \frac{325 \text{ mg acetaminophen}}{5 \text{ mL}} = 2{,}437.5 \text{ mg}/5 = 487.5 \text{ mg acetaminophen per dose}$$

If you're administering 487.5-mg acetaminophen per dose, and the patient receives six doses per day, this is a total daily acetaminophen dose of 2,925 mg, which is safely below 4 g per day. Remember that a lower total daily dose of acetaminophen may be appropriate for some patients.

As discussed earlier in this chapter, practitioners frequently use concentrated oral solutions to administer opioids to patients with advanced illnesses who have difficulty swallowing, or other reasons why swallowing the solution is not possible. In this situation, the best option may be to instill the drug in the buccal or sublingual cavity. Although it was hoped that administering an opioid such as morphine or oxycodone by the sublingual or buccal route of administration would show a faster onset of action (as is seen with other medications such as nitroglycerin), this has not been seen. This is probably because morphine, oxycodone, and hydromorphone are more water soluble, which does not favor true oral transmucosal absorption. Highly lipid-soluble opioids, such as methadone, fentanyl, and buprenorphine, are better absorbed (e.g., oral transmucosal fentanyl products are commercially available).

Having said all that, when morphine or oxycodone are administered in the sublingual or buccal cavity, the clinical effect is approximately equal to oral or rectal administration of the same dose. Most practitioners are comfortable administering up to 1 mL in the sublingual or buccal cavity with a few caveats. If the patient has copious oral secretions, the opioid may be washed away in the tide and have little hope for absorption. Patients with diminished consciousness may be given oral concentrated solutions in the sublingual or buccal cavity, but it would be prudent to prop the patient's upper body up about 30 degrees and administer no more than 1 mL at a time. Probably only a small portion of the dose is absorbed transmucosally; the majority of the oral solution trickles down the throat and is swallowed. The dose can be repeated when the initially administered volume has dissipated if necessary.

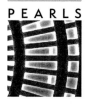 **P E A R L S** **Administering Oral Concentrated Solutions**

For patients with an impaired level of consciousness, it is important to prop the upper body up a bit (approximately a 30-degree elevation) to minimize the risk of aspiration before administering up to 1 mL of concentrated oral solution in the buccal cavity. And remember, higher volumes (> 1 mL), and all suspensions should be administered only to patients who can swallow, or be administered via feeding tube if the patient has one in place; otherwise a different formulation and route must be chosen.

Calculating the volume of oral concentrated opioid solution to be administered transmucosally is the same process as we've been discussing throughout this chapter. ***Consider the example in Case 8.3.***

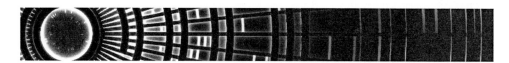

C A S E 8 . 3
•••
Calculating the Volume of a Concentrated Oral Solution

GW is a 92-year-old man with end-stage dementia. He was receiving oxycodone extended-release tablets, 15 mg every 12 hours, for generalized discomfort. He has become confused and intermittently somnolent, and is not reliably swallowing the oxycodone tablets. His provider wants to switch him to oxycodone oral solution, 5 mg every 4 hours, instilled in the buccal cavity. Using the commercially available oxycodone 20 mg/mL oral solution, what volume should you administer?

Set up your ratio as described earlier in this chapter:

$$\frac{20\ mg}{1\ mL} = \frac{5\ mg}{X\ mL}$$

Cross-multiply:

$20\ mg \times X\ mL = 5\ mg \times 1\ mL$

Solve for X by dividing both sides of the equation by 20 mg and canceling units that appear in both the numerator and denominator, as follows:

$$\frac{\cancel{20\ mg} \times X}{\cancel{20\ mg}} = \frac{5\ \cancel{mg} \times 1\ mL}{20\ \cancel{mg}}$$

$X = 5\ mL/20$

$X = 0.25\ mL$

You would administer 0.25 mL of oral oxycodone 20-mg/mL solution. You can accomplish this with an oral syringe or a calibrated dropper. Most oral concentrated solutions come with a calibrated dropper, and this would be the preferred medication administration tool.

Check your math. First, use the "does this make sense" approach. You're trying to administer 5 mg from a 20-mg/mL solution. Five milligrams is ¼ of 20 mg, so the appropriate volume should be ¼ of a mL, or 0.25 mL. *But don't rely on this method!* Do the second step to make *sure* you are on firm ground. You really don't want to make a mistake with an oral concentrated opioid solution, so sharpen that pencil my friend!

$$0.25\ mL \times \frac{20\ mg}{1\ mL} = dose$$

Solve by canceling units that appear in both the numerator and denominator as follows:

$$0.25\ \cancel{mL} \times \frac{20\ mg}{1\ \cancel{mL}} = 0.25 \times 20\ mg = 5\ mg$$

This leaves an answer of 5 mg, the correct prescribed dose. If GW is obtunded, be sure to prop him up a bit, and gently place the 0.25 mL of 20-mg/mL oral oxycodone solution in the buccal cavity. After approximately 30 minutes, check to make sure the volume has dissipated, and you can return GW to a more supine position if desired.

PITFALLS "Intensol" is NOT a Drug Name!

Roxane Pharmaceuticals manufactures several drug products as **Intensols** (see text). However, use of the term *Intensol* may lead to medication errors. One error reported to the USP Medication Error Reporting (MER) Program was an incident where a nursing supervisor didn't realize that the term *Intensol* could refer to several different medications, and the after-hours order for dexamethasone Intensol was inadvertently filled with chlorpromazine Intensol. The term *Intensol* refers to Roxane Pharmaceutical's "system of concentrated solutions of drugs with calibrated dropper." Be sure you have the right *drug. Always double check the actual drug name on the medication label.*

Source: Multiple drugs including "Intensol" in names cause confusion. Nurses.com Website. http://www.nurses.com/doc/multiple-drugs-including-intensol-in-names-ca-0001. Accessed August 26, 2017.

What do you do when you need to give an opioid dose that requires administration of more than 1 mL of oral solution in the buccal or sublingual cavity? You have a couple of options. First, you could administer a smaller volume more often (e.g., 1 mL every 2 hours, in lieu of 2 mL every 4 hours), but this becomes a labor-intensive regimen, frequently unsuitable for family caregivers. Second, you could talk to your friendly neighborhood pharmacist who may be able to compound a more highly concentrated oral solution (e.g., morphine 50 mg/mL). Pharmacists who are able to draw on an evidence base of knowledge and prepare extemporaneous products to facilitate medication administration in patients with advanced illnesses are worth their weight in gold! Of course, this excludes this author (too much like cooking!).

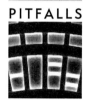

PITFALLS Writing the Right Prescription with Oral Solutions!

Oral solutions and suspensions should be prescribed using mg, not mL. In the past, pharmaceutical manufacturers have been mandated by the Food and Drug Administration (FDA) to advise prescribers how to correctly write a prescription for a highly concentrated oral solution to minimize medication errors. The correct way to write an order or prescription for an oral solution, most especially a highly concentrated solution, is as follows:

Oral morphine concentrate 20 mg/mL

Sig: 15 mg (0.75 mL) by mouth every 4 hours as needed for pain

Dispense: 30 mL

Frequently we administer co-analgesics in hospice and palliative care that are *suspensions*. A *suspension* is a liquid formulation of a medication where the drug itself is "suspended" in the liquid phase. Examples include phenytoin suspension and naproxen suspension. Suspensions must be shaken prior to administration to ensure the medication is equally distributed in the preparation, and each dose is consistent. The calculations are exactly as you've been doing throughout this chapter. Just for kicks, let's do one more example, shall we?

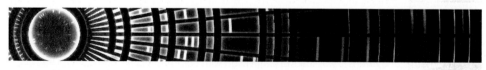

CASE 8.4

Calculating the Volume of an Oral Suspension

DS is a 72-year-old woman with breast cancer that has spread to the bone. She has become debilitated, and struggles to swallow her Aleve tablet (220 mg naproxen sodium). Her prescriber would like to switch her to naproxen suspension, which is available in a concentration of 125 mg per 5 mL. The prescribed regimen is 250 mg by mouth (po) every 12 hours. *How much volume should you administer?*

Set up your ratio as described previously.

$$\frac{125 \text{ mg}}{5 \text{ mL}} = \frac{250 \text{ mg}}{X \text{ mL}}$$

Cross-multiply:

$$125 \text{ mg} \times X \text{ mL} = 250 \text{ mg} \times 5 \text{ mL}$$

Solve for X by dividing both sides of the equation by 125 mg and canceling units that appear in both the numerator and denominator, as follows:

$$\frac{\cancel{125 \text{ mg}} \times X}{\cancel{125 \text{ mg}}} = \frac{250 \cancel{\text{ mg}} \times 5 \text{ mL}}{125 \cancel{\text{ mg}}}$$

$$X = \frac{1,250 \text{ mL}}{125} = 10 \text{ mL}$$

You would administer 10 mL of the 125-mg/5 mL naproxen suspension. Obviously, the patient would need to be able to *swallow* this volume; this could *not* be administered in the buccal or sublingual cavity.

Before you tell the patient "bottoms up," let's check that math. First, think it through. If 5 mL of the naproxen suspension gives you 125 mg, then double that volume would give you double the dose, or 250 mg. So, your mental math works out. No offense, but let's put pencil to paper just to make sure you're firing on all burners!

$$10 \text{ mL} \times \frac{125 \text{ mg}}{5 \text{ mL}}$$

Solve by canceling units that appear in both the numerator and denominator as follows:

$$10 \cancel{\text{ mL}} \times \frac{125 \text{ mg}}{5 \cancel{\text{ mL}}} = 10 \times \frac{125 \text{ mg}}{5} = \frac{1,250 \text{ mg}}{5} = 250 \text{ mg}$$

This leaves 250 mg, the prescribed dose. Go ahead and give DS 10 mL of the naproxen suspension; you'll both feel much better!

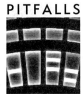

PITFALLS **Don't Mix Your Metaphors!**

In Chapter 6, you learned about methadone dosing, but it is important to recognize the benefits and risks associated with using a concentrated solution such as methadone. Methadone is the *only* opioid that is inherently long acting (dosed two or three times daily) and available as an oral solution (and even a concentrated oral solution). Palliative care providers frequently use methadone concentrated oral solution (10 mg/mL) for baseline pain control, with morphine or oxycodone 20 mg/mL concentrated oral solution for breakthrough pain. When prescribed in this way, these different oral solution concentrations can be confusing for patients and caregivers likely because different volumes of each will be required. Be very clear when providing instruction on how to use these products.

Could I Get That to Go, Please? Bottom Line It for Me . . .

▶ A *solution* is a homogeneous mixture (uniform in composition throughout) prepared by mixing two or more substances.

▶ To calculate the appropriate volume of an oral solution to give a specific prescribed dose, use the following equation:

$$\frac{\text{Concentration of oral solution in } \textbf{milligrams}}{\text{per } \textit{milliliters}} = \frac{\text{desired dose of medication in } \textbf{milligrams}}{\text{unknown (X) volume of medication in } \textit{milliliters}}$$

▶ Cross-multiply and solve for the unknown (X); check your answer by multiplying the volume you calculated by the solution concentration—your units should cancel and leave you with your intended dose with the correct units (e.g., milligrams).

▶ Make sure you use a calibrated measuring device (not a household teaspoon).

▶ You can administer an Intensol (highly concentrated oral solution) to a patient with an impaired level of consciousness. Prop the upper body up to a 30-degree elevation, and instill up to 1 mL in the buccal cavity.

▶ Calculating the volume of an oral suspension is done the same way. However, a suspension cannot be administered in the buccal or sublingual cavity; it must be swallowed.

▶ Be sure to carefully educate patients, families, and caregivers when *two* different concentration oral solutions are ordered. For example, morphine is available as a 20-mg/mL oral solution (which may be ordered for breakthrough pain), and methadone is available as a 10-mg/mL oral solution (which may be the scheduled, long-acting opioid). Be clear to be safe!

PRACTICE PROBLEMS

Here are a few practice problems for you to work on. The answers are shown at the end of the chapter. Be sure to check your math!

P8.1. Calculating the Volume of an Oral Solution

BJ is a 3-year-old boy with a sprained ankle (you *told* him not to ride his tricycle *down* the hill). The pediatrician has recommended acetaminophen 10 to 15 mg/kg every 4 hours. BJ weighs 35 pounds. The parents have selected an acetaminophen elixir that is 160 mg/5 mL. What volume do you recommend the parents administer per dose?

P8.2. Calculating the Volume of a Concentrated Oral Solution

PZ is a 62-year-old man with liver cancer. The hospice nurse would like to switch him to an oral solution because she anticipates he will not be able to swallow tablets for much longer. After consultation with the hospice medical director, they decide to switch from his previous dose of morphine sulfate extended-release tablets, 60 mg po every 12 hours, with morphine sulfate immediate-release tablets 15 mg (using about two per day) to methadone solution, 10 mg/mL. You have calculated a recommended methadone dose of 5 mg po every 8 hours (yes, that was magical—refer to Chapter 6 to see how I came up with that conversion!). What volume of methadone 10-mg/mL solution should the nurse instruct the family to administer?

P8.3. Calculating the Volume of a Co-analgesic Oral Solution

HG is a 54-year-old woman with end-stage HIV. She is complaining of very painful burning in her legs and feet, which you determine to be neuropathic pain. You would like to start nortriptyline therapy, starting with 25 mg po at bedtime, then increasing to 50 mg on day 3, and again to 75 mg on day 6. Unfortunately, HG has significant esophagitis, and she finds it very difficult to swallow tablets. Fortunately, you knew that, and that's why you selected nortriptyline because you know it is available as an oral solution, 10 mg/5 mL. What volume should you administer for the 25-mg dose? The 50-mg dose? The 75-mg dose? You should have this down pat after all that math!

P8.4. Calculating the Volume of an Oral Solution

PA is an 82-year-old woman with end-stage dementia and several large sacral pressure ulcers. She becomes quite agitated with wound care, and you decide it would be a quality idea to premedicate her with oral morphine solution. She has a feeding tube in place. The prescriber gives you an order for morphine 2.5 mg 30 minutes before wound care, administered via feeding tube. Your pharmacy carries morphine solution in the 20 mg/5 mL strength. What volume of oral morphine solution should you administer prior to PA's wound care? By the way, nice pick-up on using a preemptive opioid in this situation. PA is much appreciative!

RECOMMENDED READING

American Academy of Pediatrics Committee on Drugs. Alternative routes of drug administration: advantages and disadvantages (subject review). *Pediatrics.* 1997;100:143-152.

Coluzzi PH. Sublingual morphine: efficacy reviewed. *J Pain Symptom Manage.* 1998;16:184-192.

Gilbar PJ. A guide to enteral drug administration in palliative care. *J Pain Symptom Manage.* 1999;17:197-207.

Kestenbaum MG, Vilches AO, Messersmith S, et al. Alternative routes to oral opioid administration in palliative care: a review and clinical summary. *Pain Med.* 2014;15:1129-1153.

Leppert W, Krajnik M, Wordliczek J. Delivery systems of opioid analgesics for pain relief: a review. *Curr Pharm Des.* 2013;19(41):7271-7293.

Lugo RA, Kern SE. Clinical pharmacokinetics of morphine. *J Pain Palliat Care Pharmacother.* 2002;16:5-18.

Reisfield GM, Wilson GR. Rational use of sublingual opioids in palliative medicine. *J Palliat Med.* 2007;10:465-475.

SOLUTIONS TO PRACTICE PROBLEMS

P8.1: BJ weighs 35 pounds, and you must first convert this to kilograms because the acetaminophen is dosed by weight in kilograms. There are approximately 2.2 pounds per kilogram; or to be precise, there are 2.20462262 pounds per kilogram for you purists out there!

$$35 \text{ pounds} \times \frac{\text{kilogram}}{2.2 \text{ pounds}} = 15.9 \text{ kilograms}$$

Let's go with the 10 mg/kg dose; he weighs 15.9 kilograms, so we must next figure out the dose:

$$\frac{10 \text{ mg}}{\text{kg}} \times 15.9 \text{ kilograms} = 159 \text{ mg (let's be bold and round the dose to 160 mg) kilogram}$$

Using the 160 mg/5 solution we must now determine how much volume to advise the parents administer to little Evel Knievel.

Well this is pretty straightforward – it would be 5 mL!

You would instruct the parents to administer 5 mL of the 160-mg/5 mL oral acetaminophen solution, using a calibrated measuring device.

Check your work before you turn them loose! First, does this make sense? If 160 mg are delivered in 5 mL, and we advise the parents to administer 5 mL, it should equal 160 mg.

$$5 \text{ mL} \times \frac{160 \text{ mg}}{5 \text{ mL}}$$

Solve by canceling units that appear in both the numerator and denominator, and solve for mg dose:

$$5 \text{ mL} \times \frac{160 \text{ mg}}{5 \text{ mL}} = 160 \text{ mg}$$

This leaves an answer of 160 mg, the correct, intended dose. And be sure to give little BJ a stern talking to about listening to his parents! And don't forget the helmet!

P8.2: You need to determine how much methadone oral solution to give a patient for a 5-mg dose, using the 10-mg/mL solution.

Set up your ratio:

$$\frac{10 \text{ mg}}{\text{mL}} = \frac{5 \text{ mg}}{X \text{ mL}}$$

Cross-multiply:

$$10 \text{ mg} \times X = 5 \text{ mg} \times 1 \text{ mL}$$

Solve for X by dividing both sides of the equation by 10 mg and canceling units that appear in both the numerator and denominator, as follows:

$$\frac{10 \text{ mg} \times X}{10 \text{ mg}} = \frac{5 \text{ mg} \times 1 \text{ mL}}{10 \text{ mg}}$$

$$X = 5 \text{ mL}/10$$

$$X = 0.5 \text{ mL}$$

So, as Dr. Phil would say, "How's that working for ya?" If the methadone is 10 mg per milliliter, and you want to administer 5 mg, it would be *half* that, or 0.5 mL.

Check your math:

$$0.5 \text{ mL} \times \frac{10 \text{ mg}}{\text{mL}} = 5 \text{ mg}$$

This is the correct, intended dose. Don't forget: If PZ is becoming too weak to swallow tablets, keep a sharp eye out for when he has difficulty swallowing oral solutions as well. You can still use the methadone 10-mg/mL oral solution, but you will need to instill it in the buccal cavity, and make sure he is propped up about 30 degrees to minimize aspiration.

P8.3: We need to determine how much of the 10-mg/5 mL nortriptyline oral solution to administer to give a 25-, 50- and 75-mg dose. Let's do the 25-mg dose first:

$$\frac{10\ mg}{5\ mL} = \frac{25\ mg}{X\ mL}$$

Cross-multiply:

$10\ mg \times X = 25\ mg \times 5\ mL$

Divide both sides of the equation by 10 mg to solve for X:

$$\frac{\cancel{10\ mg} \times X}{\cancel{10\ mg}} = \frac{25\ \cancel{mg} \times 5\ mL}{10\ \cancel{mg}}$$

$X = 125\ mL/10$

$X = 12.5\ mL$

This makes sense. If every 5 mL gives you 10 mg, and you want two and a half times the 10 mg, you need two and a half times the 5 mL, or 12.5 mL.

Checking your math also shows you are correct!

$12.5\ \cancel{mL} \times \dfrac{10\ mg}{5\ \cancel{mL}} = 125\ mg/5 = 25\ mg$

If you use this same process, you will find that the 50-mg dose requires 25 mL of the 10-mg/5 mL solution be administered, and the 75-mg dose requires 37.5 mL. Obviously, for all *three* of the doses and volumes you calculated, you would have to make sure HG could *swallow* the oral solution; the volume is too high for buccal administration.

P8.4: You want to administer 2.5 mg of morphine prior to wound care for PA using a 20-mg/5 mL oral morphine solution.

$$\frac{20\ mg}{5\ mL} = \frac{2.5\ mg}{X\ mL}$$

Cross-multiply:

$20\ mg \times X = 2.5\ mg \times 5\ mL$

Solve for X:

$$\frac{\cancel{20\ mg} \times X}{\cancel{20\ mg}} = \frac{2.5\ \cancel{mg} \times 5\ mL}{20\ \cancel{mg}}$$

$X = 12.5\ mL/20 = 0.625\ mL$

Does this make sense? If 20 mg is in 5 mL, that's 4 mg per mL. We want to give a little more than half of 4 mg (2.5 mg); therefore our volume should be a little more than half of 1 mL, which it is (0.625 mL). Unfortunately, this is a tough dose to give *exactly*. You actually might want to talk to the prescriber about reducing the dose to 2 mg, which would be precisely 0.5 mL, and much easier to accurately measure.

APPENDIX 8-A

Selected Oral Solution and Suspension Nonopioid, Opioids, and Co-analgesics

Nonopioid Analgesics

Medication	Dosage Formulations
Acetaminophen (Tylenol, various)	**Solution/liquid:** 160 mg/5 mL, 325 mg/5 mL, 325 mg/10.15 mL, 500 mg/15 mL, 650 mg/20.3 mL
	Suspension: 80 mg/0.8 mL, 160 mg/5 mL, 325 mg/10.15 mL, 650 mg/20.3 mL
	Elixir: 160 mg/5 mL
	Syrup: 160 mg/5 mL
Diclofenac potassium (Cambia)	**Powder for oral solution:** 50 mg
Ibuprofen (Motrin, Advil, various)	**Oral suspension:** 40 mg/mL, 50 mg/1.25 mL, 100 mg/5 mL
Indomethacin (various)	**Oral suspension:** 25 mg/5 mL
Naproxen (Naprosyn, various)	**Oral suspension:** 125 mg/5 mL

Opioid Analgesics

Medication	Dosage Formulations
Hydromorphone (various)	**Oral solution:** 1 mg/mL
Methadone	**Oral solution:** 5 mg/5 mL, 10 mg/5 mL
	Oral concentrate: 10 mg/mL
Morphine (various)	**Oral solution:** 10 mg/5 mL, 20 mg/5 mL
	Oral concentrate: 100 mg/5 mL
Oxycodone (various)	**Oral solution:** 5 mg/5 mL
	Oral concentrate: 100 mg/5 mL

Selected Combination Opioid Analgesics

Medication	Dosage Formulations
Codeine with acetaminophen (various)	**Oral suspension, solution:** 12-mg codeine plus 120-mg acetaminophen/5 mL
Hydrocodone with acetaminophen (various)	**Oral solution:** 7.5-mg hydrocodone plus 325-mg acetaminophen/15 mL; 10-mg hydrocodone plus 300-mg acetaminophen/15 mL; 10-mg hydrocodone plus 325-mg acetaminophen/15 mL
Oxycodone with acetaminophen	**Oral solution:** 5-mg oxycodone plus 325-mg acetaminophen/5 mL

Selected Co-analgesics

Medication	Dosage Formulations
Carbamazepine (Tegretol, various)	**Oral suspension:** 100 mg/5 mL
Dexamethasone (various)	**Oral solution/elixir:** 0.5 mg/5 mL
	Oral concentrate: 1 mg/mL
Gabapentin (Neurontin)	**Oral solution:** 250 mg/5 mL
Pregabalin (Lyrica)	**Oral solution:** 20 mg/mL
Levetiracetam (Keppra)	**Oral solution:** 100 mg/mL
Nortriptyline (various)	**Oral solution:** 10 mg/5 mL
Phenytoin (various)	**Oral suspension:** 125 mg/5 mL
Valproic acid (various)	**Oral syrup:** 250 mg/5 mL

CHAPTER 9

Lagniappe: A Little Something Extra in Conversion Calculations

INTRODUCTION

What a crazy ride it's been through eight chapters—switching from one route of administration or dosage formulation using the same opioid, converting between opioids regardless of route or pharmaceutical formulation, dosage titrations, solution calculations, and more. What could possibly be left to talk about? Well, there's always room for dessert! So, what the heck is *Lagniappe* (pronounced *lan-yap*)? Of Louisiana French origin, it means "something given as a bonus or gratuity."[1] Okay, it's not a beignet, but it IS a bonus chapter!

OBJECTIVES

After reading this chapter and completing all practice problems, the participant will be able to:

1. Describe the relative potency of the fentanyl derivatives (alfentanil, sufentanil, and remifentanil), levorphanol, and nalbuphine to more traditional opioids.

2. Given a scenario that results from an opioid conversion miscalculation, analyze the situation and suggest an alternate strategy to improve therapeutic outcomes.

There are two important happenings in this chapter:

1. A review of the lesser-used opioids (the fentanyl cousins [alfentanil, remifentanil, and sufentanil], nalbuphine, and levorphanol)

2. A baker's dozen of the most common mistakes made in opioid conversion calculations (present company excepted)

Those of you who bought this book for staff development purposes can use the mistake examples to stump YOUR chumps!

ISLAND OF ORPHAN OPIOIDS

The Fentanyl Backup Singers—Alfentanil, Sufentanil, and Remifentanil

Fentanyl, alfentanil, sufentanil, and remifentanil are synthetic mu-opioid agonists that are 4-anilidopiperidine derivatives.[2] These agents are widely used as primary anesthetic agents, or more commonly as sedatives and to supplement general anesthesia, as well as several other special situations (e.g., electroconvulsive therapy, carotid endarterectomy, craniotomy).[3] In addition to intravenous (IV) delivery, the fentanyl(s) have been given by other routes including epidural, intrathecal, transdermal, and transmucosal.

Pharmacokinetics and pharmacodynamics

Fentanyl and sufentanil undergo phase I metabolism (oxidative N-dealkylation via cytochrome P450 [CYP3A4]). Sufentanil also undergoes O-demethylation and aromatic hydroxylation with sufentanil.[2] Alfentanil is primarily metabolized by the cytochrome P450 (CYP) system (CYP3A4 and CYP3A3), and remifentanil is rapidly metabolized by blood and tissue esterases, and to a minor degree, by N-dealkylation.[2] The pharmacological and physiochemical properties of fentanyl, sufentanil, alfentanil, and remifentanil are shown in Table 9-1.[4] Alfentanil has the shortest time to onset and peak effect,

Table 9-1
Overview of Pharmacological Properties of Fentanyl and Its Derivatives[8-19]

	Fentanyl[8,10-18]	Sufentanil[6,8,11-14,16-18]	Alfentanil[7,8,11-14,19]	Remifentanil[8,9,11-14,16-18]
Potency compared with morphine	100–300	800–1,000	40–50	100–200
IV induction dose (mcg/kg)	2–6	0.25–2.0	25–100	1–2
IV maintenance dose (mcg/kg)	0.5–2	2.5–10	5–10	0.1–1.0
IV infusion rate (mcg/kg/hr)	0.5–5	0.5–1.5	30–120	0.1–1.0
Other routes of administration than IV	Transdermal, transmucosal (buccal, nasal, sublingual), epidural	Epidural, sublingual		
Time to onset (min)	1.5	1	0.75	<1
Time to peak effect (min)	4.5–8	2.5–5	1.5	1.5
Duration of peak effect (min)	20–30	30	15	
Duration of analgesic effect (min)	60–120	100–150	30–60	5–10
Analgesic plasma concentration (ng/mL)	0.6–3.0	0.5–2.5	50–300	0.3–3
Plasma concentration associated with loss of consciousness (ng/mL)	>20.0	>2.5	>400	>4
$t_{1/2a}$ (min)	1.7 ± 0.1	1.4 ± 0.3	1.31 ± 0.48	1
$t_{1/2b}$ (min)	13.4 ± 1.6	17.7 ± 2.6	9.4 ± 2.7	6
$t_{1/2c}$ (min)	219 ± 10 (120–240)	164 ± 22 (120–180)	93.7 ± 8.3 (60–120)	10–20 (6–14)
Vd_C (L/kg)	0.36 ± 0.07	0.16 ± 0.02	0.12 ± 0.04	0.1
V_{dss} (L/kg)	4.0 ± 0.4 (3–5)	1.7 ± 0.2 (2.5–3.0)	1.0 ± 0.3 (0.4–1.0)	0.35 (0.2–0.4)
CL (mL/min/kg)	13 ± 2 (10–20)	12.7 ± 0.8 (10–15)	7.6 ± 2.4 (3–9)	40 (30–60)
Protein binding (%)	80–84	91–92.5	88.7–92.1	70
pKa	8.4	8.0	6.5	7.1
Non-ionized fraction at pH 7.40 (%)	8.5	20	89	67
Metabolism	CYP3A	CYP3A	CYP3A	Plasma and tissue esterases
Lipid solubility (octanol/water distribution coefficient)	813–816	1,727–1,778	128	18

Italic numbers indicate information from the Summary of Product Characteristics.

CL = clearance; CYP = cytochrome P450; IV = intravenous; $t_{1/2a}$ = distribution half-life; $t_{1/2b}$ = redistribution half-life; $t_{1/2c}$ = terminal elimination half-life; Vd_c = volume of distribution of the central compartment; V_{dss} = volume of distribution at steady state.

Source: Reprinted from Ziesenitz VC, Vaughns JD, Koch G, et al. Pharmacokinetics of fentanyl and its derivatives in children: a comprehensive review. *Clin Pharmacokinet.* 2018;57:393-417; Copyright ©2018. Used with permission from Springer/Nature.

and sufentanil has the longest duration of peak and analgesic effect. It is important to recognize that many factors affect the pharmacokinetics of the fentanyls such as age, body mass, plasma protein content, acid-base status, presence of liver or renal disease, and the use of cardiopulmonary bypass.[5]

Comparative potency/equianalgesic dosing

There are no data to provide definitive equianalgesic dosing among fentanyl and its derivatives. Hall and Hardy's data summarize the potency of fentanyl and derivatives based on the rat tail flick test and dog intubation (Table 9-2).[2]

Data from the animal models are consistent with Ziesenitz and colleague's data,[4] as follows:

- Alfentanil is 40 to 50 times more potent than morphine (and approximately one-fifth as potent as fentanyl).

- Sufentanil is substantially more potent than fentanyl (5- to 10-fold more potent).

- Ziesenitz proposes remifentanil is approximately equipotent to fentanyl.

Despite these data, it is insufficient to calculate conversion doses between fentanyl and derivatives. This is not a common clinical scenario; however, if the occasion arises and you have to perform this calculation, it is recommended to use the most conservative conversion possible and titrate to effect. Or better, use the recommended starting dose and titrate the dose as needed.

A Blast from the Past—Levorphanol!

Often referred to as "the forgotten opioid," levorphanol is another option for the treatment of severe pain. Pharmacologically, levorphanol has many similarities to methadone such as a strong affinity for the mu- (delta, kappa 1, and kappa 3) opioid receptor, it's an NMDA (N-methyl-D-aspartate) receptor antagonist, and it blocks the reuptake of serotonin and norepinephrine.[20] Pasternak and colleagues carefully evaluated the pharmacologic similarities and differences between morphine and levorphanol on a range of various opioid receptors.[21] Their evaluation disclosed subtle differences between morphine and levorphanol, which account for incomplete cross-tolerance of levorphanol with morphine and oxycodone, and diminished respiratory depressant activity. Given these multiple mechanisms, levorphanol may be an attractive option for neuropathic or difficult-to-treat pain syndromes.

For opioid-naïve patients, dosing should be initiated at 1 to 2 mg every 6, 8 (most common), or 12 hours. It may be increased to 3 mg every 6 to 8 hours.[22] Dosage increases should not occur before 72 hours (half-life is 11 to 16 hours), although weekly titration is preferable.[23]

Table 9-2
Potency Ratio of Fentanyl and Derivatives

	Morphine	Fentanyl	Alfentanil	Sufentanil	Remifentanil
Rat tail flick test[2]	1	292	73	4,521	
Dog intubation[2]	1	125	30	625	
Ziesenitz[4]	1	100–300	40–50	800–1,000	100–200

So, the $64,000 question is how to switch to levorphanol? Levorphanol is considered to be four to eight times more potent than morphine and has a longer half-life. Due to incomplete cross-tolerance, the package insert recommends when converting from another opioid to levorphanol, a further 33% dose reduction be implemented (e.g., 1/12 to 1/15 or less that of the total daily dose [TDD] of oral morphine).[24,25] McNulty reported on a series of 31 patients in a palliative care practice who were treated with levorphanol.[25] They reported their suggested morphine:levorphanol conversions as follows: the conversion from the oral morphine equivalent (OME) to levorphanol ranges from 12:1 to 25:1 (<100 mg OME → 12:1 [morphine:levorphanol]; 100 to 299 mg OME → 15:1; 300 to 599 mg OME → 20:1; 600 to 799 mg OME → 25:1; > 801 mg OME → no data).

Others have suggested using the most conservative estimates published (such as those above) and further reducing the starting dose by 25% to 50%.[23] Although it's nice to have an additional therapy option, this older-than-dirt opioid is quite expensive (Sentynl Therapeutics, approximately $5,000/month).

Nalbuphine

Nalbuphine is a semisynthetic phenanthrene mu receptor antagonist/kappa receptor agonist used to treat mild-to-moderate pain. It is structurally related to oxymorphone and the opioid antagonist naloxone. It is often lumped in with other agonist/antagonist opioids such as pentazocine, butorphanol, and buprenorphine; however, nalbuphine distinguishes itself as having greater antagonist activity and fewer behavioral effects at equivalent doses (e.g., the psychotomimetic effects seen with pentazocine).[26] Nalbuphine is a weak mu receptor antagonist, approximately 0.03 as potent as naloxone.[27] Nalbuphine is a neutral antagonist as compared to inverse mu receptor agonists (e.g., naloxone and naltrexone that cause an abstinence syndrome and withdrawal symptoms). Nalbuphine is much less likely to cause opioid withdrawal and may be used to reduce adverse effects from potent opioid agonists (e.g., pruritus) without causing withdrawal or reducing the analgesic effect.

Parenteral nalbuphine crosses the blood-brain barrier readily with onset of analgesia seen within 5 minutes. It undergoes extensive hepatic metabolism, and inactive metabolites are primarily excreted in the stool (approximately 7% of the unchanged drug and metabolites are eliminated renally).[28] The elimination half-life is approximately 3 hours (longer with oral administration, which is not available in the United States).[28]

Nalbuphine use is generally limited to acute pain or serving in an adjunctive role to reduce adverse effects from other opioids. There are few data available evaluating the role of nalbuphine in chronic pain. When given parenterally, nalbuphine has been either administered as a clinician bolus, by patient-controlled analgesia (PCA), and by intrathecal injection (including epidural) to manage labor and postoperative pain.[28]

Nalbuphine provides several benefits when compared to other opioids, including not causing biliary spasm or colic, urinary retention, hypotension, reduced cardiac output, prolonged QTc interval, and less likelihood of causing respiratory depression.[29] Zeng and colleagues compared nalbuphine with morphine in terms of analgesia and safety. The relative risk of adverse effects of nalbuphine as compared to morphine was as follows: nausea 0.78, vomiting 0.65, pruritus 0.17, and respiratory depression 0.27.[30]

In a meta-analysis of 820 patients, Zeng concluded that nalbuphine provides comparable analgesia to morphine.[30] A study comparing intramuscular (IM) nalbuphine with morphine in postoperative patients showed that nalbuphine was up to 0.9 times the potency of morphine, with a slightly longer duration of action.[31] Zacny and colleagues demonstrated that 10 mg of IV nalbuphine produced subjective, psychomotor, and physiologic effects similar to that of 10 mg of IV morphine.[32]

Dosing strategies for nalbuphine are as follows:[28-29]

- Adjunctive dosing to reverse opioid toxicity such as urinary retention, respiratory depression, and pruritus: 2.5 to 5 mg

- Intermittent IV dosing: 0.3 to 3 mg/kg IV over a 10- to 15-minute period with maintenance doses of 0.25 to 0.5 mg/kg in single IV injections

- Maximum single doses: 20 mg; maximum daily doses: 160 mg

- PCA dosing: 1 to 3 mg/hr with 1 mg patient demand bolus every 20 minutes as needed

If a patient is rotated from nalbuphine to morphine, higher than equianalgesic doses of morphine may be required due to the effect of nalbuphine as a mu receptor antagonist; however, this evidence is anecdotal.[28] As stated earlier, it is inadvisable to use nalbuphine for breakthrough pain, or to rotate from morphine to nalbuphine, as this may cause opioid withdrawal. Two reports of patients on chronic opioid therapy (methadone 10 mg twice daily, and morphine SR [slow release] 360 mg twice daily) who were given nalbuphine 10 mg IM experienced opioid withdrawal symptoms fairly quickly.[33]

Nalbuphine may be a preferred opioid in several clinical situations such as patients at increased risk for morphine-related adverse effects, patients in the intensive care unit, cardiac patients, and patients with renal failure.[28] Importantly, nalbuphine is a valuable therapeutic option when other parenteral opioids are in short supply (e.g., morphine, hydromorphone, and fentanyl).[29]

Next Generation (Third Edition?)

We have spent a LOT of time in this book talking about equianalgesic dosage calculations—how to switch from one opioid regimen to a different opioid regimen. *But, is this the whole story?* Interestingly, a whole body of literature has been emerging describing the "utility" of mu-opioid receptor agonists. Sheiner and Melmon describe the utility function (UF) of a medication as follows: $UF = benefit - harm$.[34] Henthorn and colleagues ask if the guidance recently issued by the Centers for Disease Control and Prevention (CDC) regarding the prescription of opioids to "prescribe the lowest effective dose . . . (and) incorporate into the management plan strategies to mitigate risk" might be best determined by defining the utility of an opioid.[35,36] Using pharmacokinetic and pharmacodynamic data, the utility factor can be determined for an opioid by assessing the probability of achieving a 25% increase (or 50% increase) in pain tolerance without significant respiratory depression versus plasma opioid concentration.[36] This might represent a new strategy for treating pain, by determining the probability of treating pain successfully while reducing risk of adverse outcomes. These data can then be compared with opioid regimens to determine equivalent, superior, or inferior utility.[37,38] For example, in this book, you learned that fentanyl and buprenorphine have similar potency, but respiratory depression is less likely to occur with buprenorphine. Nalbuphine and morphine are approximately equipotent, but nalbuphine is less likely to cause respiratory depression. Could the UF (aiming to maximize pain relief while minimizing risk) be the future of opioid selection and opioid switching? Well, keep your eyes peeled as we learn more about the opioid UF. We'll likely revisit this in the third edition of this book!

A BAKER'S DOZEN OF OPIOID CONVERSION CALCULATION MISTAKES

Before we even get to the calculation boo-boos, first we must get to the bottom of WHERE did the *baker's dozen* (referring to 13 items) *come from*? It's a legitimate question! Apparently, dishonest 13th-century bakers are to blame! In the 1260s, King Henry, III, grew sick and tired of British breadmakers making skimpy loaves of bread and short-sheeting customers. The King implemented a new law standardizing the weight of a loaf. Many bakers didn't own a scale; however, to meet the letter of the law (which was punishable by beatings or jail time), they gave 13 loaves to anyone buying a dozen. Hence, a "baker's dozen" refers to 13 objects.[39]

Let's explore this baker's dozen of commonly committed opioid conversion calculation mistakes!

Scenario 1

What's the sitch?

Mr. Harley is admitted to the hospital for spinal fusion surgery. Postoperatively, Dr. Sturgeon prescribed a morphine PCA pump, 1 mg IV every 10 minutes as needed, and a nurse-clinician bolus of morphine 2.5 mg IV every 10 minutes up to five doses. Ninety minutes later, the recovery room nurse contacts Dr. McLaughlin, the pharmacist on the pain team. "He's a big guy, and he's screaming in pain. Frankly, he's scaring me a little bit because he's being so demanding. I've given him four boluses of morphine 2.5 mg IV. Can you come take a look?" Dr. McLaughlin hustles right down to the recovery room to interview Mr. Harley. She finds that he is in a very aggressive mood and quite vocal about his out-of-control pain. Mr. Harley keeps asking, "When can I get my OxyContin?" Dr. McLaughlin asks what he means by that. "Oh, I've been taking OxyContin 80 mg three times a day for several years." Well, hello, apparently that's fresh information!

What's wrong with this picture?

Dr. McLaughlin realizes the problem—Dr. Sturgeon's PCA prescription for Mr. Harley was for an opioid-naïve patient, and Mr. Harley is no stranger to opioids! Mr. Harley's TDD of 240-mg oral oxycodone is approximately equivalent to 300-mg oral morphine per day, or 120-mg IV morphine per day (or 5 mg/hr continuous infusion IV morphine). Dr. Sturgeon should have increased the bolus dose and considered providing a continuous infusion to compensate partially for the oxycodone.

Play it again, Sam

Dr. McLaughlin recommends increasing the nurse-clinician bolus to 5 mg hourly and increasing the patient demand dose to 2-mg IV bolus every 10 minutes. Seven hours later, the patient is still quite vociferous about his opioid needs. Over the past 8.5 hours in total, Mr. Harley has received about 15 mg/hr of IV morphine. His pain control is better, but he (and the nurse) complain about frequent dosing. "How in the heck am I going to get any rest when I have to stay up and hit this darned button every 10 minutes all night long?" asks an exasperated Mr. Harley. Dr. McLaughlin recommends a continuous infusion of 5 mg/hr, keeping both the patient demand dose and nurse-clinician as-needed bolus in place. Hopefully, the surgical procedure itself will help reduce the pain, and the pain team can reduce the continuous infusion tomorrow. *To review these principles, refer to Chapter 7.*

Scenario 2

What's the sitch?

Mr. Krank is a 76-year-old irascible man admitted to hospice with end-stage colon cancer. His pain is fairly well controlled on Kadian 40 mg by mouth every 12 hours for the persistent pain, and his physician, Dr. Fletcher, prescribed morphine 5 mg by mouth every 8 hours as needed for additional pain. Mr. Krank tells his hospice nurse, Molly, that five or six times a day his abdominal pain "goes through the roof" (he rates it as greater than 10 [on a 0–10 scale; 0 = no pain, 10 – worst imaginable pain]), which he finds unbearable. In between these episodes, his pain is completely controlled. Mrs. Krank volunteers that it makes her life unbearable when Mr. Krank has these episodes of pain. Mr. Krank asks Molly, "Why can't you increase the Kadian?" Molly admits that's a fair question, so she contacts Dr. Fletcher with a request. "Is he taking the morphine 5 mg that's available to him every 8 hours?" asks Dr. Fletcher. "No," says Molly. "He says it doesn't do any darned good; he says it's too little too late. Can't we just increase the Kadian?" "Absolutely not," says Dr. Fletcher. "His pain is well controlled aside from these pain flares. That's what the breakthrough morphine order is for." Molly is between a rock and a hard place. She asked Dr. Fletcher, "Can we increase the short-acting morphine instead from 5 mg to 10 mg?" "No," says Dr. Fletcher. "I'm not increasing the morphine until he gives the 5-mg dose a fair shake." Awesome; Mr. Krank won't bother with the morphine 5 mg for breakthrough pain, and Dr. Fletcher won't increase the breakthrough dose until Mr. Krank tries the 5-mg morphine dose for some unspecified period of time. *Tell me, do Mr. Krank and Dr. Fletcher need THEIR heads knocked together? Don't'cha love it when two grown-ups play chicken?*

What's wrong with this picture?

Aside from dealing with two very strong-willed people, Mr. Krank's dose of morphine for breakthrough pain is a bit on the low side, and it's being offered too infrequently. Importantly, it would be preferable to optimize the dose of breakthrough opioid, instead of increasing the Kadian because he is pain free between these episodes. Of course, if he uses the breakthrough analgesia more than three to four times a day, it may be appropriate to increase the Kadian (as well as using adjuvant analgesics, of course). Molly wants to bang her head on the desk but being of that hardy breed—hospice nurse—Molly is the queen of a work-around. Let's watch Molly work her magic.

Play it again, Sam

Molly calls Dr. Fletcher again. "Dr. Fletcher, you and I both know Mr. Krank is a little on the cranky side, and he's just not going to do as you ask. He is clearly miserable when he has these episodes, and Mrs. Krank is beside herself. I was reading in that amazing book, *Demystifying Opioid Conversion Calculations: A Guide for Effective Dosing*, about breakthrough pain, and apparently it's a standard of practice to offer 10% to 20% of the total daily scheduled opioid as the breakthrough analgesic. So, if Mr. Krank is taking 80-mg oral morphine scheduled per day, 10% to 20% would be 8 to 16 mg. Because he seems to want to be in control of the situation, can I suggest you give me TWO orders—one for morphine 10 mg for moderate pain, and one for morphine 15 mg for severe pain, and allow him to select the best dose based on his pain severity? And I'd really like to have this available to him more often than every 8 hours. As you know, short-acting morphine only lasts 4 hours at the most. So, can we go with every 2 or 3 hours? I'll make sure Mrs. Krank keeps a medication administration record (MAR), and I'll keep a close eye on him. I'll keep you posted; in a couple of days you can decide whether you want to increase the Kadian. Does this sound like a good plan to you?" Dr. Fletcher recognizes that Molly is trying hard to take the high road—making everyone happy, but most important getting the best possible care for her patient. "Okay," says Dr. Fletcher. "But if he doesn't use THESE breakthrough doses, he's up the creek." "Awesome," says Molly. "I'll keep you posted on his progress!" Molly institutes the orders (every 2 hours because she's nobody's fool), and Mrs. Krank agrees to keep the MAR. Over the next few days, Mr. Krank uses three to four doses of the short-acting morphine, using on average 50 mg a day. He rates his pain as an 8 to 10 prior to taking the morphine, and as a 3 or 4 one hour later. Success! Molly offers to call Dr. Fletcher to suggest increasing the Kadian, but Mr. Krank says, "No thanks, I'm very happy with how things are now. I can take it when I need it, but no more than that." Molly is nominated for and wins employee of the year! *To review the principles discussed in this sitch, refer to Chapter 4.*

Scenario 3

What's the sitch?

Holly the hospice nurse reaches out to Kristina, the advance practice nurse, about Mrs. Delaney, a 58-year-old woman admitted with lung cancer with a primary complaint of pain. Mrs. Delaney was started on long- and short-acting morphine with fair effect (pain intensity goal is <4 [on a 0–10 scale; 0 = no pain, 10 = worst imaginable pain], average pain rating is 5 to 6), but this regimen has caused widespread, unrelenting itching. At first, Holly recommended soaking in a bath with Aveeno, followed by good moisturizing. Mrs. Delaney now has skin like a baby but still complains about the fire ants crawling around under her skin. Next, nurse practitioner Kristina ordered diphenhydramine, and then hydroxyzine for the itching, but it only made Mrs. Delaney super sleepy (well, there's a surprise!).

Finally, Holly and Kristina decide that switching from morphine to oxycodone might be a good idea (Eureka!). Kristina asks Holly what Mrs. Delaney is getting, and Holly responds, "Well, she takes the MS Contin 15 mg every 12 hours and she has the Roxanol 10 mg every 2 hours as needed." Kristina does some quick calculations. "MS Contin 15 mg every 12 hours is 30-mg oral morphine, and Roxanol 10 mg 12 times a day is 120-mg oral morphine, for a total of 150-mg oral morphine per day." Kristina and Holly agree that switching to oxycodone is a fabulous idea.

Kristina sets up her equation:

$$\frac{\text{"X" mg oral oxycodone}}{\text{150-mg oral morphine}} = \frac{\text{20-mg oral oxycodone}}{\text{25-mg oral morphine}}$$

$(X)(25) = (20)(150)$

$X = 120$-mg oral oxycodone per day

Because Holly shared that Mrs. Delaney's pain wasn't totally controlled, Kristina decides to go with her calculated dose, and orders OxyContin 60 mg by mouth every 12 hours with OxyIR 15 mg by mouth every 2 hours as needed for moderate pain, or OxyIR 30 mg by mouth every 2 hours as needed for severe pain. Kristina tells Holly to keep her updated on how Mrs. Delaney does on the new regimen. Hopefully, the itching will be a thing of the past!

The oxycodone is delivered at 6 p.m., and Mrs. Delaney takes her first dose of OxyContin 60 mg at 9 p.m. When Holly visits the next morning, Mrs. Delaney is ecstatic! "Wow, I slept like a top! My pain is a 1. I'm a little sleepy even now, but it's probably because I wasn't sleeping well when I was on the morphine with the itching. Thank goodness that seems to be going away!"

Holly is delighted, and she calls Kristina to share the happy news. "Nailed it!" cries Kristina. "Keep up the good work!" Holly advises Mrs. Delaney to stay on this regimen and to call if she has any problems. Around 1 p.m. that day, Mr. Delaney calls Holly to say his wife is EXTREMELY hard to wake up. "She's snoring, and even though I've tried to wake her up, she falls asleep in the middle of a sentence. I think something's wrong." Did Holly or Kristina make a mistake?

What's wrong with this picture?

Because you're smarter than the average bear, you already KNOW what's wrong! Holly told Kristina the ORDER for breakthrough pain—Roxanol 10 mg by mouth every 2 hours as needed—but that doesn't mean Mrs. Delaney TOOK 12 doses a day. Kristina made an assumption (and you know how well that generally turns out!), but Holly didn't correct Kristina either. Had Kristina asked explicitly "How many milligrams of the oral morphine solution is Mrs. Delaney taking on average per day?" Holly would have told her "No more than twice a day." Well . . . that's a horse of a different color! Important points are to determine the AVERAGE (especially over the past 24 to 48 hours) use of breakthrough opioid the patient has received. Your first choice would be to consult the patient's MAR if the patient is in a facility, and calculate the TDD of short-acting opioid administered. Second best would be to review any MARs the patient or family have been keeping. If that's not available, ask the patient or family how much the patient was receiving per day on average (to confirm, factor in how much of the drug has been used since the medication was dispensed). If no records are available or no one can give any accounting, don't include it in your calculation at all!

Play it again, Sam

Holly tells Kristina that Mrs. Delaney is taking MS Contin 15 mg by mouth every 12 hours (30-mg oral morphine per day) and two doses of oral morphine solution per day (10-mg each, so 20-mg oral morphine per day) for a grand total of 50-mg oral morphine per day.

Kristina would have set up her equation as follows:

$$\frac{\text{"X" mg oral oxycodone}}{\text{50-mg oral morphine}} = \frac{\text{20-mg oral oxycodone}}{\text{25-mg oral morphine}}$$

$$(X)(25) = (20)(50)$$

X = 40-mg oral oxycodone per day

Kristina decides to reduce the dose by only 25% because Mrs. Delaney's pain control could be a bit better so she prescribes OxyContin 15 mg by mouth every 12 hours with oxycodone 5 mg by mouth every 2 hours as needed for moderate pain, or oxycodone 10 mg by mouth every 2 hours as needed for severe pain. Kristina orders a 4- to 5-day supply so she can increase the OxyContin to 20 mg by mouth every 12 hours within a few days as necessary. **Refer to Chapters 3, 4, and 8 to review the concepts covered in this scenario.**

Scenario 4

What's the sitch?

Mr. Daley is an 82-year-old Texan who has advanced esophageal cancer. He has been experiencing pain, which had been well controlled with oral morphine until the past few days. For the past 48 hours, the patient's pain has been about 7 (on a 0–10 scale; 0 = no pain, 10 = worst imaginable pain), and the nurse suspects disease progression. Nurse Albert contacts Dr. Kostkowski to discuss the situation. Because Mr. Daley has a hard time swallowing tablets or capsules, he has been taking oral morphine solution every 4 hours. Dr. Kostkowski asks Nurse Albert how much morphine Mr. Daley is getting at this time, and Nurse Albert responds, "Oh, a whole mL every 4 hours." Dr. Kostkowski decides to be aggressive and says, "Let's increase it 50%, to 1.5 mLs every 4 hours." "Roger that," says Nurse Albert, "1.5 mLs every 4 hours. I'll let you know how it goes."

Nurse Albert instructs Mr. Daley to increase his dose of oral morphine solution to 1.5 mL every 4 hours around the clock. Twenty-four hours later Mr. Daley tells Albert, "Dude, that increase in morphine didn't do squat. My pain is just as bad as ever." Albert briefly wonders if Mr. Daley is a drug-seeker or diverter, or if someone else in the family is taking some of Mr. Daley's oral morphine solution from the bottle and diluting the remainder so it will look like nothing was withdrawn. However, the nurse quickly discards that notion—Mr. Daley has been a straight shooter all along and was even reluctant to take the morphine to begin with. Nurse Albert decides to call Dr. Kostkowski to report the lack of progress. "That's so odd," says Dr. Kostkowski. "I thought going up to 30 mg would really do the job." "Wait—what?" asks Nurse Albert. "He's not getting 30 mg—his morphine is 10 mg/5 mL. The pharmacy was out of our normal 20-mg/mL oral morphine solution, and as he was getting a low dose, I figured it didn't matter. We started with 2-mg oral morphine because when he was in the hospital 5 mg of oral morphine knocked him out. You said to increase by 50% so I increased it to 3 mg by mouth every 4 hours. What do you want to do now?" *Ok, so who are we taking to the woodshed—Albert or Dr. K? I say off with BOTH their heads!*

What's wrong with this picture?

Albert, Albert, ALBERT, you KNOW back in nursing school they taught you to speak in doses, not volume, especially if you don't provide the concentration as well! Oral morphine solution is available as 10 mg/5 mL, 20 mg/5 mL, and 100 mg/5 mL. Because hospice programs are fond of using the 100 mg/5 mL (which is 20 mg/mL), Dr. K assumed Mr. Daley was taking 20-mg oral morphine every 4 hours. ***Take a look at this chart:***

Morphine Dose	What Dr. Kostkowski Assumed (100 mg/5 mL)	What Mr. Daley Was Actually Receiving (10 mg/5 mL)
Original morphine dose	20 mg	2 mg
Increased dose	30 mg	3 mg

If there's one saving grace here, it's that Dr. Kostkowski didn't say "Ok, let's increase it to oral morphine 30 mg every 4 hours." That's because I'm not feeling lucky that Albert would have said "WHAT?" to that! If 5-mg oral morphine knocked Mr. Daley out, 30 mg would have put him 6 feet under.

Play it again, Sam

When Dr. Kostkowski asked Nurse Albert how much oral morphine Mr. Daley was getting, Nurse Albert should have said, "He uses an oral syringe and takes 1 mL of the 10 mg/5 mL morphine solution, which is 2 mg. So he's getting 2-mg oral morphine every 4 hours around the clock." Dr. K. probably would have responded with "I think he can handle a 100% increase in the dose since he's having severe pain so let's double it; go up to 4 mg and see how he does. If you or the patient feels it's too much, you can back it down to 3 mg by mouth every 4 hours. If it's not enough, you can increase to 5 mg after a couple doses. Let me know the status in 24 to 48 hours." *Bottom line—don't just talk in "mLs"*—that's a disaster waiting to happen! ***For more information related to this scenario, refer to Chapters 4 and 8.***

Scenario 5

What's the sitch?

Physician Assistant Geneviève (yes, pronounced with an ADORABLE French accent)[40] is doing palliative care rounds at Sunny Days Retirement Community. She is visiting Mrs. Rodriguez, a 78-year-old stroke victim who has been taking MS Contin 30 mg by mouth every 12 hours for pain control. Mr. Rodriguez tells Geneviève that he's having a hard time getting the Mrs. to swallow a tablet due to her history of worsening swallowing difficulties. Geneviève says, "No problem. Let's put your wife on oral morphine solution around the clock. Are you ok with that?" Mr. Rodriguez says, "Sure, I can give it during the day, and we have a paid caregiver at night because my wife tries to get out of bed and wanders." "Très bien," says Geneviève. "So, 60 mg a day, every 4 hours, let's go with oral morphine solution, 15 mg every 4 hours. I'll order the 20-mg/mL oral morphine solution so the dose will be just a tiny volume you would put in her mouth. I will swing by this afternoon after the morphine solution is delivered and show you how to prepare a dose." She comes back at the end of the day and shows Mr. Rodriguez how to prepare and give the dose. "You did a great job," says Geneviève. "I'll be back in 2 days to check in."

When Geneviève visits in 2 days, she asks Mr. Rodriguez how things are going. "Well, okay I guess, but she is zonked—all she does is sleep. I feel like I'm giving her too much medicine. I don't want to kill her," he exclaims while wringing his hands. "Oh my," says Geneviève. "Of course, you don't. I don't understand—she was taking 60 mg of oral morphine a day by tablet before and all we did was switch to the oral solution." Geneviève looks mystified. Mr. Rodriguez, who is Professor Emeritus, retired head of the Division of Mathematics at Stamford University said, "Actually that's not true. We're giving her 15 mg every 4 hours now—six times in 24 hours, which is 90 mg. I thought perhaps you increased it on purpose because the solution didn't work as well as the tablets. And by the way, it's Dr. Rodriguez." "Je suis tellement gênée," thought Geneviève (which means "I'm so embarrassed").

What's wrong with this picture?

Geneviève immediately realized her mistake. While she was thinking oral morphine solution is dosed every 4 hours, she accidently divided the TDD of morphine (60 mg) by 4, instead of 6. This is a very common mistake, dividing the TDD by 4 for an every-4-hour drug, or 6 for an every-6-hour drug. Luckily, although Mrs. Rodriguez is sleepy, her respiratory rate is 16, and she does not have periods of apnea or constricted pupils. Geneviève asked Dr. Rodriguez to hold the next dose and call her in 4 to 6 hours to determine when to restart the oral morphine.

Play it again, Sam

There is really no difference in the bioavailability of oral morphine tablets versus oral morphine solution, so Geneviève should have ordered oral morphine solution (20 mg/mL), 10 mg (0.5 mL) by mouth every 4 hours. The good news is no harm was done to Mrs. Rodriguez. Geneviève will remember this the rest of her natural born days, and Dr. Rodriguez is thinking, "Yep, I still got it!" *To review the principles discussed in this scenario, refer to Chapter 8.*

Scenario 6

What's the sitch?

Mr. Morgan is a 44-year-old man diagnosed with a giant tumor (18 cm × 15 cm × 14 cm) in the left thoracic cavity. He underwent surgery, and the tumor (which was adherent to the left upper lobe of the lung), mediastinal pleura, and parietal pleural was completely resected with combined resection of part of the left upper lobe of lung. The surgeon was generous with the postoperative analgesic plan, knowing that post-thoracotomy pain can be profound. *Mr. Morgan's use of IV hydromorphone is as follows:*

Hours Post-surgery	12-Hour Use of IV Hydromorphone
0–12	24 mg
12–24	20 mg
24–36	17 mg
36–48	14 mg
48–60	10 mg
60–72	8 mg
72–84	6 mg

On the morning of postoperative day 4, the surgeon is discharging Mr. Morgan home. The surgeon is mindful of the CDC recommendations for the management of acute pain. Specifically, the guidelines state, "Clinicians should prescribe the lowest effective dose of immediate-release opioids and should prescribe no greater quantity than needed for the expected duration of pain severe enough to require opioids. Three days or less will often be sufficient; more than seven days will rarely be needed."[41] Keeping this in mind, the surgeon gives Mrs. Morgan a prescription for her husband for oxycodone 5 mg/acetaminophen 325 mg, one tablet every 4 hours as needed, quantity 18. The surgeon also reminds Mrs. Morgan to pick up some polyethylene glycol while she's at the pharmacy. After all, nobody wants to be straining to stool post-thoracotomy!

The next morning, Mrs. Morgan contacts the surgeon's office demanding to speak to the surgeon. "My husband is in EXCRUCIATING pain. He's screaming and crying, and we've been up all night. What kind of monster are you? These pills barely touch the pain. I even gave him two at a time during the night, and it didn't really help. He's complaining of stomach pain now, too. Should I bring him to the emergency department (ED) or what?" The surgeon is taken aback. He wonders if Mr. Morgan (or maybe even Mrs. Morgan) is a drug-seeker, or if the patient had a history of illicit drug use of which the surgeon was unaware.

What's wrong with this picture?

Well, this is a fine kettle of fish. Mr. Morgan is clearly in pain crisis (possibly opioid withdrawal), the surgeon is trying to be a good citizen and follow the CDC guidelines, and Mrs. Morgan wants to throw them both in the river. Of course, practitioners today must practice good risk mitigation such as considering the use of illicit opioids, or opioid misuse, or diversion. However, the CDC guidelines were intended for the majority of postsurgical cases, not all cases. A thoracotomy is considered one of the most painful surgical procedures there is. Let's consider what Mr. Morgan received in the 12 hours immediately prior to discharge: 6-mg IV hydromorphone. We consider the opioid use in 12-hour increments because the acute pain should be improving as time goes on. However, if we double the 6-mg IV hydromorphone, this would be the equivalent of 12-mg IV hydromorphone in 24 hours. This would be equivalent to 120-mg oral oxycodone, as shown by this calculation:

$$\frac{\text{"X" mg oral oxycodone}}{\text{12-mg IV hydromorphone}} = \frac{\text{20-mg oral oxycodone}}{\text{2-mg IV hydromorphone}}$$

(X)(2) = (20)(12)

X = 120-mg oral oxycodone in 24 hours

The surgeon sent Mr. Morgan home on a maximum of 30-mg oral oxycodone per day—this is a dramatic reduction and insufficient opioid. He is even complaining of nausea, which could be a sign of opioid withdrawal. But hey—thanks for remembering the bowels!

Play it again, Sam

What should the surgeon have done instead? Although we usually use a short-acting opioid postoperatively, the surgeon could have chosen to use either short- or long-acting oxycodone. If she chose long-acting oxycodone, she could have prescribed OxyContin 10 mg, and advised Mr. Morgan to take it in a declining fashion as follows:

- Day 1 at home—three tablets every 12 hours (OxyContin 30 mg by mouth every 12 hours)
- Day 2 at home—two tablets every 12 hours (OxyContin 20 mg by mouth every 12 hours)
- Day 3 at home—one tablet every 12 hours (OxyContin 10 mg by mouth every 12 hours)

In addition, supplement with oxycodone 10 or 15 mg every 4 hours as needed. Alternately, the surgeon could have chosen to go with OxyIR 15 mg, one or two tablets every 4 hours as needed, and explain that the patient may need to take the oxycodone fairly regularly the first day or two, then would expect to decrease use. The surgeon could also recommend acetaminophen 4 g per day to supplement the oxycodone in either case. If this is insufficient, the surgeon could also consider providing a bit more opioid, depending on how Mr. Morgan responds. Most important, let's remember that guidelines are just that—guidelines. We must meet our patients' needs, and first *"do no harm!" **Read all about it—refer to Chapter 3 for a refresher on the principles discussed in this sitch.***

Scenario 7

What's the sitch?

Ms. Evans is a 48-year-old woman with breast cancer. Thankfully, she has had minimal pain, and she is well controlled on acetaminophen 1,000 mg every 6 hours, with an occasional ibuprofen 400 mg as needed. She's at home with her daughter one day when the family golden retriever, Buttercup, grabs Ms. Evans' slipper and starts to abscond with it. Ms. Evans makes a grab to rescue her slipper and experiences a SEARING pain in her right humerus. The pain is so horrific it literally takes her breath away, but when she can breathe, she starts screaming. Ms. Evans daughter immediately loads Mom into the car and off they go to the ED with Ms. Evans screaming hysterically the whole way. When she gets to the ED, she is immediately taken into an exam room, and she tells the ED doctor (Dr. Marcus Welby) that her pain is so horrific, she can't even rate it. Dr. Welby sits by Ms. Evans' bed and begins to administer IV morphine, 1 mg every minute for 10 minutes. After a 5-minute respite, Ms. Evans rates her humerus pain as a 9 or 10 (on a 0–10 scale; 0 = no pain, 10 = worst imaginable pain). Dr. Welby proceeds through another cycle, administering morphine 1 mg IV every minute for 10 minutes. After another 5-minute respite, Ms. Evans says the pain is a 6 or 7, but could certainly be better. Dr. Welby commences with the third cycle of morphine 1 mg IV every minute for 10 minutes. Five minutes after that cycle, Ms. Evans smiles at Dr. Welby and says, "No wonder everyone loves you Dr. Welby. My pain is a 2 now. You're an angel." Dr. Welby smiles avuncularly at Ms. Evans and orders an x-ray of her humerus now that she's comfortable. Off Ms. Evans goes to radiology. She has to wait in the hall for 30 minutes because radiology is backed up; as they wheel her in to have her x-ray done, the x-ray technician notices that Ms. Evans is nonresponsive. "Holy moly," cries the x-ray technician, who pulls the ripcord to initiate a code. People come running from all over, and Ms. Evans requires two doses of naloxone to bring her back. "Wow, that was a close one," says the shaky x-ray technician. Dr. Welby, what did you do?

What's wrong with this picture?

What's wrong is that Dr. Welby was TOO darned nice. By giving 1 mg of IV morphine every minute for 10 minutes, he was "dose-stacking" the morphine. When he started the second cycle of morphine, the first morphine injection was just then starting to peak. By the time he had administered 30 mg of IV morphine, only a small portion of that dose had reached the peak clinical effect. Unfortunately, it reached a critical peak effect while she was unattended in the hall outside radiology.

Play it again, Sam

Dr. Welby should have stopped after two cycles of the morphine 1 mg every minute. At that point, Ms. Evans' pain was 6 or 7, which would have allowed her to have the x-ray without too much discomfort (especially since the morphine serum level was still on the way up). By the way, the humerus pain was a pathologic fracture from metastatic breast cancer. *For a review of this topic, refer to Chapter 4*.

Scenario 8

What's the sitch?

Mrs. Madderhorn is an 82-year-old woman with multiple comorbidities, including uterine cancer; post-stroke pain; diabetes; heart disease; osteoarthritis of the knees, hips, and spine; and Alzheimer's dementia. The patient's usual blood pressure is 105/70 mm Hg, heart rate 68 bpm, and respiratory rate 16. She is 5'0" and weighs 86 pounds. Her appetite is poor and she appears to be malnourished. She has been admitted to hospice under the uterine cancer diagnosis. She was receiving MS Contin 15 mg by mouth every 12 hours with oral morphine solution for breakthrough pain (not using) on admission, but as her dementia has worsened, she started to forget to take her medication. She was switched to transdermal fentanyl (TDF) 12 mcg/hr with morphine oral solution for breakthrough pain, 5 mg every 2 hours as needed. The hospice nurse, Stephanie, observes that Mrs. Madderhorn is exhibiting signs of pain, even though the patient isn't verbal. Stephanie uses the Checklist for Nonverbal Pain Indicators and decides the patient is in moderate pain. The TDF is increased to 25 mcg/hr on day 3, and again to 50 mcg/hr on day 5. Stephanie visits daily, and reports at the hospice team meeting that she just doesn't think the patient is getting the relief you would expect from the TDF. Dr. North, the hospice team physician agrees and recommends switching back to MS Contin since the family hired a full-time caregiver who can give the morphine to Mrs. Madderhorn. She calculates TDF 50 mcg/hr ≈ 100-mg oral morphine per day, but she is still showing signs of pain so she prescribes MS Contin 60 mg by mouth every 12 hours with oral morphine solution 15 mg every 2 hours as needed. Dr. North advises Stephanie to remove the TDF patch and start the MS Contin 12 hours later. Within 24 to 36 hours, Mrs. Madderhorn is completely zonked and very hard to wake up. The paid caregiver says she can't sufficiently awaken the patient to administer the next dose of MS Contin. Now what? Switch to around-the-clock oral morphine solution instead?

What's wrong with this picture?

Wow, there's a whole lot wrong in this red-hot mess. First, was Mrs. Madderhorn an appropriate candidate for TDF? As you recall, a patient needs to be receiving 60 mg of oral morphine equivalent a day for at least a week prior to starting TDF. She had only been receiving MS Contin 15 mg by mouth every 12 hours on admission to hospice (and unsure how long she'd been getting that), which is far short of the 60-mg oral morphine mark. Another HUGE red flag is the patient's cachexia. As you read in Chapter 5, cachectic patients frequently don't seem to get the response you would expect from TDF. This could be due to a poorly selected application site or the transcapillary leak associated with hypoalbuminemia, which causes fentanyl to be sequestered in the extravascular interstitial spaces and NOT in the systemic circulation. Next, the manufacturer's guidelines state you can increase TDF after 3 days after the initial application, then every 6 days subsequently. This patient was increased on day 3 and again on day 5, which is too soon. Probably the most egregious error in this case was basing the calculation off TDF from the most recent dose—TDF 50 mcg/hr (which Dr. North correctly determined is usually equivalent to 100-mg oral morphine) but this patient weighs 86 pounds! THEN Dr. North increased the dose further! Clearly, Dr. North is out of control. Last, even though we are unsure how much fentanyl the patient was absorbing or retaining, it takes up to 24 hours for the fentanyl serum level to decrease. To be completely safe, it is wise to wait 24 hours before starting the full replacement dose of a different long-acting opioid (e.g., MS Contin).

Play it again, Sam

Well, life would have been much simpler if the family had hired the paid caregiver at the time of hospice admission, then we could have avoided the whole TDF issue. We could have continued the MS Contin, titrating that appropriately, and, of course, adding adjuvant analgesics when needed. If the patient was switched to TDF regardless, we could have increased at appropriate intervals (3 days after initial application, then every 6 days). Most important, once the team realized the TDF just wasn't cutting the mustard, it would have been far more appropriate to go back to the MS Contin 15-mg dose by mouth every 12 hours (which was the last known effective dose), or preferably, go with morphine 5 mg every 4 hours around the clock, and 5 mg every 2 hours as needed for additional pain. We could start the "as needed" dose immediately after removing the patch, and start the around-the-clock morphine in 24 hours. *For a review of the principles discussed in this sitch, please refer to Chapter 5.*

Scenario 9

What's the sitch?

Ms. Ives is a 32-year-old woman with end-stage cervical cancer, referred to hospice. On admission, she is receiving IV morphine, 30 mg/hr, with a 10-mg bolus every 15 minutes as needed (using at least once, often twice, per hour). Her 24-hour use of IV morphine is 1,080 mg, which is about equivalent to 2,700 mg oral morphine per day. *Wow, that's a whole lotta morphine!* The attending physician, Dr. Rosenthal says, "This dose of morphine is ridiculous! She can swallow; she has a fair prognosis—let's switch her to methadone." Dr. Rosenthal asks you to do the conversion calculation. Oh my—where to start—so many methods recommended in the literature. You decide to use the Ayonrinde method,[42] which calls for a 20:1 (oral morphine:oral methadone) conversion for TDDs in excess of 1,001 mg per day. Dividing 2,700-mg oral morphine per day by 20, you calculate 135-mg oral methadone per day. The patient declines to be admitted as an inpatient (she is a single mother with three small children at home), so you decide to do this as a rapid switch at home. You stop the morphine infusion, start methadone

45 mg by mouth every 8 hours, and you decide to use morphine 60 mg by mouth every 2 hours as needed for breakthrough pain. For the first couple of days, things are a little rough; the patient uses the morphine breakthrough pain dose frequently. Then by days 2 and 3, things are starting to look up. The patient has achieved a reasonable level of pain control, and she's happy to not be dragging the IV pump around with her. Day 4 she complains of being sleepy, and day 5 she can't get out of bed. *What's the scoop?*

What's wrong with this picture?

Although the mathematical calculation was correct, we know that there probably should be a maximum starting dose line-in-the-sand with methadone. *As discussed by Dr. Eduardo Bruera, there are several reasons for this:* The morphine:methadone relationship is not linear because methadone may have slight binding differences at the opioid receptor, methadone has multiple mechanisms of action, and the high dose of morphine this patient was receiving may be proalgesic (increasing the pain).[43] Chatham and colleagues reported a series of 10 patients receiving very high-dose morphine, and the vast majority were converted to and stabilized on methadone 10 mg by mouth every 8 hours.[44] The American Pain Society guidelines on methadone use suggest starting no higher than 30- to 40-mg oral methadone per day.[45]

Play it again, Sam

First, this is an enormous conversion, which would really be better accomplished in an inpatient setting. The team should try a bit harder to convince the patient to initiate dosing as an inpatient for a few days. Alternately, the team could have replaced a PORTION of the IV morphine with methadone, and done this in a couple of steps over a week or two. Last, the maximum starting dose of methadone should not exceed 30 to 40 mg a day. For example, methadone 10 mg by mouth every 8 hours, or perhaps 12.5 mg by mouth every 8 hours (a 10-mg tablet plus half a 5-mg tablet). Close follow-up is critically important. ***For more information on this sitch, refer to Chapter 6***.

Scenario 10

What's the sitch?

Mrs. Gladson is a 78-year-old woman diagnosed with end-stage hepatic cancer. She was admitted to hospice on MS Contin 15 mg by mouth every 12 hours, with oral morphine solution 5 mg every 3 hours as needed for additional pain. The hospice nurse reports that the patient is having a pain crisis; she is taking her MS Contin as directed and has taken several doses of the oral morphine solution with no relief. The patient says the pain is greater than 10 (on a 0–10 scale; 0 = no pain, 10 = worst imaginable pain), and her family is insistent that she be admitted to the hospice inpatient unit. She is transported to the inpatient unit, arriving at 6 p.m. The attending on call is Dr. Doogie Howser (he's so excited—this is his first position post-fellowship!). Dr. Howser calculates that the patient was receiving approximately 40-mg oral morphine in the past 24 hours, which he figures is about 16-mg IV morphine per day. This is about 0.6 mg/hr of IV morphine so he orders a 2.5-mg IV morphine loading dose, and a continuous morphine infusion to begin at 1.2 mg/hr, with an order to titrate to comfort per nursing judgment. The family stays with the patient and keeps the nurse informed of the patient's response to the morphine infusion. The family is concerned that she is still complaining of pain that she rates as 9 or 10 at 8:00 p.m., so the nurse increases the infusion to 3 mg/hr and the clinician bolus to 5 mg. At 10 p.m., the family reports the patient is still grimacing and crying out, so the nurse repeats the 5-mg IV morphine-loading dose and increases the infusion to 5 mg/hr. The patient seems to settle down, and the family leaves around midnight. When the nurse checks on Mrs. Gladson at 3 a.m., she is nonresponsive, even to sternal rub. Her respiratory rate is 6 breaths per minute with periods of apnea. She has pinpoint pupils, and the nurse calls Dr. Howser in a panic.

What's wrong with this picture?

Clearly Mrs. Gladson has been overdosed on her morphine infusion. *Where did we go wrong?* Did Dr. Howser order an incorrect starting dose of morphine (bolus or infusion)? Was his order to "titrate to comfort" inappropriate? No, and yes. Dr. Howser correctly calculated the patient's at-home oral morphine TDD (40 mg) and correctly converted to TDD of parenteral morphine (16; which is 0.6 mg/hr). He appropriately ordered a clinician bolus dose of 2.5 mg to get the patient's serum level of morphine up, and he doubled the TDD because the patient was complaining of severe pain, starting the infusion at 1.2 mg/hr. Dr. Howser derailed with the order to "titrate to comfort per nursing judgment." The infusion was started at 6 p.m., increased at 8 p.m. and again at 10 p.m. If the patient had a normal half-life of morphine (2 hours), it would take 6 hours to be 87.5% of the way to steady state, or 8 hours to be 93.75% of the way to steady state. Mrs. Gladson, however, is elderly, and has a terminal illness—hepatic cancer. Her morphine half-life is probably closer to 5 hours. To get 87.5% or 93.75% of the way to steady state, it would take 15 to 20 hours. Her morphine was increased at 2 and 4 hours after beginning the infusion—WAY too early! *As stated in Chapter 7, we have two issues at play here:*

- We need to FULLY appreciate the clinical impact of the current continuous opioid infusion dose when it achieves a steady-state serum level (both therapeutic gain and potential toxicity) BEFORE we increase the dose (and make the situation worse, and that always seems to happen at 3 a.m. when no one is really paying close attention).

- We don't want the patient to suffer with pain while we are waiting for the magical moment of steady state to make sure we haven't overdosed the patient.

Doogie, Doogie, DOOGIE—this is why we never let 14-year-olds be a doctor—EVER! *So, how should Dr. Howser have handled this situation?*

Play it again, Sam

Dr. Howser calculated the patient's at-home oral morphine TDD (40 mg) and correctly converted to a TDD of parenteral morphine (16 mg; which is 0.6 mg/hr). Was his calculation of a clinician loading dose correct? Well, the National Comprehensive Cancer Network (NCCN) 2018 Guidelines state for moderate-to-severe pain in an opioid-tolerant patient, to administer 10% to 20% of the total opioid taken in the previous 24 hours.[46] Mrs. Gladson has received the equivalent of 16-mg IV morphine in the past 24 hours, so 10% would be 1.6 mg, 20% would be 3.2 mg. Dr. Howser ordered a 2.5-mg IV morphine bolus, which is right in the middle. He started the continuous infusion at 1.2 mg/hr (double the TDD she was receiving at home). However, instead of ordering "titrate to comfort per nursing judgment," he should have provided more precise guidance to the nurse. For example, the guidelines further state that the practitioner should reassess for efficacy and adverse effects at 15 minutes, and if the pain is unchanged or worsens to increase the bolus dose by 50% to 100%. Dr. Howser could have written, "Administer

2.5-mg IV morphine now. Begin continuous morphine infusion at 1.2 mg/hr. Reassess pain every 30 minutes × 3 and if pain decreased but is not adequately controlled, repeat 2.5-mg IV bolus dose of morphine. If pain is unchanged or increased, increase the dose to 5 mg. If pain is not adequately controlled after three IV bolus doses, contact prescriber. Do not increase continuous infusion before 8 a.m. (morning rounds)." *For a review of this sitch, refer to Chapters 4 and 7.*

Scenario 11

What's the sitch?

This is a real case from my practice. I was on vacation with my family in West Palm Beach, and one of the hospice nurses I worked with called me. "You have to help me—I can't figure out what's going on with this guy. Mr. Rogers is an 82-year-old man with us for prostate cancer, mets to the brain and bone. He's been doing so well on methadone 5 mg by mouth every 12 hours, with oxycodone 5 or 10 mg as needed for breakthrough pain. Over the past few days, he's been acting very peculiarly, almost like a drunk monkey. His pain control has significantly deteriorated. His ataxia has caused him to fall, and he hurt his wrist. I'm not at all sure what's going on, but I don't think it's related to his disease process. Do you have any great ideas?" Hmmmm . . . . I asked if the prescriber started any new medications. *Nope.* I asked if the prescriber stopped any other medications. *Nope.* Okay, this is a stumper. Did ANYTHING change in the medication regimen at all? "Well," said the nurse, "The only thing that changed is the doctor ordered a phenytoin level, and it came back below the therapeutic range (it was 7.8 mcg/mL) so the doctor increased the phenytoin from 300 mg once daily to 500 mg once daily." *Holy moly, cue the orchestra, I've figured it out!* Mr. Rogers was a frail, slight man, and I suspected he was slightly malnourished. So, what's that got to do with anything? *What would you have done in this situation?*

What's wrong with this picture?

Phenytoin is 90% bound to serum albumin, which is why the preferred therapeutic range is 1 to 2 mcg/mL of UNBOUND phenytoin (instead of a total phenytoin concentration of 10 to 20 mcg/mL). If Mr. Rogers was hypoalbuminemic, his unbound phenytoin may have been therapeutic, despite a subtherapeutic total phenytoin level. I asked the nurse to hold the phenytoin and get a stat total and unbound phenytoin level. She did, and the unbound was 2.86 mcg/mL and the total was 12.4 mcg/mL. The prescriber probably would have thought he did an awesome job adjusting the phenytoin based on a total serum level of 12.4 mcg/mL (therapeutic range is 10 to 20 mcg/mL). However, the truth is, the patient was NOW phenytoin toxic, with an unbound level of 2.86 mcg/mL (which, in someone with a normal albumin would be like a total phenytoin concentration of 28.6 mcg/mL—toxic). The patient WAS showing clinical signs of toxicity with the ataxia. We held the phenytoin for several days, and then lowered the dose back down to 300 mg once a day. *A couple things to note here:* We generally don't give 500-mg phenytoin as one dose for fear of bezoar formation and, more important, this patient had never had a seizure and guidelines recommend NOT using an anticonvulsant prophylactically for primary or metastatic disease to the brain. I digress.

The reason the patient was likely having increased pain was the increase in phenytoin dose further induced the metabolism of methadone. I encouraged the nurse to use the breakthrough oxycodone until the phenytoin serum level came back down, and the metabolism of methadone would then go back to baseline. Everything resolved with these interventions, and the patient was back to his prephenytoin dose increase in about 5 days.

Play it again, Sam

Well, I pretty much already explained what SHOULD have been done. Checking the unbound phenytoin level would have confirmed the patient was fine, and no phenytoin dose adjustment was needed. However, if the prescriber was aware and realized the patient didn't need to be on an anticonvulsant, we would need to be cognizant that stopping the phenytoin would take away the increased methadone metabolism, likely increasing the risk for sedation from the higher methadone serum level. *The bottom line is that we must always be aware of the impact of starting, stopping, or adjusting medications that interact with methadone (or any medication for that matter).* One last important little tidbit: Enzyme inhibition occurs quickly (1 or 2 days); enzyme induction takes about a week to see the full effect. Of course, the same is true in reverse! *Refer to Chapter 6 for more edge-of-the seat excitement about methadone and drug interactions!*

Scenario 12

What's the sitch?

You're cruising around the beltway one day when your mobile phone rings. You answer (on your blue tooth—safety first!); it's Amanda, one of the hospice nurses you work with. "I've got this older woman who I think would really benefit from methadone. Can you help me do the conversion?" "Sure," you say. "Tell me about your patient." "Well, she's 78-years-old, and cared for by her son. She's only receiving morphine oral solution as needed for pain, taking 5 mg per dose. He tells me he's giving it to her every 4 hours around the clock, occasionally giving 10 mg, but she's still having a lot of pain." The patient, Mrs. Stevenson, has a diagnosis of colon cancer but no other conditions or medications that would preclude the use of methadone. The nurse tells you that she observes the patient grimacing, guarding, and bracing when she provides care to the patient. The patient frequently moans and groans as well, so the nurse believes the patient is having significant pain. You recommend methadone 3 mg by mouth every 12 hours and ask the nurse to follow up and let you know how things go. The methadone is delivered by midday and started immediately. After receiving methadone for 24 hours, Amanda calls you to say "YOU are a rock star! Mrs. Stevenson is calm, exhibiting NO signs of pain or distress. She's a little bit sleepy, but wakes up right away. The son is delighted!" You're delighted too and ask the nurse to keep you posted. The next day, the nurse calls you and says, "Well, her pain is REALLY well controlled, but she's really getting sleepy. Maybe she was sleep deprived before and she's just catching up." You agree that's probably the situation, and tell Amanda to stay the course. The next day Amanda calls you and says, "So, you're really nice and all, but are you SURE you did the math right with this methadone dose? Mrs. Stevenson's respiratory rate is down to 10 to 12, and I can't wake her up. What's going on?" Assailed with self-doubt, you review your calculations and can't find fault with what you did. However, you tell Amanda to hold methadone until further notice, and you get continuous care nursing in the home to monitor the patient closely to determine if naloxone therapy is required.

What's wrong with this picture?

Did you incorrectly calculate the methadone dose? No, not incorrectly; it might have been preferable to start methadone a little lower (e.g., 2 mg by mouth every 12 hours), but the 3 mg by mouth every 12 hours isn't a crazy pants dose. Three days later, Amanda calls you and says, "You're not going to believe this, but that 30 to 40 mg of oral morphine per day I told you the son was giving Mrs. Stevenson? Turns out he wasn't giving her ANY morphine, but he didn't want me to think he was a bad son so he made it up!" Holy moly! That's insane! *What should have been a clue that you were in over your head though?* When you were a rock star on day 2. You don't want to be a rock star until day 3, 4, or 5.

Play it again, Sam!

You have no reason to suspect Amanda was giving you misinformation about the use of morphine, as told to her by the son. Amanda could have asked to see any MARs the son was keeping, although he may not have had any. The only clue is probably the complete and total relief of pain within 24 hours, and the fact that the patient was a little sleepy. You could have asked Amanda to ask the evening nurse to follow up later that day, even if by phone, to determine the patient's level of consciousness and to assess for opioid intoxication. Even though this is a low dose of methadone, we have seen older adults zonked by these very low doses. Someone 78 years old who was opioid-naïve would probably be better treated with methadone 1 mg by mouth every 12 hours to start. *For more information on this topic, refer to Chapter 6.*

Scenario 13

What's the sitch?

Mr. Morganstern is a 58-year-old man with end-stage lung cancer being discharged from the hospital to home hospice. He is receiving a complex opioid regimen, and Dr. Davis wants to switch the whole mess to long- and short-acting morphine. The patient is 5'8", 150 pounds and can swallow tablets and capsules. The patient is currently receiving TDF 50 mcg/hr, OxyContin 20 mg by mouth every 12 hours, hydromorphone 4 mg IV every 4 hours as needed (about five doses per day), and hydrocodone/acetaminophen 5/325 mg every 4 hours as needed (not using). Dr. Davis decides this is a complex calculation, so he whips out his smartphone and uses an opioid conversion app. *The app provides the following conversion information to oral morphine:*

- TDF 50 mcg/hr → 100 mg oral morphine per day
- OxyContin 20 mg by mouth every 12 hours → 60-mg oral morphine per day
- Hydromorphone 4-mg IV every 4 hours as needed (5 doses → 20 mg) → 400-mg oral morphine per day

This totals 560-mg oral morphine, so Dr. Davis puts the patient on MS Contin 200 mg by mouth every 8 hours with MSIR 30 mg, one or two capsules every 4 hours as needed. The patient starts on this regimen, but within a day or so, he is extremely lethargic and according to Mrs. Morganstern, "Nobody likes a drunk monkey, and that's what he is right now!" (Thank you Dr. Doolittle!). Dr. Davis is shocked. "I used an app—the calculation is impeccable!"

What's wrong with this picture?

Dr. Davis returns to the website. *He finds the equianalgesic conversion ratio used by the app, as follows:*

Drug	Equianalgesic Doses (mg) Parenteral	Oral
Morphine	10	30
Hydromorphone	1.5	7.5
Oxycodone	10	20
Transdermal fentanyl (TDF)	TDF in mcg/hr × 2 = TDD oral morphine	

These data are somewhat different from the data used in this book (which is way cooler and based on cutting-edge data). **Let's compare:**

Drug	App-Derived Data (Oral Morphine per Day)	Equianalgesic Data Used in this Text (Oral Morphine per Day)
TDF 50 mcg/hr	100 mg	100 mg
OxyContin 20 mg by mouth every 12 hours	60 mg	50 mg
Hydromorphone 20 mg IV	400 mg	250 mg
TOTAL	**560 mg**	**400 mg**

The problem with apps is that they are "plug-and-chug" calculators. Some of the opioid conversion apps will allow the user to build in a percent reduction in the calculated dose to allow for lack of complete cross-tolerance, but not all do. Some users tend to lose all sense of *"does that LOOK right?"* when using an app. I had a pharmacy student on rotation with me when a nurse asked me to do a calculation. So, I turned to my student and said, "Hey, this is a great exercise for you. Can you do the calculation?" "Sure," he said. "I've got an app for that!" (Of course, he had an app for that. When he was born, he probably took a selfie 10 minutes later.) He crunches through the calculation, leans back, and whispers, *"Whoa."* Being the astute preceptor that I am, I said "What, whoa?" "Jeez, it calculates to close to 5,000 mg of oral morphine per day." Knowing that one of us had just suffered brain damage, I asked, "So what do YOU think of that?" He looks me right in the eye and says, "Well, we're going to have to order more morphine!" Shoot me now. *Clearly, clearly, he had NO sense of "does this LOOK right?"*

Play it again, Sam

It would be preferable for Dr. Davis to use the equianalgesic data presented in this book (see Chapter 1). Using an app is fine for checking your math, but I would be careful about relying solely on the app. The reason you went to your professional school of choice is what makes YOU smarter than the app—you know your patient! Young, old, frail, robust, in pain or pain well-controlled, organ dysfunction or not, and so forth. *Use that big old brain you have, dude!* **Your homework is to reread this entire book!**

REFERENCES

1. *English Oxford Living Dictionaries.* Lagniappe. https://en.oxforddictionaries.com/definition/lagniappe. Accessed May 7, 2018.

2. Hall T, Hardy JR. The lipophilic opioids: fentanyl, alfentanil, sufentanil, and remifentanil. In: Davis MP, Glare PA, Hardy J, et al., eds. *Opioids in Cancer Pain.* Oxford: Oxford University Press; 2009:173-190.

3. Beers R, Camporesi E. Remifentail update: Clinical science and utility. *CNS Drugs.* 2004;18(15):1085-1104.

4. Ziesenitz VC, Vaughns JD, Koch G, et al. Pharmacokinetics of fentanyl and its derivatives in children: a comprehensive review. *Clin Pharmacokinet.* 2018;57:125-149.

5. Scholz J, Steinfath M, Schulz M. Clinical pharmacokinetics of alfentanil, fentanyl and sufentanil. *Clin Pharmacokinet.* 1996;31(4):275-292.

6. Bovill JG, Sebel PS, Blackburn CL, et al. The pharmacokinetics of sufentanil in surgical patients. *Anesthesiology.* 1984;61(5):502-506.

7. Bower S, Hull CJ. Comparative pharmacokinetics of fentanyl and alfentanil. *Br J Anaesth.* 1982;54(8):871-877.

8. Westmoreland CL, Hoke JF, Sebel PS, et al. Pharmacokinetics of remifentanil (GI87084B) and its major metabolite (GI90291) in patients underqoinq elective inpatient surgery. *Anesthesiology.* 1993;79(5):881-892.

9. Egan TD, Lemmens HJ, Fiset P, et al. The pharmacokinetics of the new short-acting opioid remifentail (GI87084B) in healthy adult male volunteers. *Anesthesiology.* 1993;79(5):881-892.

10. McClain DA, Hug CC Jr. Intravenous fentanyl kinetics. *Clin Pharmacol Ther.* 1980;28(1):106-114.

11. Meuldermans WE, Hurkmans RM, Heykants JJ. Plasma protein binding and distribution of fentanyl, sufentanil, alfentanil and lofentanil in blood. *Arch Int Pharmacodyn Ther.* 1982;257(1):4-19.

12. Freye E. Pharmakokinetik der Opioide: bedeutung fur den praktischen Einsatz. In: Freye E, ed. *Opioide in der Medizin.* 6th ed. Berlin: Springer; 2004:229-235.

13. Freye E. Opioide im Rahmen der Allgemeinanasthesie. In: Freye E, ed. *Opioide in der Medizin.* 6th ed. Berlin: Springer; 2004:193-228.

14. Kretz F-J, Schaffer J, Gleiter CH, et al. Pharmakologie: grundlagen und klinisch-praktische. In: Kretz F-J, Schaffer J, Gleiter CH, et al., eds. *Anasthesie Intensivemedizin.* Heidelberg: Springer; 2011:3-69.

15. Peng PW, Sandler AN. A review of the use of fentanyl analgesia in the management of acute pain in adults. *Anesthesiology.* 1999;90(2):576-599.

16. Schäfer M. Opioide. In: Tonner PH, Hein L, eds. *Pharmakotherapie in der Anasthesie und Intensivmedizin.* Heidelberg: Springer; 2011:109-130.

17. Schäfer M, Zöllnler C. Opioide. In: Rossaint R, Werner C, Zwissler B, eds. *Die Anasthesiologie: Allgemeine und spezielle Anasthesiologie, Schmerztherapie und Intensivmedizin.* 3rd ed. Berlin: Spring; 2012:240.

18. Scholz J, Steinfath M, Schulz M. Clinical pharmacokinetics of alfentanil, fentanyl and sufentail: an update. *Clin Pharmacokinet.* 1996;31(4):275-292.

19. Bovill JG, Sebel PS, Blackburn CL, et al. The pharmacokinetics of alfentail (R39209); a new opioid analgesic. *Anesthesiology.* 1982;57(6):439-443.

20. Prommer E. Levorphanol: Revisiting an underutilized analgesic. *Palliat Care.* 2014;8:7-10.

21. Le Rouzic V, Narayan A, Hunkle A, et al. Pharmacological characterization of levorphanol, a G-protein based opioid analgesic. *Anesthesia & Analgesia,* 2018; Apr 11.

22. DailyMed. Levorphanol tartrate. https://dailymed.nlm.nih.gov/dailymed/drugInfo.cfm?setid=77f4a54a-6901-46d9-93db-ad4be7eae6c3. Accessed May 7, 2018.

23. Pham TC, Fudin J, Raffa RB. Is levorphanol a better option than methadone? *Pain Med.* 2015;16:1673-1679.

24. Nalamachu SR, Gudin JA. Levorphanol: an optimal choice for opioid rotation. *Pract Pain Manage.* 2016;16:20-23.

25. McNulty JP. Can levorphanol be used like methadone for intractable refractory pain? *J Palliat Med.* 2007;10(2):293-296.

26. De Souza EB, Schmidt WK, Kuhar MJ. Nalbuphine: an autoradiographic opioid receptor binding profile in the central nervous system of an agonist/antagonist analgesic. *J Pharm and Exp Ther.* 1988;244(1):391-402.

27. Schmidt WK, Tam SW, Shotzberger GS, et al. Nalbuphine. *Drug Alcohol Depend.* 1985;14:339-362.

28. Davis MP, Fernandez C, McPherson ML. Does nalbuphine have a niche in managing pain? *J Opioid Manage.* 2018;14(2):143-151.

29. Davis MP, McPherson ML, Mehta Z, Fernandez C. What parenteral opioids to use in face of shortages of morphine, hydromorphone, and fentanyl. *Am J Hospice Palliat Care.* 2018; Jan 1:1049909118771374. doi: 10.1177/1049909118771374. [Epub ahead of print].

30. Zeng Z, Lu J, Shu C, et al. A comparison of nalbuphine with morphine for analgesic effects and safety: meta-analysis of randomized controlled trials. *Sci Rep.* 2015;3;5:1-8.

31. Beaver WT, Feise GA. A comparison of the analgesic effect of intramuscular nalbuphine and morphine in patients with postoperative pain. *J Pharmacol Exp Ther.* 1978;204(2):487-496.

32. Zacny JP, Conley K, Marks S. Comparing the subjective, psychomotor and physiological effects of intravenous nalbuphine and morphine in healthy volunteers. *J Pharmacol Exp Ther.* 1997;280(3):1159-1169.

33. Hartree C. Caution with nalbuphine in patients on long-term opioids. *Palliat Med.* 2005;19(2):168.

34. Sheiner LB, Beal SL. The utility function of antihypertensive therapy. *Ann NY Acad Sci.* 1978;30-4:112-127.

35. Frieden TR, Hourty D. Reducing the risks of relief—the CDC opioid-prescribing guideline. *N Engl J Med.* 2016;374:1501-1504.

36. Henthorn TK, Mikulich-Gilbertson SK. μ-Opioid receptor agonists: do they have utility in the treatment of acute pain? *Anesthesiology.* 2018;128(5):867-870.

37. Boom M, Olofsen E, Neukirchen M, et al. Fentanyl utility function: a risk-benefit composite of pain relief and breathing responses. *Anesthesiology.* 2013;119(3):663-674.

38. Roozekrans M, van der Schrier R, Aarts L, et al. Benefit versus severe side effects of opioid analgesia: novel utility functions of probability of analgesia and respiratory depression. *Anesthesiology.* 2018;128(5):932-942.

39. Trex E. Why is a baker's dozen 13? Mental Floss, 2013 Jan 10. http://mentalfloss.com/article/32259/why-bakers-dozen-13. Accessed May 7, 2018.

40. Pronounce names. PronounceNames.com. https://www.youtube.com/watch?v=qnKoUFNNZbk. Accessed May 7, 2018.

41. Centers for Disease Control and Prevention. CDC Guideline for Prescribing Opioids for Chronic Pain—United States, 2016. *MMWR.* 2016;65(1):1-49. https://www.cdc.gov/mmwr/volumes/65/rr/rr6501e1.htm. Accessed May 7, 2018.

42. Ayonrinde OT, Bridge DR. The rediscovery of methadone for cancer pain management. *Med J Aust.* 2000;173:536-540.

43. Bruera E, Sweeney C. Methadone use in cancer patients in pain: a review. *J Palliat Med.* 2002;5:127-138.

44. Chatham MS, Dodds Ashley ES, SVengsouk JS, et al. Dose ratios between high dose oral morphine or equivalents and oral methadone. *J Palliat Med.* 2013;16(8):947-950.

45. Chou R, Cruciani Ra, Fiellin DA, et al. Methadone safety guidelines: a clinical practice guideline from the American Pain Society and College on Problems of Drug Dependence, in collaboration with the Heart Rhythm Society. *J Pain.* 2014;1594:321-337.

46. National Comprehensive Cancer Network. NCCN Clinical Practice Guidelines in Oncology. Adult Cancer Pain, v.1.2018. https://www.nccn.org/professionals/physician_gls/pdf/pain.pdf. Accessed May 7, 2018.

Glossary

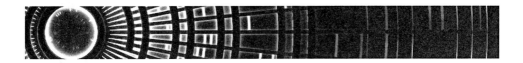

Abuse-deterrent opioid formulation—specially formulated tablets or capsules designed to deter dosage form manipulation that allows crushing for purposes of snorting or dissolving in order to inject the opioid.

Basal dose—opioid administered around the clock; usually refers to a continuous parenteral infusion or a regularly scheduled long-acting oral opioid.

Bioavailability—a term relating to the percentage of drug that is detected in the systemic circulation after its administration. Also defined as the rate and extent to which the active ingredient or active moiety (the active part of the drug molecule) is absorbed from a drug product and becomes available at the site of action.

Breakthrough pain—pain that "breaks through" controlled persistent pain.

Buccal—a term referring to the cheeks or to the sides of the mouth.

Cytochrome P450 system—an enzyme system involved in the biosynthesis of steroids, fatty acids, and bile acids, and the metabolism of endogenous and exogenous substances including toxins and drugs.

Drug formulation—the active medication combined with other pharmaceutical ingredients in a form that is stable, efficacious, appealing, easy to administer, and safe. Examples include tablets, capsules, lotions, ointments, transdermal patches, rectal suppositories, and injectable formulations.

Drug interaction—process by which one drug alters the pharmacokinetic or pharmacodynamic properties of another drug, potentially changing the pharmacological effect (therapeutic or toxic).

Drug moiety—the active part of a drug molecule.

Dysphagia—difficulty in swallowing.

Dyspnea—shortness of breath or an uncomfortable awareness of breathing.

End-of-dose pain—pain that recurs before the next regularly scheduled dose of an analgesic.

Epidural space—also known as the extradural space; also, the area outside the dura mater.

Equianalgesic—two opioid regimens that provide the same degree of pain relief.

Equipotent—having equivalent potency.

Excipient—ingredients in a drug formulation aside from the active drug designed to solubilize, suspend, thicken, dilute, emulsify, stabilize, preserve, color, flavor, and fashion medications into useful drug products.

First-pass effect—the metabolism of orally administered drugs by gastrointestinal and hepatic enzymes, resulting in a significant reduction in the amount of unmetabolized drug reaching the systemic circulation.

Immediate-release formulation—an unmodified tablet, capsule, or other dosage formulation that begins to dissolve and be absorbed after administration.

Incident pain, nonvolitional—pain that occurs from an identifiable cause that is not under the patient's control.

Incident pain, volitional—pain that occurs from an identifiable cause that is under the patient's control.

Incomplete cross-tolerance—increased sensitivity to the new opioid when switching opioids.

Intensol—a highly or "intensely" concentrated oral solution of medication.

Intranasal—a route of administration in which drugs are insufflated (blown into a body cavity) through the nose.

Lipophilic—fat-soluble.

Neuraxial—a term referring to administering drugs (such as opioids) into the spaces or potential spaces surrounding the spinal cord; also referred to as intraspinal.

Odynophagia—pain with swallowing.

Opioid-naïve—a term characterizing a patient who has not been regularly taking opioids; the opposite of an opioid-tolerant patient.

Opioid responsiveness—the degree of analgesia achieved as the dose is titrated to an endpoint defined by either intolerable side effects or the occurrence of acceptable analgesia.

Opioid rotation—transitioning a patient from one opioid or route of administration to another opioid and/or route of administration.

Opioid substitution—transitioning a patient from one opioid or route of administration to another opioid and/or route of administration.

Opioid switching—transitioning a patient from one opioid or route of administration to another opioid and/or route of administration.

Parenteral—situated or occurring outside the intestine; usually referring to administration of a drug by intravenous, intramuscular, or subcutaneous injection.

Patient-controlled analgesia—a system that allows self-administration of analgesics (usually parenteral) using a programmable infusion pump.

Persistent pain—continuous pain; pain that is always present, around the clock.

Pharmacodynamics—the branch of pharmacology having to do with the effects of a drug, including both therapeutic and toxic effects.

Pharmacokinetics—the branch of pharmacology having to do with what the body does to a drug: absorption, distribution, metabolism, excretion.

Physiochemistry—the physical and chemical processes of a drug binding to a receptor.

Potency—the intensity of the analgesic effects of a given dose, which is dependent on access to the opioid receptor and binding affinity at the receptor site.

Proalgesic effect—a pain-producing effect.

Sleep apnea—periods of breathing cessation during sleep.

Solute—substance that is added for dissolution in a solution; usually present in an amount smaller than the solvent.

Solution—a homogeneous mixture (uniform in composition throughout) prepared by mixing two or more substances.

Solvent—volume to which a solute is added; usually a liquid.

Spontaneous pain—pain that involves no precipitating stimulus.

Steady state—a state of equilibrium in which the rate of the drug going into the body is equal to the rate coming out of the body, resulting in a "steady" serum concentration of the drug in the blood.

Subarachnoid space—space between the arachnoid mater and the pia mater.

Subdural space—cavity between the dura and the arachnoid mater.

Sublingual—a term referring to the area under the tongue.

Suspension—a mixture in which solid particles are suspended in a fluid. The particles are prone to settle on standing; therefore, the mixture must be shaken prior to administration.

Sustained-release formulation—a pharmaceutically modified tablet, capsule, or other dosage formulation designed to provide sustained or repeated release of the drug, allowing a longer dosing interval.

Tolerance—a phenomenon whereby continued exposure to a drug reduces its effectiveness, occasionally necessitating an increase in dosage.

Transcutaneous electrical nerve stimulation (TENS)—a device that provides electrical stimulation to the skin to relieve pain; it is thought to act by interfering with the neural transmission of pain.

Transdermal—a term referring to the absorption of a drug across the skin, usually intending a systemic effect. It most commonly refers to a drug-soaked adhesive patch applied to the skin.

Transmucosal—a term referring to the administration of a drug through the mucous membrane.

Transmucosal immediate-release fentanyl (TIRF)—a fast-onset formulation of fentanyl administered by the transmucosal route of administration (buccal, sublingual, or intranasal).

Index

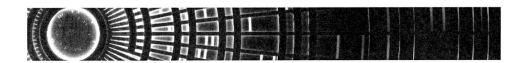

Note: IR indicates immediate release; SR, sustained release. Page numbers followed by f indicate figure; t, table.